Emergency and Trauma Radiology

Editor

SAVVAS NICOLAOU

RADIOLOGIC CLINICS OF NORTH AMERICA

www.radiologic.theclinics.com

Consulting Editor
FRANK H. MILLER

July 2015 • Volume 53 • Number 4

ELSEVIER

1600 John F. Kennedy Boulevard • Suite 1800 • Philadelphia, Pennsylvania, 19103-2899

http://www.theclinics.com

RADIOLOGIC CLINICS OF NORTH AMERICA Volume 53, Number 4
July 2015 ISSN 0033-8389, ISBN 13: 978-0-323-39117-7

Editor: John Vassallo (j.vassallo@elsevier.com)
Developmental Editor: Donald Mumford

Radiologic Clinics of North America (ISSN 0033-8389) is published bimonthly by Elsevier Inc., 360 Park Avenue South, New York, NY 10010-1710. Months of issue are January, March, May, July, September, and November. Periodicals postage paid at New York, NY and additional mailing offices. Subscription prices are USD 460 per year for US individuals, USD 709 per year for US institutions, USD 220 per year for US students and residents, USD 535 per year for Canadian individuals, USD 905 per year for Canadian institutions, USD 660 per year for international individuals, USD 905 per year for international institutions, and USD 315 per year for Canadian and foreign students/residents. To receive student and resident rate, orders must be accompanied by name of affiliated institution, date of term and the signature of program/residency coordinator on institution letterhead. Orders will be billed at individual rate until proof of status is received. Foreign air speed delivery is included in all *Clinics* subscription prices. All prices are subject to change without notice. **POSTMASTER:** Send address changes to *Radiologic Clinics of North America*, Elsevier Health Sciences Division, Subscription Customer Service, 3251 Riverport Lane, Maryland Heights, MO63043. **Customer Service: Telephone: 1-800-654-2452** (U.S. and Canada); **1-314-447-8871** (outside U.S. and Canada). **Fax: 1-314-447-8029. E-mail: journalscustomerservice-usa@elsevier.com (for print support);** journalsonlinesupport-usa@elsevier.com **(for online support)**.

Reprints. For copies of 100 or more of articles in this publication, please contact the Commercial Reprints Department, Elsevier Inc., 360 Park Avenue South, New York, New York 10010-1710. Tel.: +1-212-633-3874; Fax: +1-212-633-3820; E-mail: reprints@elsevier.com.

Radiologic Clinics of North America also published in Greek Paschalidis Medical Publications, Athens, Greece.

Radiologic Clinics of North America is covered in *MEDLINE/PubMed (Index Medicus), EMBASE/Excerpta Medica, Current Contents/Life Sciences, Current Contents/Clinical Medicine, RSNA Index to Imaging Literature, BIOSIS, Science Citation Index,* and *ISI/BIOMED.*

Printed in the United States of America.

Contributors

CONSULTING EDITOR

FRANK H. MILLER, MD
Chief, Body Imaging Section and Fellowship
Program and GI Radiology; Medical Director
MRI; Professor, Department of Radiology,
Northwestern Memorial Hospital,
Northwestern University, Feinberg School of
Medicine, Chicago, Illinois

EDITOR

SAVVAS NICOLAOU, MD, FRCPC
Vice Academic Chair of Undergraduate
Education and Continued Professional
Development; Director of Emergency Trauma
Imaging, Department of Radiology, Vancouver
General Hospital; Associate Professor,
University of British Columbia, Vancouver,
British Columbia, Canada

AUTHORS

ISIDRO ALVARO HUETE GARIN, MD
Associate Professor of Radiology, Department
of Radiology, Catholic University, Santiago,
Chile

GORDON T. ANDREWS, MD, FRCPC
Department of Radiology, Vancouver General
Hospital, University of British Columbia,
Vancouver, British Columbia, Canada

JAYSON L. BENJERT, DO
Department of Radiology, VA Puget Sound
Health Care System, Seattle, Washington

SANJEEV BHALLA, MD
Professor of Radiology, Mallinckrodt Institute
of Radiology, Washington University School of
Medicine, St Louis, Missouri

UTTAM K. BODANAPALLY, MBBS
Assistant Professor, Department of Diagnostic
Radiology and Nuclear Medicine, University of
Maryland Medical Center, Baltimore, Maryland

KIM CABAN, MD
Assistant Professor, Department of Radiology,
Jackson Memorial Hospital/Ryder Trauma
Center, University of Miami Miller School of
Medicine, Miami, Florida

KATHRYN DARRAS, MD
University of British Columbia, Vancouver,
British Columbia, Canada

ANTHONY M. DURSO, MD
Assistant Professor, Department of Radiology,
Jackson Memorial Hospital/Ryder Trauma
Center, University of Miami Miller School of
Medicine, Miami, Florida

KATHLEEN R. FINK, MD
Department of Radiology, University of
Washington, Seattle, Washington

BRUCE B. FORSTER, MD, FRCPC
Department of Radiology, Vancouver General
Hospital, University of British Columbia,
Vancouver, British Columbia, Canada

DANIEL B. GREEN, MD
Cardiothoracic Imaging Fellow, Mallinckrodt
Institute of Radiology, Washington University
School of Medicine, St Louis, Missouri

JOEL A. GROSS, MD
Department of Radiology, Harborview Medical
Center, University of Washington School of
Medicine, Seattle, Washington

MARTIN L. GUNN, MBChB, FRANZCR
Associate Professor, Department of
Radiology, University of Washington, Seattle,
Washington

STEPHEN F. HATEM, MD
Staff Radiologist, Department of Radiology,
Imaging Institute, Cleveland Clinic, Cleveland,
Ohio

**NIVMAND KHORRAMI-ARANI, BSc, BMBS,
FRANZCR, FRCPC**
Department of Radiology, St Joseph's
Hospital, Comox, British Columbia, Canada

DIGNA R. KOOL, MD
Nijmegen, The Netherlands

WAYNE SCOTT KUBAL, MD
Professor of Medical Imaging, University of
Arizona, Tucson, Arizona

CHRISTINA A. LeBEDIS, MD
Department of Radiology, Assistant Professor,
Boston University Medical Center, Boston,
Massachusetts

BRUCE E. LEHNERT, MD
Associate Professor, Department of
Radiology, University of Washington, Seattle,
Washington

KEN F. LINNAU, MD
Department of Radiology, Harborview Medical
Center, University of Washington School of
Medicine, Seattle, Washington

LUCK LOUIS, MD, FRCPC
Department of Radiology, Vancouver General
Hospital, University of British Columbia,
Vancouver, British Columbia, Canada

PEDRO LOURENCO, MD
Department of Radiology, Vancouver General
Hospital, University of British Columbia,
Vancouver, Canada

MICHAEL M. MAHER, MD
Professor, Department of Radiology,
University College Cork, Cork University
Hospital, Wilton, Cork, Ireland; Department
of Radiology, Mercy University Hospital,
Cork, Ireland

PAUL MALLINSON, FRCPC
Department of Radiology, Vancouver General
Hospital, University of British Columbia,
Vancouver, Canada

**PATRICK D. McLAUGHLIN, MB BCh BAO,
FFR RCSI, FRCPC**
Emergency and Trauma Radiology,
Department of Radiology, Vancouver General
Hospital, University of British Columbia,
Vancouver, British Columbia, Canada

KIRA MELAMUD, MD
Department of Radiology, Radiology Resident,
PGY5, Boston University Medical Center,
Boston, Massachusetts

FELIPE MUNERA, MD
Professor of Radiology, Department of
Radiology, Jackson Memorial Hospital/Ryder
Trauma Center; Medical Director, Radiology
Services, University of Miami Hospitals,
University of Miami Miller School of Medicine,
Miami, Florida

KEVIN P. MURPHY, MB
Department of Radiology, University College
Cork, Cork University Hospital, Wilton, Cork,
Ireland; Department of Radiology, Mercy
University Hospital, Grenville Place, Cork,
Ireland

SAVVAS NICOLAOU, MD, FRCPC
Vice Academic Chair of Undergraduate
Education and Continued Professional
Development; Director of Emergency Trauma
Imaging, Department of Radiology, Vancouver
General Hospital; Associate Professor,
University of British Columbia, Vancouver,
British Columbia, Canada

OWEN J. O'CONNOR, MD
Department of Radiology, University College
Cork, Cork University Hospital, Wilton, Cork,
Ireland; Department of Radiology, Mercy
University Hospital, Grenville Place, Cork,
Ireland

CONSTANTINE A. RAPTIS, MD
Assistant Professor of Radiology, Mallinckrodt Institute of Radiology, Washington University School of Medicine, St Louis, Missouri

ALEXANDRA ROSTON, BA
Zanvyl Krieger School of Arts and Sciences, Johns Hopkins University, Washington, DC

CLAIRE K. SANDSTROM, MD
Department of Radiology, Harborview Medical Center, University of Washington School of Medicine, Seattle, Washington

PAMELA W. SCHAEFER, MD, FACR
Clinical Director of MRI; Associate Director of Neuroradiology, Massachusetts General Hospital; Associate Professor of Radiology, Harvard Medical School, Boston, Massachusetts

KATHIRKAMANATHAN SHANMUGANATHAN, MD
Professor, Department of Diagnostic Radiology and Nuclear Medicine, University of Maryland Medical Center, Baltimore, Maryland

JORGE A. SOTO, MD
Department of Radiology, Professor, Boston University Medical Center, Boston, Massachusetts

CHANDLER SOURS, PhD
Postdoctoral Research Associate, Department of Diagnostic Radiology and Nuclear Medicine, University of Maryland Medical Center, Baltimore, Maryland

MARIA TWOMEY, MB
Department of Radiology, University College Cork, Cork University Hospital, Wilton, Cork, Ireland

SCOTT TYSON, MD
Department of Radiology, Imaging Institute, Cleveland Clinic, Cleveland, Ohio

BEHROZE A. VACHHA, MD, PhD
Fellow, Neuroradiology, Massachusetts General Hospital, Harvard Medical School, Boston, Massachusetts

BRYAN B. VOELZKE, MD, MS
Department of Urology, Harborview Medical Center, University of Washington School of Medicine, Seattle, Washington

JOSEPH S. YU, MD
Vice Chair for Academic Affairs and Education; Professor of Radiology and Orthopedic Surgery; Director of Musculoskeletal Imaging, Department of Radiology, The Ohio State University Wexner Medical Center, Columbus, Ohio

JIACHEN ZHUO, PhD
Assistant Professor, Department of Diagnostic Radiology and Nuclear Medicine, University of Maryland Medical Center, Baltimore, Maryland

Contents

pleura, diaphragm, and mediastinum. The mechanism of injury in ballistic and nonballistic trauma and the impact the injury trajectory has on imaging evaluation of penetrating injuries to the chest are discussed. The article presents the broad spectrum of imaging findings a radiologist encounters with penetrating injuries to the chest, with emphasis on injuries to the lungs and pleura, diaphragm, and mediastinum.

Imaging plays an important role in the management of patients with traumatic brain injury (TBI). Computed tomography (CT) is the first-line imaging technique allowing rapid detection of primary structural brain lesions that require surgical intervention. CT also detects various deleterious secondary insults allowing early medical and surgical management. Serial imaging is critical to identifying secondary injuries. MR imaging is indicated in patients with acute TBI when CT fails to explain neurologic findings. However, MR imaging is superior in patients with mild TBI and also predicts neurocognitive outcome.

Radiographs remain the mainstay for initial imaging of suspected fracture in the emergency setting. Missed fractures potentially have significant negative consequences for patients, referring physicians, and radiologists. Most missed fractures are owing to perceptual errors. In this review, we emphasize knowledge of 3 categories of pitfalls as they pertain to the upper extremity: the common but challenging; the out of mind, out of sight; and those related to satisfaction of search. For specific injuries, emphasis is placed on helpful radiographic signs and important additional radiographic views to obtain.

As long as radiography remains cheap and provides value in patient care, it will continue to be widely used as a front-line imaging technique. There are limitations to what a radiograph can depict, however. It is imperative to understand the limitations of radiography to avoid pitfalls owing to the overlap of numerous osseous structures. This article reminds the reader of the association between certain radiographic abnormalities and the anatomic relevance in the patient. Although interpretive errors occur in fast-paced, high-volume emergency settings, meticulous attention to changes in the cortex and medullary bone may help to keep errors to a minimum.

Pancreatic and duodenal injuries are rare but life-threatening occurrences, often occurring in association with other solid organ injuries. Findings of pancreatic and duodenal trauma on computed tomography and MR imaging are often nonspecific, and high levels of clinical suspicion and understanding of mechanism of injury are imperative. Familiarity with the grading schemes of pancreatic and duodenal injury is important because they help in assessing for key imaging findings that directly influence management. This article presents an overview of imaging of blunt and penetrating pancreatic and duodenal injuries, including pathophysiology, available imaging techniques, and variety of imaging features.

Computed tomography (CT) imaging of the kidney, ureter, and bladder permit accurate and prompt diagnosis or exclusion of traumatic injuries, without the need to move the patient to the fluoroscopy suite. Real-time review of imaging permits selective delayed imaging, reducing time on the scanner and radiation dose for patients who do not require delays. Modifying imaging parameters to obtain thicker slices and noisier images permits detection of contrast extravasation from the kidneys, ureters, and bladder, while reducing radiation dose on the delayed or cystographic imaging. The American Association for the Surgery of Trauma grading system is discussed, along with challenges and limitations.

Computed tomography pulmonary angiography (CTPA) is the principal means of evaluating dyspnea in the emergency department. As its use has increased, the number of studies positive for pulmonary embolism (PE) has decreased to less than 20%. Many of the negative PE studies provide an alternative explanation for dyspnea, most commonly pneumonia, pulmonary edema, pleural effusion, or atelectasis. Nonthrombotic emboli may also be suggested. Airway and obstructive lung disease may be detected on CTPA. Pleural and pericardial disease may also explain the dyspnea, but more detailed evaluation of the serosal surfaces may be limited on the arterial phase of a CTPA.

Neuroimaging plays a key role in the initial work-up of patients with symptoms of acute stroke. Understanding the advantages and limitations of available CT and MR imaging techniques and how to use them optimally in the emergency setting is crucial for accurately making the diagnosis of acute stroke and for rapidly determining appropriate treatment.

An overview of the imaging of face and neck infections is presented. Most of the imaging presented is contrast-enhanced computed tomography. The emphasis of this presentation is to enable the emergency radiologist to accurately diagnose face and neck infections, to effectively communicate the imaging findings with emergency physicians, and to function as part of a team offering the best care to patients.

Intestinal ischemia is a serious condition that continues to be associated with mortalities in excess of 70%. Intestinal obstruction and gastrointestinal tract sepsis are

PROGRAM OBJECTIVE

The objective of the *Radiologic Clinics of North America* is to keep practicing radiologists and radiology residents up to date with current clinical practice in radiology by providing timely articles reviewing the state of the art in patient care.

TARGET AUDIENCE

Practicing radiologists, radiology residents, and other health care professionals who provide patient care utilizing radiologic findings.

LEARNING OBJECTIVES

Upon completion of this activity, participants will be able to:

1. Review recent advances in MR techniques.
2. Discuss advances in Diffusion Weighted Imaging and T1- and T2-weighted imaging.
3. Recognize the basic techniques and clinical applications of Perfusion Imaging in Neuro-Oncology.

ACCREDITATION

The Elsevier Office of Continuing Medical Education (EOCME) is accredited by the Accreditation Council for Continuing Medical Education (ACCME) to provide continuing medical education for physicians.

The EOCME designates this enduring material for a maximum of 15 *AMA PRA Category 1 Credit*(s)™. Physicians should claim only the credit commensurate with the extent of their participation in the activity.

All other health care professionals requesting continuing education credit for this enduring material will be issued a certificate of participation.

DISCLOSURE OF CONFLICTS OF INTEREST

The EOCME assesses conflict of interest with its instructors, faculty, planners, and other individuals who are in a position to control the content of CME activities. All relevant conflicts of interest that are identified are thoroughly vetted by EOCME for fair balance, scientific objectivity, and patient care recommendations. EOCME is committed to providing its learners with CME activities that promote improvements or quality in healthcare and not a specific proprietary business or a commercial interest.

The planning committee, staff, authors and editors listed below have identified no financial relationships or relationships to products or devices they or their spouse/life partner have with commercial interest related to the content of this CME activity:

Gordon T. Andrews, MD, FRCPC; Jayson L. Benjert, DO; Sanjeev Bhalla, MD; Uttam K. Bodanapally, MBBS; Kim Caban, MD; Kathryn E. Darras, MD; Anthony M. Durso, MD; Anjali Fortna; Daniel B. Green, MD; Joel A. Gross, MD; Stephen F. Hatem, MD; Kristen Helm; Isidro Alvaro Huete Garin, MD; Nivmand Khorrami-Arani, BSc, BMBS, FRANZCR, FRCPC; Wayne Scott Kubal, MD; Christina A. LeBedis, MD; Bruce E. Lehnert, MD; Ken F. Linnau, MD; Luck Louis, MD, FRCPC; Pedro Lourenco, MD; Michael M. Maher, MD; Paul Mallinson, FRCPC; Kira Melamud, MD; Frank H. Miller, MD; Felipe Munera, MD; Kevin P. Murphy, MB; Owen J. O'Connor, MD; Constantine A. Raptis, MD; Alexandra Roston, BA; Claire K. Sandstrom, MD; Pamela W. Schaefer, MD, FACR; Kathirkamnathan Shanmuganathan, MD; Jorge A. Soto, MD; Chandler Sours, PhD; Karthikeyan Subramaniam; Maria Twomey, MB; Scott Tyson, MD; Behroze A. Vachha, MD, PhD; Isidro Alvaro Huete Garin, MD; Bryan B. Voelzke, MD, MS; Joseph S. Yu, MD; Jaichen Zhuo, PhD.

The planning committee, staff, authors and editors listed below have identified financial relationships or relationships to products or devices they or their spouse/life partner have with commercial interest related to the content of this CME activity:

Kathleen R. Fink, **MD**'s spouse has research support from Bayer AG, Guerbet Group, and Bracco Diagnostics, Inc.

Bruce B. Forster, **MD, FRCPC** is a consultant/advisor for Toshiba America Medical Systems and Siemans Corporation, and is on the speakers' bureau for Bayer AG.

Martin L. Gunn, **MBChB, FRANZCR** has stock ownership in TransformativeMed, research support from Philips Healthcare and Medical Imaging Technology Alliance, a division of National Elecrical Manufacturers Association, and has an employment affiliation with Wolters Kluwer.

Digna R. Kool, **MD** has stock ownership in Stryker; CVS Health; and Sarepta Therapeutics.

Patrick D. McLaughlin, **MB BCh, BAO, FFR, RCSI, FRCPC** is on the speakers' bureau for an event for Siemens Corporation.

Savvas Nicolaou, **MD, FRCPC** is a consultant/advisor for Siemens Corporation.

UNAPPROVED/OFF-LABEL USE DISCLOSURE

The EOCME requires CME faculty to disclose to the participants:

1. When products or procedures being discussed are off-label, unlabelled, experimental, and/or investigational (not US Food and Drug Administration [FDA] approved); and
2. Any limitations on the information presented, such as data that are preliminary or that represent ongoing research, interim analyses, and/or unsupported opinions. Faculty may discuss information about pharmaceutical agents that is outside of FDA-approved labelling. This information is intended solely for CME and is not intended to promote off-label use of these

medications. If you have any questions, contact the medical affairs department of the manufacturer for the most recent prescribing information.

TO ENROLL
To enroll in the *Radiologic Clinics of North America* Continuing Medical Education program, call customer service at 1-800-654-2452 or sign up online at http://www.theclinics.com/home/cme. The CME program is available to subscribers for an additional annual fee of USD 315.

METHOD OF PARTICIPATION
In order to claim credit, participants must complete the following:
1. Complete enrolment as indicated above.
2. Read the activity.
3. Complete the CME Test and Evaluation. Participants must achieve a score of 70% on the test. All CME Tests and Evaluations must be completed online.

CME INQUIRIES/SPECIAL NEEDS
For all CME inquiries or special needs, please contact elsevierCME@elsevier.com.

RADIOLOGIC CLINICS OF NORTH AMERICA

ISSUE OF RELATED INTEREST

Neuroimaging Clinics August 2014 (Vol. 24, No. 3)
Craniofacial Trauma
Deborah R. Shatzkes, *Editor*
Available at: http://www.neuroimaging.theclinics.com/

THE CLINICS ARE AVAILABLE ONLINE!
Access your subscription at:
www.theclinics.com

Preface
Emergency Radiology: The New Frontier of Imaging

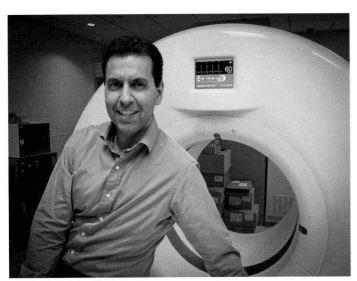

Savvas Nicolaou, MD, FRCPC
Editor

It is an exciting time for radiologists involved in acute patient imaging since the birth of Emergency Room (ER)/Trauma Radiology over 20 years ago. Never before have the expertise, training, and education in imaging of acute conditions been so in demand as it is presently. ER/Trauma Radiology as a recognized and expanding subspecialty worldwide has been driven by rapidly evolving innovations in imaging, such as dual-energy, ultra-low-dose, and cardiac and dynamic perfusion imaging. Thus, this collection of work was undertaken as a contribution to the rapidly expanding and dynamic field of Emergency and Trauma Radiology. This issue seeks to distill the knowledge and experience gained through the creation of the first ER/Trauma Radiology program in Canada at Vancouver General Hospital for the past 15 years and in conjunction with the knowledge, support, and experience of other leaders in the field of ER/Trauma Radiology. The increasing ability to intervene therapeutically in many conditions that were previously difficult to image and manage, such as acute stroke, severe whole-body polytrauma, acute pulmonary embolism, and vascular/nonvascular emergencies in

the chest, abdomen, and pelvis, has led to an increased need for an accurate, rapid detection and classification of these conditions by designated radiologists subspecializing in acute imaging (ie, emergency/trauma radiologists).

This issue of *Radiologic Clinics of North America* aims to provide a real-world unique and methodical approach to commonly encountered conditions by all radiologists involved in the assessment and evaluation of acute conditions. In addition, it addresses new innovative diagnostic techniques, such as dual-energy computed tomography, in the acute setting, as methods to further enhance patient care and outcomes.

I am hopeful this issue will be of practical benefit to acute imaging specialists in real-world practice in the Emergency Department setting.

A special and deep thanks is extended to Dr Patrick McLaughlin for his dedicated efforts and hard work in assisting and contributing his expertise to this issue, also for his belief in Emergency/Trauma Radiology as a subspecialty, and his energetic desire to expand the subspecialty. I want to express my thanks and appreciation to

Radiol Clin N Am 53 (2015) xv–xvi
http://dx.doi.org/10.1016/j.rcl.2015.04.001
0033-8389/15/$ – see front matter © 2015 Published by Elsevier Inc.

my ER/Trauma team at Vancouver General Hospital, particularly Dr Luck Louis, Dr Tim O'Connell, and Dr Patrick McLaughlin, for their support and commitment to our program past, present, and future. An additional thank-you to Dr David Tso and Dr Teresa Liang for their ongoing commitment, support, and research efforts. And great thanks is also extended to Dr Shamir Rai for his contributory efforts to this work.

Savvas Nicolaou, MD, FRCPC
Department of Radiology
Vancouver General Hospital
University of British Columbia
895 West 12th Avenue
Vancouver, British Columbia V5Z 1M9, Canada

E-mail address:
savvas.nicolaou@vch.ca

Dual-Energy Computed Tomography
Advantages in the Acute Setting

Patrick D. McLaughlin, MB BCh BAO, FFR RCSI, FRCPC*,
Paul Mallinson, FRCPC, Pedro Lourenco, MD, Savvas Nicolaou, MD, FRCPC

KEYWORDS

• Dual energy • Computed tomography • Trauma • Gout • Uric acid • Marrow edema

---

KEY POINTS

- The fundamental principle of dual-energy (DECT) and spectral CT imaging is that certain materials with a high atomic weight have significantly higher attenuation values when exposed to an x-ray beam of low rather than high mean kV values.
- Dual-energy (DECT) and spectral CT post processing allows for material specific display and subtraction. Material specific identification of uric acid crystals can greatly benefit patients who present with acute articular pain and acute flank pain.
- Material specific subtraction of calcium allows for accurate detection of bone marrow hemorrhage and edema. Material specific subtraction and quantification of iodine allows more accurate characterization of abdominal incidentalomas.
- Image quality optimization is possible using energy specific display techniques.

INTRODUCTION

Since its first public unveiling in 1973, computed tomography (CT) has played a profound role in medical diagnosis, greatly enhancing the depth of understanding of many disease processes. Academic and industry collaboration has resulted in unparalleled evolution of CT technology and techniques over the past 40 years. The first CT system produced by Electric and Musical Industries produced one 80 × 80-pixel axial image after 5 minutes of scanning, whereas state-of-the-art CT technology today can acquire 1200 axial images of 512 × 512 pixels in 1 second, representing an increase in efficiency of 1.5 billion percent.[1]

The concept of acquiring 2 sets of CT images with different x-ray spectra to enhance material differentiation was conceived and tested only 5 years after the initial public unveiling of CT.[2] Original attempts at dual-energy imaging involved the acquisition of 2 separate, contemporaneous CT scans and clinical results were greatly impacted by variability in phase of contrast enhancement, patient motion, limited spatial resolution, instability of CT attenuation values, and postprocessing difficulties. These limitations were addressed with the introduction of dual-source CT in 2006 and in the subsequent 9 years dual-energy CT (DECT) has regained clinical significance and widespread application.[3] Today, several CT vendors have implemented DECT with different technical approaches, and integration into the diagnostic pathways of emergency medicine continues to grow. For in-depth

---

Disclosures: P.D. McLaughlin – Speaker, Innovations Conference 2014 (Siemens Healthcare).
Department of Radiology, Vancouver General Hospital, University of British Columbia, 899 West 12th Avenue, Vancouver V5Z 1M9, Canada
* Corresponding author.
E-mail address: mclaughlin.paddy@gmail.com

Radiol Clin N Am 53 (2015) 619–638
http://dx.doi.org/10.1016/j.rcl.2015.02.016
0033-8389/15/$ – see front matter © 2015 Elsevier Inc. All rights reserved.

information regarding the technical characteristics of single-source fast kV switching, single-source dual-layer detector, and dual-source implementations of DECT, the reader is directed to an excellent summary of the topic by Marin and colleagues.[4]

The fundamental principle of DECT and spectral CT imaging is that certain materials can have significantly higher or lower attenuation values when exposed to an x-ray beam of different mean kV values. Elements with a high atomic number (Z), such as iodine, xenon, and calcium (Z = 53, Z = 54, and Z = 20), attenuate a greater proportion of low kV rather than high kV photons due to photoelectric effect. The photoelectric effect occurs because the k-edge of these elements (I = 33 keV, Xe = 34.6 keV, Ca = 4.03 keV) is more closely matched to the mean energy of the low-kV source. Elements such as hydrogen, oxygen, carbon, and nitrogen, os which the human body primarily consists, have low atomic numbers (Z = 1, Z = 8, Z = 6, and Z = 7) and therefore attenuate low kV and high kV photons in a more equal manner given that neither beam is sufficiently matched to their very low k-edge values. This characteristic and reproducible behavior provides the basis for material differentiation achieved by postprocessing software that maps different tissues according to their unique dual-energy index (DEI).[5]

$$DEI = \frac{x_{80} - x_{140}}{x_{80} + x_{140} + 2000},$$

In parallel with the aforementioned technical advances, the medical community has witnessed an exponential increase in the use of CT in the acute care setting over the past 20 years. A retrospective study conducted in the United States involving 1.29 billion weighted emergency department visits found that CT use in the emergency department has increased from 3% of visits in 1996 to 14% of visits in 2007.[6] This study found that increased CT usage has been driven primarily by expanded indications in patients with acute flank pain, acute abdominal pain, trauma, and acute chest pain. The unique demands that are placed on CT in the emergency and trauma settings play well to the strengths of DECT. In our experience, the ability of DECT to successfully differentiate densely organized uric acid crystals or uric acid–containing calculi from calcium-containing compounds is pivotal to the management of many patients presenting to the emergency department. The manipulation of dual-energy data to enhance, quantify, and subtract iodine-based contrast agents is an exciting and rapidly evolving field of research with great potential to increase diagnostic yield over single-energy CT (SECT) in the setting of acute chest and abdominal pain and also to help reduce the number of costly follow-up examinations of abdominal incidentalomas. The aim of this article is to inform and update emergency radiologists in respect of the clinically relevant benefits that DECT contributes over conventional CT in the emergency setting using practical imaging examples. The relevant scientific literature will be summarized and limitations of the technique also will be emphasized to provide the reader with a rounded concept of the current state of technology.

GOUT
Clinical Characteristics

Gout is the most common crystal-induced arthritis. It is characterized by extracellular fluid saturation, with the final product of purine metabolism, uric acid, which densely precipitates into rodlike crystals within soft tissues after binding with sodium ions to form monosodium urate (MSU) ($NaC_5H_3N_4O_3$ H_2O). Deposition of MSU crystals within articular and synovial soft tissues as well as ligaments and tendons can result in well-described clinical manifestations, including recurrent attacks of acute inflammatory arthritis, chronic arthropathy, and importantly, from the perspective of DECT imaging, macroscopic accumulation of MSU crystals in the form of tophaceous deposits.[7]

Patients typically present to the emergency department with severe pain, redness, warmth, and swelling of a joint. Maximal severity of the attack is usually reached within 12 to 24 hours with complete resolution of pain almost always occurring within a few days to several weeks, even in untreated individuals. When a patient presents to the emergency department with suspected gout, a definitive diagnosis should be sought given the clinical and laboratory overlap with septic arthritis.[8] Acute monoarticular gout can cause fever, leukocytosis, and elevated erythrocyte sedimentation rate and therefore can be clinically indistinguishable from acute septic arthritis.[9]

At least 80% of initial attacks of gout involve a single joint, most frequently the first metatarsophalangeal joint and second most commonly the knee. A potential explanation for preferential involvement of the lower limb and in particular the first metatarsophalangeal joint is temperature. A reduction of temperature by 2°C, from 37 to 35°C has been shown in in vitro studies to lower the solubility point of urate from 6.8 to

6.0 mg/dL.[10] The first metatarsophalangeal joint has both a relatively reduced blood flow and increased surface-to-volume ratio, promoting heat loss, and similarly the knee is more vulnerable to heat loss than the spine or joints in the upper limb. It is proposed that the heat produced during the acute inflammatory episode may contribute to the subsequent dissolution of crystals, potentially accounting for why acute gout is typically self-limiting.[11]

Serum uric acid levels are difficult to interpret and generally not helpful when a patient presents to the emergency department with acute joint pain.[12] Patients with gout will by definition have hyperuricemia at some point in their disease process; however, most hyperuricemic patients never experience an episode of acute inflammatory arthritis. Normal to low serum urate values have been noted in 12% to 43% of patients with acute episodes of gout.[13] Definitive diagnosis of gout therefore requires polarized light microscopic analysis of fluid aspirated from the involved joint demonstrating needle-shaped, negatively birefringent MSU crystals. The sensitivity of arthrocentesis for gout is in the range of 85% to 95% with specificity of 100%.[14] Although aspiration is considered the diagnostic gold standard, it is invasive and carries a risk of potential complications. In clinical practice, only 11% of patients undergo arthrocentesis; therefore, there is great interest in noninvasive strategies for the diagnosis of gout given that currently most cases are diagnosed on clinical grounds alone.[15] Features of gout, such as punched out, juxta-articular erosions, and soft tissue tophi, can be found on conventional plain radiographs but these are usually not apparent until the chronic stage of disease. Earlier changes can be found using ultrasound, MR imaging, and most recently DECT.[16]

Imaging Characteristics

When accumulated in sufficient density, the highly organized crystalline deposits of MSU that precipitate within joint and periarticular soft tissues can be observed on CT. Using DECT, these macroscopic MSU deposits can be differentiated from calcium-containing compounds within joints (**Fig. 1**) and periarticular soft tissues such as tendons (**Fig. 2**), given that MSU crystals have slightly negative DEI values. This is to say that MSU crystals, which are composed of hydrogen, oxygen, carbon, nitrogen, and sodium ($Z = 1$, $Z = 8$, $Z = 6$, $Z = 7$, and $Z = 11$) do not have higher attenuation values on 80-peak kilovoltage (kVp) as compared with 140-kVp images irrespective of their density. The reverse is true for calcium-

containing deposits ($Z = 20$), which, due to the photoelectric effect, have significantly higher attenuation values on 80 kVp as compared with 140 kVp, allowing for accurate material decomposition with postprocessing algorithms. It is important to emphasize that postprocessing algorithms, such as the gout application on Syngo.Via (Siemens Medical Solutions, Forchheim, Germany) and Gemstone Spectral Imaging Viewer (GE Healthcare, Milwaukee, WI, USA) typically use a lower threshold value in the range of 130 HU (Syngo.Via); therefore, if MSU deposits are not of sufficient density, then they will be excluded from the analysis using current techniques. It is therefore possible that early MSU deposits could remain undetected by DECT in some patients who present with acute monoarticular pain; the available literature examining the diagnostic accuracy of the technique will be reviewed as follows.

Diagnostic Accuracy

A recently published systematic literature review and meta-analysis comparing the ultrasound and DECT diagnosis of gout by Ogdie and colleagues[17] found 9 articles and 2 meeting abstracts that were methodologically acceptable for inclusion. A pooled analysis of 3 DECT studies, which used arthrocentesis as the gold standard, demonstrated a sensitivity of 87% and specificity of 84% (**Table 1**). Importantly, each included study was set in the secondary care setting with a mean gout disease duration of at least 7 years. In 20 patients who presented with a first flare of inflammatory arthritis, Bongartz and colleagues[18] found that MSU deposits were not demonstrated on DECT in 4 patients (20%) who were found to be positive for MSU crystals after joint aspiration. The diagnostic performance of DECT during the first presentation of suspected acute gout in the emergency department therefore has yet to be adequately established. MSU deposits that have not reached threshold density for inclusion in the postprocessing algorithm could result in false-negative interpretations and imaging artifacts can result in false positives, therefore the emergency radiologist needs to consider steps to improve their specificity and sensitivity.

How to Improve Specificity

Specificity of the technique can be improved by recognition of imaging artifacts that mimic MSU deposits, which may be found in up to 90% of DECT studies.[19] Nail bed artifacts are the most commonly encountered mimics of MSU; they are frequently found in the feet (42% of patients) but rarely in the hands (4.3% of patients). Artifacts mimicking

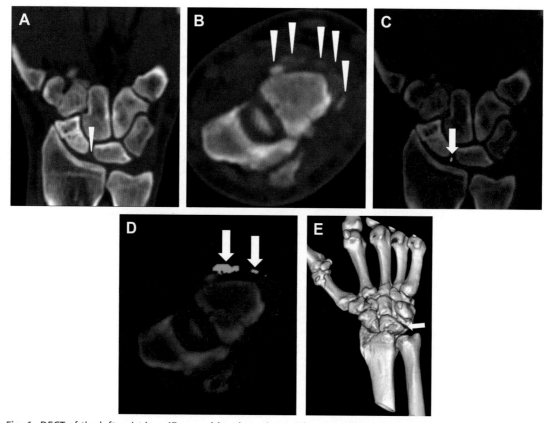

Fig. 1. DECT of the left wrist in a 47-year-old male patient with acute wrist pain. Gray-scale mixed images (*A, B*) show a long-standing nonunited scaphoid fracture and numerous intra-articular "calcific" densities that were felt likely to be posttraumatic (*arrowheads*). Color-coded images from the DECT gout application (*C–E*) show that some of the presumed calcific densities had negative dual-energy indices in keeping with MSU deposits (*arrows*).

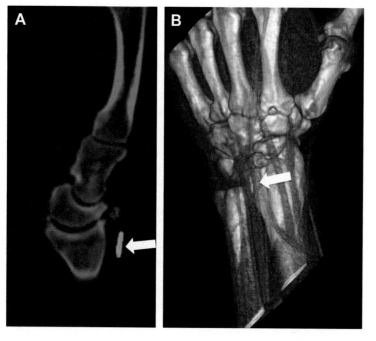

Fig. 2. DECT of the left wrist in a 47-year-old male patient with acute wrist pain. (*A*) Sagittal 2-material decomposition color-coded images and (*B*) VRT images from the DECT gout application confirm the presence of small-volume MSU deposits in the extensor digitorum tendon. Arrow points to urate deposits color-coded in green present within extensor digitorum tendon.

Table 1
Results from a systematic literature review and meta-analysis evaluating the diagnostic performance of DECT in patients with gout

	True Positive	False Positive	False Negative	True Negative	Sensitivity	Specificity	DECT: MSU Crystal Deposition Meta-Analysis Results		
							Sensitivity	Specificity	AUC
Glazebrook et al[78] {Glazebrook:2011ij}	12	4	0	15	1	0.79	0.87 (0.79–0.93)	0.84 (0.75–0.90)	0.90
Bongartz et al[18] {Bongartz:2014ec}	36	7	4	34	0.90	0.83			
Choi z et al[79] {Choi:2012cc}	34	3	6	37	0.78	0.93			

Abbreviations: AUC, area under the curve; DECT, dual-energy computed tomography; MSU, monosodium urate.
Adapted from Ogdie A, Taylor WJ, Weatherall M, et al. Imaging modalities for the classification of gout: systematic literature review and meta-analysis. Ann Rheum Dis 2014; http://dx.doi.org/10.1136/annrheumdis-2014-205431 [Epub ahead of print].

MSU also can be seen at the skin interfaces, surrounding metallic jewelry, and cortical bone secondary to beam hardening and artifacts can be created if a patient moves during scan acquisition. Increased image noise can result in more troublesome pixilated foci of apparent MSU deposition; however, these can be differentiated from true deposits by their nonanatomic distribution. **Table 2** outlines the routine CT parameters used at our institution using the Definition FLASH dualsource, DECT system (Siemens Healthcare) with suggested protocol adjustments that can reduce MSU mimicking artifacts outlined on **Table 3**.

How to Improve Sensitivity

Sensitivity of the technique potentially could be improved by routinely scanning multiple body parts, such as the elbows, wrists, hands, knees, and feet in any individual presenting with acute monoarthritis. Sensitivity for detection of gout is likely to be increased by this approach, particularly in cases in which the episode of acute monoarthritis in question does not involve joints of the foot. This rationale is supported by a retrospective single-center analysis by Mallinson and colleagues,[20] who report that 68.2% of patients had MSU deposits in the foot, most commonly in the first metatarsophalangeal joint; 56.1% of patients had MSU deposits in the knee, 53.4% in the ankle, 27.7% in the elbow, and 16.9% in the wrist and hand, respectively, when 148 patients with gout were imaged using a standardized 4-limb DECT protocol. Of note, tendons were also frequently involved including the Achilles in 35.8% of patients and triceps tendon in 23.0%.[20,21] MSU deposits also were found in the menisci of the knee in 21.0% of patients and in the cruciate ligaments

in 16.2% of cases. The elbow joint, suprapatellar bursa, and ankle collateral ligaments were among the least common of the affected sites. Adapted results from this valuable study are adapted for

Table 3
Dual-energy computed tomography gout application artifacts and how to reduce them

Artifact Type	Reduction Measures
Motion	• Use of tape/blocks to immobilize the patient's limbs • Increase the speed of the gantry from 1 rotation/s to 1 rotation every 0.3 s
Single pixels	• Use D24 Kernel or Q34 (ItR) • Increase range from 3 to 5
Beam-hardening/metal artifacts	• Use D24, D34, or Q34 Kernel to reconstruct. • Remove metal (eg, jewelry) where possible
Nail bed, skin, plantar fascia	Use settings: • Increase air distance from 5 to 10 • Decrease bone distance from 10 to 5 • Kernel D33 to reduce skin artifact
Vascular	• Increase Minimum and Range parameter • Add new reconstruction with softer kernel (D20/D24) or ItR such as Q 30

Adapted from Mallinson PI, Coupal T, Reisinger C, et al. Artifacts in dual-energy CT gout protocol: a review of 50 suspected cases with an artifact identification guide. AJR Am J Roentgenol 2014;203(1):W105; with permission.

Table 2
Dual-source dual-energy computed tomography for gout: suggested protocol

Parameter	Body Part							
	Elbows		Wrists/Hands		Knees		Ankles/Feet	
	Tube A	Tube B	Tube A	Tube B	Tube A	Tube B	Tube A	Tube B
CTDIw Effective	8.7442	8.7442	10.2119	10.2119	11.503	11.503	11.503	11.503
Effective mAs	202	101	236	118	248	124	248	124
Pitch Factor	0.70	0.70	0.70	0.70	0.70	0.70	0.70	0.70
Quality Reference (mAs)	202	101	202	101	249	124	249	124
Rotation Time	0.330	0.330	0.330	0.330	1.000	1.000	1.000	1.000
Slice Width	0.60	0.60	0.60	0.60	0.60	0.60	0.60	0.60
Voltage	80	140	80	140	80	140	80	140

Abbreviations: CTDIw, weighted computed tomography dose index; mAs, milliamperes/second.
Adapted from Mallinson PI, Coupal T, Reisinger C, et al. Artifacts in dual-energy CT gout protocol: a review of 50 suspected cases with an artifact identification guide. AJR Am J Roentgenol 2014;203(1):W104; with permission.

review on **Table 4**. On the basis of these findings, patients who present with acute monoarticular arthritis at our institution are most frequently imaged with a 4-limb DECT protocol.

BONE MARROW EDEMA
Background

Traumatic bone marrow edema results in small but measurable increases in CT attenuation values due to the presence of hemorrhage and increased interstitial fluid within the bone marrow cavity. Bone marrow edema is readily visualized on MR imaging as regions of reduced signal intensity on T1-weighted MR imaging and increased signal intensity on T2-weighted fat-suppressed or short tau inversion recovery (STIR) sequences, reflecting the increase in water content of the marrow cavity as a result of hemorrhage. However, MR imaging may not always be immediately available as an investigative modality due to potential time and resource constraints in the emergency setting. Furthermore, its use may be contraindicated in some patients. Detection of bone marrow edema using SECT has been attempted, and although attenuation-based algorithms remove many bone structures, SECT methods are still unable to remove fine trabecular bone with sufficient quality to reliably reveal density changes in the bone marrow.[22]

Evidence

Given its relatively high atomic number (Z = 20) and high DEI, the calcium in trabecular bone can be successfully removed in DECT images using a process termed virtual noncalcium subtraction (VNCa) (**Fig. 3**).[23] Pache and colleagues[22] were the first to successfully evaluate the presence of bone marrow edema in patients with acute knee trauma using a DECT VNCa. The investigators reported a sensitivity of 86.4% and specificity of 95.0% in a cohort of 21 patients with acute knee trauma (mean age = 36 years) using fat-suppressed MR images as the reference standard. Subsequent studies show that traumatic marrow lesions in the knees as demonstrated on VNCa images persist for at least 10 weeks[24] and conspicuity is not significantly reduced with a CT dose reduction of 28%.[25] Guggenberger and colleagues[26] performed a similar study in 30 consecutive young patients using DECT VNCa for detection of bone marrow edema in the ankle following trauma. Interreader agreement for qualitative grading of DECT images was substantial (k = 0.66) with reported sensitivity of 90.0% and specificity of 80.5% respectively. Wang and colleagues[27] demonstrated that DECT VNCa can be

Table 4
Urate distribution ranked by anatomic structure in order of prevalence (highest to lowest) reported in a retrospective single-center analysis involving 148 patients using a standardized 4-limb DECT protocol

	No of patients (N = 148)	Patients (%)
1st MTP	85	57.4
Achilles tendon	53	35.8
Ankle joint	38	25.7
Triceps tendon	34	23
Other MTP	34	23
Meniscii	31	21
Popliteus	30	20.3
Tarsal joint	28	18.9
Carpus	24	16.2
Cruciate ligaments	24	16.2
Quadriceps tendon	24	16.2
Pre patella bursa	24	16.2
Hand tendons	16	15.6
Peroneal tendon	22	14.9
Patellar ligament	18	12.2
MCP	13	8.8
Collateral ligaments (knee)	13	8.8
Hand IP joints	12	8.1
Olecranon bursa	13	7.2
Foot IP joints	10	6.8
Wrist tendon	8	5.4
Ankle MCL	8	5.4
Other tendon foot	7	4.7
Knee articular cartilage	5	3.4
Elbow joint	4	2.7
Knee other	4	2.7
Elbow other	3	2
Ankle LCL	2	1.4
Suprapatellar bursa	2	1.4

"Elbow other" composed of 1 radial collateral ligament, 2 biceps insertions and bilateral collateral ligaments. "Foot other" composed of 3 unilateral flexor tendon and 1 bilateral and 1 extensor tendon and 2 in the plantar fascia. "Knee other" composed of 2 synovial-based deposits and 1 flexor tendon and 1 in the iliotibial band.

Abbreviations: DECT, dual-energy computed tomography; IP, interphalangeal; LCL, lateral collateral ligament; MCL, medial collateral ligament; MCP, metacarpophalangeal; MTP, metatarsophalangeal.

Adapted from Mallinson PI, Reagan AC, Coupal T, et al. The distribution of urate deposition within the extremities in gout: a review of 148 dual-energy CT cases. Skeletal Radiol 2014;43(3):279; with permission.

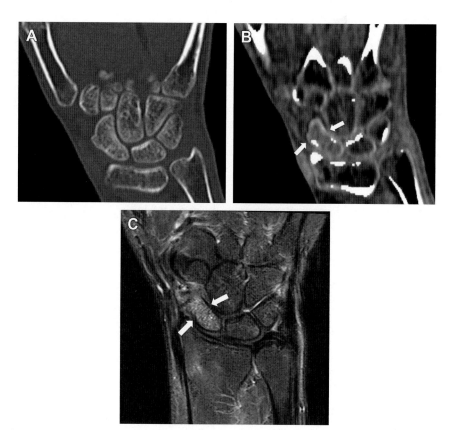

Fig. 3. (*A–C*) DECT of the left wrist in a 54-year-old female patient with anatomic snuffbox tenderness after a fall. Gray-scale mixed image (*A*) shows no signs of scaphoid fracture. Virtual noncalcium-subtracted image (*B*) shows homogeneous increased soft tissue attenuation within the marrow cavity of the left scaphoid (*arrows*). The appearances are out of keeping with fat-attenuation values noted within the marrow cavities of the remainder of the carpal bones. This would be in keeping with marrow edema suggestive of a microtrabecular fracture. (*C*) Coronal STIR MR image obtained 3 days later confirms the presence of (marrow edema) elevated T2 signal within the scaphoid bone in keeping with a nondisplaced fracture microtrabecular fracture (*arrows*).

used to accurately detect bone marrow edema in acute vertebral compression fractures. In this study, comparison was made with MR images depicting 46 edematous and 66 nonedematous vertebral compression fractures with reported VNCa sensitivity of 96.3%, specificity of 98.2%, and accuracy of 97.6% in comparison with MR imaging. Bierry and colleagues[28] published a similar study involving 20 patients with nontumoral vertebral compression fractures and report similar findings. Reddy and colleagues[29] retrospectively assessed the diagnostic accuracy of DECT VNCa in the detection of radiographically occult, undisplaced hip fractures in 25 elderly patients (mean age = 77 years). Sensitivity was 90% for 2 readers; however, there were 3 false-positive cases of a total of 5 patients without fracture, yielding a low specificity value of 40%. In this preliminary study, MR imaging was not available as a reference standard, therefore further research will be required to validate these results.

Pearls and Pitfalls

Important limitations of the DECT VNCa technique include the inability to show marrow alterations directly adjacent to cortical bone owing to incomplete masking of the cortex and spatial averaging.[22] Marrow edema related to osteochondral lesions that are confined to this area could therefore be missed. Wang and colleagues[27] encountered false-negative findings when vertebral bodies contained locules of gas or if they were overtly (>50%) sclerotic. Pache and colleagues[22] suggest that sensitivity also may be reduced due to reader inexperience when interpretation is performed using gray-scale images alone. Most investigators on the subject advise a combined review of gray-scale images and color-coded images enhanced with lookup tables, such as the "parathyroid" color overlay setting, which can accentuate visibility of the small Hounsfield unit changes observed within the marrow cavity. The recently released Syngo.Via (software version VA 30) application from Siemens Healthcare contains an enhanced, color-coded, dual-energy virtual noncalcium application that demonstrates excellent preliminary results (Fig. 4).[30] It should be noted that false-positive results could be encountered by the presence of normal red marrow, which may be present in adult patients in the hip, pelvis, spine, and shoulder girdle.[29] Similar to MR imaging, marrow edema on VNCa, when present, may be related to pathologies other than occult fractures and bone bruises, such as osteonecrosis or degenerative changes.

TENDONS AND LIGAMENTS

Tendons and ligaments are unquestionably best visualized by MR imaging and ultrasound. DECT shows promise over conventional CT in the evaluation of tendons and ligaments in the extremities, given the observed differences in atomic numbers encountered between these structures and surrounding tissues, such as bone and fat. The circuitry of many large tendons are readily displayed and pathologic conditions, such as avulsions, atrophy, compression, and thickening, can be diagnosed.[31] Individual case reports show positive results in complete tears and avulsions of large collagenous structures, such as the patellar, posterior cruciate, and triceps tendon (Fig. 5).[32] DECT when performed to evaluate comminuted fractures shows particular promise in the diagnosis of tendon entrapment. Tendinopathy also has been diagnosed in the Achilles tendon.[33] Similar positive results have been reported in large ligamentous structures, such as the anterior cruciate ligament, and initial case reports also show positive results in the diagnosis of complete tears of small ligamentous structures in the extremities, such as plantar plate injury of the foot.[34] In an animal study, Fickert and colleagues[35] compared the diagnostic accuracy of DECT and MR imaging in the detection of arthroscopically induced total and partial tears of the anterior cruciate ligament (ACL) in 20 porcine hind legs. Consensus interpretation was performed using DECT tendon color maps with reported sensitivity and specificity of 75.0% and 68.8% for the detection of complete ACL tears. In this study, both DECT and MR imaging poorly identified partial disruptions with sensitivities ranging from 0% to 33.3%. Glazebrook and colleagues[36] more recently evaluated the diagnostic performance of DECT in a total of 27 human patients with MR imaging correlation; 16 of the 27 patients had anterior cruciate ligament tears confirmed by MR imaging and 4 musculoskeletal radiologists randomly evaluated the DECT images. The investigators found the area under the curve to be greatest for reconstructed sagittal oblique dual-energy images with bone removal or conventional mixed soft tissue display (area under the curve >0.93 for all readers).

URIC ACID NEPHROLITHIASIS

Five percent to 10% of urinary tract stones in the United States and Europe are composed of uric

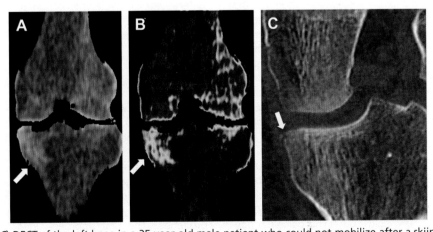

Fig. 4. (A–C) DECT of the left knee in a 35-year-old male patient who could not mobilize after a skiing accident. Gray-scale mixed images (not shown) were preliminarily reviewed by the trauma radiologist and reported as negative. Virtual noncalcium-subtracted image in gray scale (A) and with color coding (B) show elevation of marrow-attenuation values in the medial tibial plateau in keeping with marrow edema (arrows point to marrow edema within the medial tibial plateau on both gray-scale and color-coded images). (C) Subsequent scrutiny of the mixed, bone reformatted images showed a subtle nondisplaced fracture of the medial tibial plateau (white arrow points to fracture).

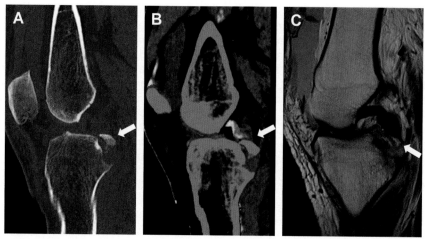

Fig. 5. DECT of the left knee in a 41-year-old male patient who suffered dashboard contact during a high-speed motor vehicle collision. Sagittal mixed, bone reformatted images (*A*) showed a displaced fracture fragment at the posteromedial tibial plateau (*arrow*). DECT tendon application (*B*) clearly demonstrates avulsion at the foot-plate of the posterior cruciate ligament (*arrow*), which was confirmed on sagittal oblique proton density MR imaging (*C*).

acid. The risk of developing uric acid–containing stones is solely related to the amount of uric acid excreted in the urine, in fact more patients with hyperuricosuria are found to have calcium-containing stones rather than uric acid–containing stones. Similarly patients with gout have a higher risk of developing calcium-containing rather than uric acid–containing stones. Having a low urine PH is the most critical biochemical driver for development of uric acid stones. The solubility of uric acid is proven to fall by more than 90% when urine pH drops from 7 to 5.[37] Medications therefore that raise urinary pH, such as potassium bicarbonate or potassium citrate, can be used to increase the solubility of uric acid, and observational studies demonstrate a dramatic reduction in recurrent stone episodes.[38] Alkalinization has been shown in one series of 8 patients who were longitudinally followed with CT and ultrasound to result in dissolution of nonobstructing uric acid calculi measuring less than or equal to 15 mm within 6 weeks to 6 months.[39]

Although measurement of stone attenuation values on SECT has been shown in some studies to correctly characterize calculi, this approach is not robust or reliable enough to be used to accurately identify uric acid–containing calculi in day-to-day practice. Uric acid–containing stones are structurally different from MSU deposits in that they are mainly composed of the protonated, anhydrous form of uric acid admixed with crystals of calcium oxalate.[11] Despite this difference, uric acid stones remain predominantly composed of

light chemical elements, such as hydrogen, nitrogen, carbon, and oxygen, therefore they have significantly smaller atomic weight than other stone types that contain elements with a higher atomic number, such as phosphorus (Z = 15), calcium (Z = 20), and sulfur (Z = 16) (**Table 3**). There is now compelling evidence that DECT can be used to reliably differentiate uric acid–containing from non–uric acid calculi in vitro and in vivo over a large range of body sizes (**Fig. 6**).[40] Evidence also suggests that it is also possible to accurately differentiate different types of non–uric acid calculi using both the second-generation dual-source[41] and single-source fast kV switching DECT systems.[42]

IODINE DISPLAY AND SUBTRACTION

The relatively high atomic number and relatively high k-edge (33.2 kiloelectron volts [keV]) of iodine results in large changes in attenuation when imaged using 2 different x-ray energies in comparison to fat, water, and soft tissue. Dedicated post-processing algorithms have been successfully implemented to measure and segment iodine content using 2 different vendor-specific approaches. The first approach involves a dual-source DECT platform; 3-material decomposition is performed in image space using modeled absorption characteristics of 3 idealized materials, including soft tissue, fat, air, calcium, and iodine using the Syngo.Via Dual-Energy application (Siemens Healthcare).[4] The concentration of

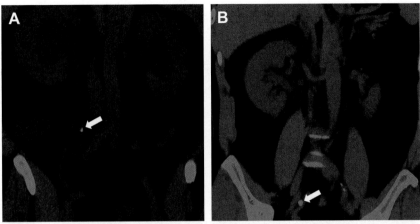

Fig. 6. (A) Noncontrast DECT of the abdomen in a 53-year-old male patient with right renal colic. An obstructing 4-mm calculus was noted in the mid right ureter with attenuation values of 279 HU on the 100-kVp images and 302 HU on the Sn140-kVp images giving DE ratio of 0.91 in keeping with a uric acid–containing calculus (*white arrow* points to uric acid stone color-coded in red in keeping with low molecular weight composition). (*B*) Non-contrast DECT of the abdomen in a 59-year-old male patient with right renal colic. An obstructing 8-mm calculus was found in the distal right ureter with attenuation values of 1518 HU on the 100-kVp images and 1129 HU on the Sn140-kVp images in keeping with a calcium-containing stone (*white arrow* points to calcium calculus color-coded in blue in keeping with high molecular weight composition).

iodine within the imaged vascular structures, organs, or masses can be quantified in milligrams per milliliter or can be superimposed as a color "iodine" map. Using this technique, it is also possible to generate robust virtual non–contrast-enhanced (VNC) images from which Hounsfield unit attenuation values of adrenal and renal lesions can be measured.[43] The second approach involves a single-source, fast kilovolt-peak switching DECT platform; 2-material decomposition is performed in the projection space, which relies on differing absorption characteristics of 2 base materials, such as iodine and water at high-kV and low-kV values. This is achieved using the Gemstone Spectral Imaging application, which generates 2 sets of material density images from which iodine concentration values, but not attenuation values, can be measured.[44]

Depending on the DECT technique and acquisition parameters used, noise is often lower on VNC images compared with true nonenhanced (NC) images; nevertheless, given the synthetic nature of postprocessing, VNC images often have a different noise texture and more grainy appearance as compared with NC images. They also can be susceptible to certain artifacts, including unsharpness, incomplete iodine subtraction, and subtraction, which can include small foci of calcification, prostheses, and renal calculi up to 3 mm in size.[45] These minor pitfalls are offset against the dose and logistical penalties of recalling emergency patients for additional noncontrast CT acquisitions, which are also vulnerable to misregistration artifacts that limit comparison of attenuation values between separate scan acquisitions.[46]

Specific Applications

Head

Noncontrast CT of the head is one of the most commonly performed CT examinations in the emergency setting to investigate complaints ranging from headaches and focal neurologic deficits to acute severe polytrauma. One of the main reasons to perform noncontract CT in this setting is to exclude intracranial hemorrhage, but occasionally a significant diagnostic dilemma can arise when indeterminate hyperdense areas with attenuation values in the same range as blood are found within the brain parenchyma on the initial study. Foci of intermediate-density amorphous calcification are potential mimics of intracranial hemorrhage and early phantom-based studies find that foci of calcification with attenuation levels of less than 100 HU can be differentiated from hemorrhage with greater than 90% accuracy using DECT.[47] Iodinated contrast staining after neurointerventional treatment of acute stroke also can obscure postprocedural intraparenchymal hemorrhage. DECT-generated iodine maps and virtual noncontrast images, as well as direct iodine quantification, are valuable to troubleshoot these situations (**Fig. 7**).[48] In patients presenting with acute

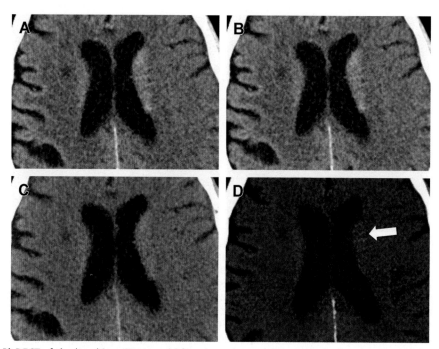

Fig. 7. (A–D) DECT of the head in a 67-year-old female patient with neurologic deterioration after recent intra-arterial thrombolysis for a left M1 segment middle cerebral artery thrombus. Gray-scale mixed image (A) shows relative hyperdensity (44 HU) of the caudate head and body in a pattern that could relate to iodine staining or petechial hemorrhage. The 80-kVp image (B) shows an increase in attenuation in comparison with the Sn140-kVp image (C) (48 vs 34 HU) in keeping with the positive appearance of the DECT iodine map for postprocedural iodine-contrast staining (D) (white arrow points to high attenuation within the left caudate on the color-coded iodine maps in keeping with iodine staining, if this was blood this would not be color coded as iodine on the color-coded iodine overlay maps).

intracerebral hemorrhage, a postcontrast DECT of the head has been shown to reveal previously un-detectable internal areas of enhancement within the hemorrhage, which can indicate an underlying neoplasm with a reported sensitivity of 94% and specificity of 97%.[49]

Chest

Iodine overlay images generated from DECT pulmonary angiograms can provide valuable information regarding lung perfusion distal to a pulmonary embolism. Regional reductions in iodine concentration in the lung parenchyma correspond to reduced blood volume in the pulmonary capillary bed and therefore are an acceptable surrogate for parenchymal perfusion.[5] Simultaneous observation of a filling defect within the pulmonary artery and distal, triangular-shaped, or segmental absence of parenchymal iodine using DECT is indicative of an occlusive PE. Changes observed on pulmonary perfusion iodine maps appear to correlate well with embolic occlusion, as demonstrated using isotope scintigraphy.[50] Preliminary evidence shows that the extent and size of perfusion defects demonstrated on iodine overlay

have a good correlation with right ventricle to left ventricle diameter ratio, which is a key predictor of early death in acute pulmonary embolism (Fig. 8).[51] Kerl and colleagues[52] advise that a triphasic injection protocol composed of iodinated contrast, part contrast-saline followed a by saline chaser should be used to suppress streak artifacts from high-density, undiluted contrast material in the SVC, which can significantly degrade DECT iodine maps of the lung.

Cardiac

Although myocardial perfusion defects can be demonstrated on conventional gray-scale image using SECT, iodine mapping and iodine quantification of the myocardium using DECT increases the conspicuity of hypoperfused segments allowing more confident identification of myocardial ischemia.[53] Early studies show 92% sensitivity and 93% specificity for the detection of myocardial perfusion defects seen on single-photon emission computed tomography (SPECT).[54] Interestingly, this study and others find that rest DECT is able to demonstrate some reversible myocardial perfusion defects that are observed only on

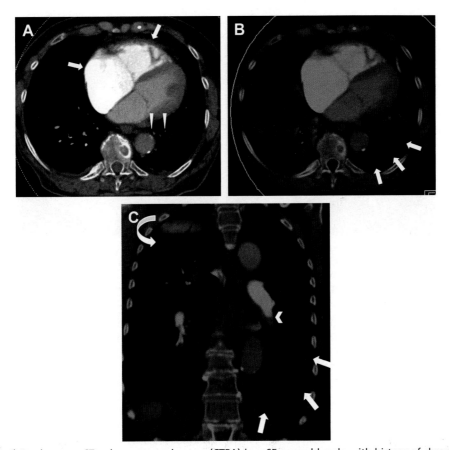

Fig. 8. (A–C) Dual-energy CT pulmonary angiogram (CTPA) in a 65-year-old male with history of chronic pulmonary thromboembolic disease. Mixed gray-scale image (A) shows occlusive thrombi in the left lower lobe (*white arrowheads*) and moderate dilation of the right heart (*white arrows*). DECT iodine maps (B, C) confirm segmental perfusion defects of the left lower lobe related to non-recannulized thrombus (*open white arrows*) (*arrowhead* points to thrombus within left lower lobe segmental artery). Apparent defect in the right upper lobe with linear margins is classic for beam-hardening artifact secondary to high attenuation contrast within the superior vena cava (*curved white arrow*).

SPECT imaging after the administration of pharmacologic stress agents, albeit with a low overall positive predictive value in the region of 26%.[53] When DECT iodine maps of the myocardium were assessed in addition to conventional images of the coronary arteries, Wang and colleagues[55] found that sensitivity for detecting significant coronary stenosis increased from 82% to 90%. Although data are limited in the emergency setting, there appears to be an incremental benefit of DECT over SECT given its ability to simultaneously evaluate the coronary arteries and assess myocardial perfusion with future potential to improve our detection of morphologically and hemodynamically significant coronary artery disease over the purely anatomic test of coronary CT angiography (CTA) alone.[56] Early evidence from a single center suggests that stress DECT perfusion may be better at detecting small areas of myocardial ischemia and balanced myocardial ischemia in multivessel disease or coronary microvascular disease, compared with rest DECT and SPECT.[57]

Cardioembolic stroke carries a major risk of stroke recurrence, which can be markedly reduced by early initiation of appropriate secondary prevention. Although transesophageal echocardiography (TEE) has been validated as an accurate tool for the detection of thrombus in the left atrial appendage, there is good evidence that cardiac CT is a reliable and noninvasive alternative, particularly when delayed imaging or a dual-phase injection (arterial and 180s delayed) is performed (**Fig. 9**).[58] An elegant use of cardiac DECT has been described by Hur and colleagues[59] in a group of 63 patients with stroke. The investigators performed a cardiac DECT in a single-detector fast kV switching system using a dual-phase injection protocol combining arterial (70 mL) and 180-second delayed (50 mL) phases

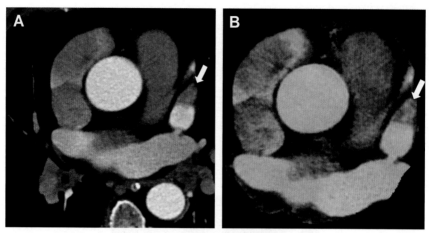

Fig. 9. Cardiac DECT in a 58-year-old female with history of atrial fibrillation. Gray-scale mixed image (A) shows white arrow points to poor mixing of contrast in the left atrial appendage with possible eccentric clot toward the apex. (B) DECT color-coded overlay iodine map reveals white arrow points to more homogeneous iodine-based contrast throughout the atrial appendage, which was considered negative for thrombus.

in a single acquisition. They compared diagnostic performance against TEE as the reference standard and found overall sensitivity, specificity, positive predictive value, and negative predictive value of DE cardiac CT for detection of left atrial appendage thrombi to be 97%, 100%, 100%, and 97%, respectively.

Abdomen

The ability to quantify and map iodine distribution and create VNC images using DECT in the abdomen and pelvis adds depth and significant insight over the routine interpretation of focal solid-organ and hollow visceral diseases using SECT. Perhaps one of the most significant contributions of DECT in the emergency setting is

the ability to better characterize adrenal, renal, and hepatic incidentalomas that are found in approximately 7%, 27%, and 52% of the adult population.[60]

A number of studies document the reliability of VNC attenuation values as compared with NC images and conclude that incidental adrenal lesions can be accurately characterized using a single contrast-enhanced DECT scan (Fig. 10).[43,61,62] Ho and colleagues[43] found a mean difference of only 1.8 HU between VNC and NC in 23 adrenal lesions. Gnannt and colleagues[62] had similar findings in a study of 51 adrenal masses; however, diagnostic accuracy was significantly better for lesions measuring greater than 1 cm in this study (78% vs 97%).

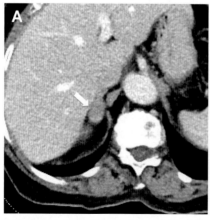
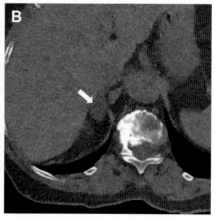

Fig. 10. (A, B) Dual-energy, contrast-enhanced CT of the abdomen in a 47-year-old male with acute appendicitis. Gray-scale mixed images (A) white arrow shows an incidental right adrenal mass with attenuation value of 63 HU. Normally this patient would return as an outpatient for an adrenal protocol CT. (B) However, further postprocessing using the DECT virtual noncontrast iodine subtraction application in this instance demonstrated VNC attenuation of 12 HU in keeping with a benign adrenal adenoma (white arrow points to adrenal adenoma).

Although most cystic renal lesions can be characterized on a single postcontrast study, some that contain septations or hyperdense debris require further workup to determine if they enhance. In a study of 72 renal masses, Ascenti and colleagues[63] found that DECT whole-tumor iodine quantification was more accurate than conventional attenuation measurements between noncontrast and postcontrast images (97% vs 89%) with histopathology or imaging follow-up serving as the reference standard. Results from a more recent study of 59 patients with 80 renal lesions assigned an iodine concentration threshold of greater than 0.5 mg/mL for positive lesions and had similar findings.[64] In a 49-patient study involving a single-detector fast kV switching system, Lv and colleagues[65] found that 21 hepatic hemangiomas could be accurately differentiated from 28 hepatocellular carcinomas based on the higher normalized iodine concentrations on arterial and portal venous phases.

In our early experience, iodine maps also may be helpful in evaluating segmental small intestinal ischemia (Fig. 11) and can improve the conspicuity of mucosal enhancement in cases of bowel obstruction. Iodine overlay images increase confidence in detecting endoleaks after aortic stent graft placement.[66] VNC images are valuable in the emergency setting to increase the conspicuity

between enhancing soft tissue and dense non–iodine-containing materials, such as hematomas in the bowel wall, peritoneal cavity, or abdominal wall (Figs. 12 and 13). Nonenhancing products of necrotic pancreatitis also can be identified on VNC images without loss of image quality over NC examinations.[67] Care should be taken, however, when interpreting VNC images from in the setting of pancreatitis, as the 3-material decomposition process assumes that each voxel in the abdomen is composed of either soft tissue, iodine, or fat, and therefore small foci of calcification are usually subtracted from the image.[67] VNC images alone are therefore not suitable to evaluate for pancreatic parenchymal calcification and pancreatic duct calculi, although an additional postprocessing step that includes calcium, iodine, and soft tissue into the 3-material decomposition algorithm has been proposed to overcome these artifacts.[46] Mangold and colleagues[45] report that renal calculi that measure greater than 2.9 mm and have attenuation values of higher than 387 HU can be reliably detected (sensitivity of 76% and specificity of 90%) in an evaluation of 87 renal calculi in which VNC images were generated from the delayed excretory phase images of DECT urograms and compared with true NC images. Performance is likely to be better if VNC subtraction is performed using portal venous phase

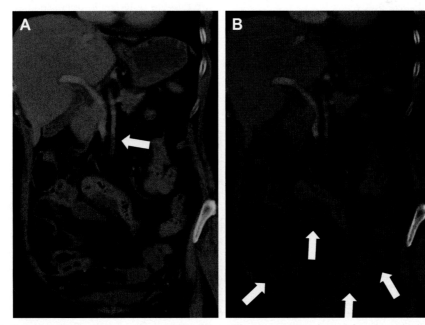

Fig. 11. (A, B) Dual-energy, contrast-enhanced CT of the abdomen in a 77-year-old female with acute abdominal pain on a background of atrial fibrillation. On the mixed gray-scale images, white arrow points to an occlusive filling defect in the proximal superior mesenteric artery (A). White arrows point to relative hypoenhancement and lack of iodine uptake of infarcted loops of ileum that is more obviously demonstrated on the DECT color-coded iodine overlay maps (B).

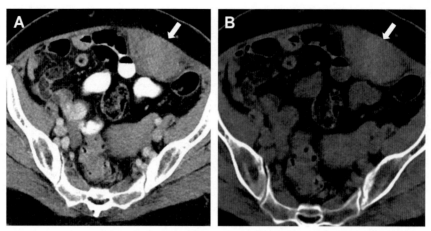

Fig. 12. Dual-energy, contrast-enhanced CT of the abdomen in a 63-year-old female with acute on chronic left lower quadrant abdominal pain. Mixed gray-scale images show marked expansion of the lower left rectus abdominis muscle (*arrow*) with possible internal enhancement and no definite hematocrit level (*A*). The differential at this point includes a mass or spontaneous hematoma. DECT virtual noncontrast iodine subtraction image was generated (*B*) in which the white arrow clearly points to hyperdense hemorrhagic debris diagnostic for a spontaneous rectus hematoma.

DECT scans, given the high concentrations of contrast medium within the collecting system on the excretory phase images that results in beam hardening and scatter radiation. An additonal unique and innovative use of DECT involves the differentiation of heroin from cocaine in body packs on the basis of their different dual energy indices and spectral curves which has been validated in one ex vivo study.[68]

ENERGY-SPECIFIC DISPLAY

Using sophisticated reconstruction algorithms, either in projection or image space, data from 2 polychromatic exposures can be processed to generate synthetic images that simulate those obtained from a true monochromatic source. Currently available algorithms allow reconstruction of virtual monochromatic images (VMIs) far beyond the range of mean kV levels available using today's CT tube technology (40–190 keV). Virtual monochromatic imaging represents one of the most widely applicable attributes of DECT, with great future potential to optimize image quality of enhanced and unenhanced CT from head to toe. One of the immediate benefits of VMI is the potential to correct HU-reducing artifacts related to preferential absorption of low-energy photons from a polychromatic source known as beam hardening. Pomerantz and colleagues[69] successfully use

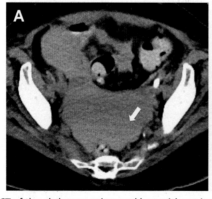
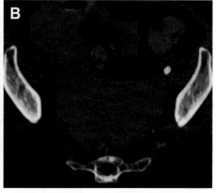

Fig. 13. DECT of the abdomen using oral but without intravenous contrast in a 65-year-old female with suspected anastomotic leak after recent ileal resection. Gray-scale mixed images (*A*) show high attenuation fluid collecting in the pelvis (*arrow*), which was initially presumed to represent a mixture of oral contrast and free fluid. DECT iodine map was generated (*B*) which shows no iodine content in keeping with postoperative intraperitoneal hematoma.

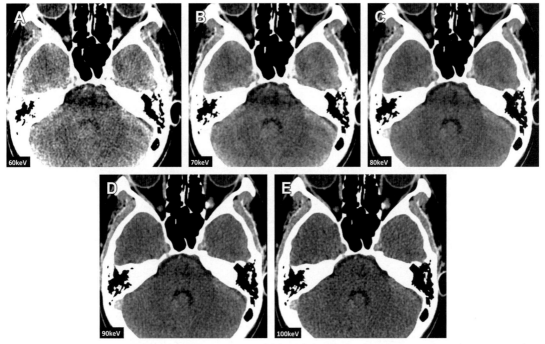

Fig. 14. Noncontrast DECT of the head in a 19-year-old female patient. Virtual monoenergetic reconstructions (*A–E*) at 60, 70, 80, 90, and 100 keV show a progressive reduction in the severity of posterior fossa beam-hardening artifact at the expense of reduced gray-white matter differentiation.

VMI reconstructed at 65 keV to maximize gray/white matter signal-to-noise ratios and 75 keV to reduce posterior fossa beam-hardening artifact (**Fig. 14**). Scheske and colleagues[70] used VMI reconstructed at 90 keV to substantially reduce myocardial beam-hardening artifacts in the basal inferior wall and midseptum using DE-coronary computed tomography angiography.

Synthetic monochromatic images reconstructed at low-keV levels maximize signal from iodinated contrast materials given that they more closely approximate the k-edge of iodine (33 keV). Low-keV VMI images can be used to improve signal-to-noise ratios in angiographic studies throughout the body and iodinated contrast dose may be reduced by 50% or more without significant loss in CTA quality.[71] Contrast-to-noise ratios in both hyperenhancing and hypoenhancing lesions of the liver, pancreas, and other solid organs also can be increased using tailored low-keV reconstructions.[72–74] Potretzke and colleagues[75] surgically induced 8 ischemic segments of bowel in 4 swine that were subsequently scanned using DECT and regular 120-kVp CT. The investigators found that attenuation difference between ischemic and perfused segments was significantly greater on DECT VMI images reconstructed at 51 keV as compared with conventional 120-kVp CT images (mean difference, 91.7 vs 47.6 HU).

Metallic implants, prostheses, and foreign bodies can severely degrade the quality of CT images due to summative artifacts, including beam hardening, photon starvation, and photon scattering.[4] Although VMI cannot correct for photon starvation and scattering, a reduction in beam-hardening artifact with high keV reconstructions is associated with significantly improved image quality,[76,77] and in our experience greatly aids in the interpretation of acute periprosthetic complications, projectile-related bone injury, and assessment of vasculature surrounding metallic stents, clips, and coils.

REFERENCES

1. Rubin GD. Computed tomography: revolutionizing the practice of medicine for 40 years. Radiology 2014;273(2 Suppl):S45–74.
2. Alvarez RE, Macovski A. Energy-selective reconstructions in X-ray computerized tomography. Phys Med Biol 1976;21(5):733–44.
3. Johnson TR, Krauss B, Sedlmair M, et al. Material differentiation by dual energy CT: initial experience. Eur Radiol 2007;17(6):1510–7.
4. Marin D, Boll DT, Mileto A, et al. State of the art: dual-energy CT of the abdomen. Radiology 2014;271(2):327–42.

5. Johnson T, Fink C, Schönberg SO, et al. Dual energy CT in clinical practice. Heidelberg: Springer; 2011.

6. Kocher KE, Meurer WJ, Fazel R, et al. National trends in use of computed tomography in the emergency department. Ann Emerg Med 2011;58(5): 452–62.e3.

7. Nicolaou S, Liang T, Murphy DT, et al. a promising new technique for assessment of the musculoskeletal system. Am J Roentgenol 2012;199(5 Suppl): S78–86.

8. Morán LM, Martínez LP. Gouty inflammation confused with septic arthritis. Reumatol Clin 2013; 9(5):324–5.

9. Suresh E. Problem based review: the patient with acute monoarthritis. Acute Med 2013;12(2):111–6.

10. Loeb JN. The influence of temperature on the solubility of monosodium urate. Arthritis Rheum 1972; 15(2):189–92.

11. Martillo MA, Nazzal L, Crittenden DB. The crystallization of monosodium urate. Curr Rheumatol Rep 2014;16(2):400.

12. Nicolaou S, Yong-Hing CJ, Galea-Soler S, et al. Dual-energy CT as a potential new diagnostic tool in the management of gout in the acute setting. Am J Roentgenol 2010;194(4):1072–8.

13. Lally EV, Zimmermann B, Ho G, et al. Urate-mediated inflammation in nodal osteoarthritis: clinical and roentgenographic correlations. Arthritis Rheum 1989;32(1):86–90.

14. Simkin PA, Campbell PM, Larson EB. Gout in Heberden's nodes. Arthritis Rheum 1983;26(1):94–7.

15. Underwood M. Diagnosis and management of gout. BMJ 2006;332(7553):1315–9.

16. Choi HK, Al-Arfaj AM, Eftekhari A, et al. Dual energy computed tomography in tophaceous gout. Ann Rheum Dis 2009;68(10):1609–12.

17. Ogdie A, Taylor WJ, Weatherall M, et al. Imaging modalities for the classification of gout: systematic literature review and meta-analysis. Ann Rheum Dis 2014. [Epub ahead of print].

18. Bongartz T, Glazebrook KN, Kavros SJ, et al. Dual-energy CT for the diagnosis of gout: an accuracy and diagnostic yield study. Ann Rheum Dis 2014. [Epub ahead of print].

19. Mallinson PI, Coupal T, Reisinger C, et al. Artifacts in dual-energy CT gout protocol: a review of 50 suspected cases with an artifact identification guide. Am J Roentgenol 2014;203(1):W103–9.

20. Mallinson PI, Reagan AC, Coupal T, et al. The distribution of urate deposition within the extremities in gout: a review of 148 dual-energy CT cases. Skeletal Radiol 2014;43(3):277–81.

21. Dalbeth N, Kalluru R, Aati O, et al. Tendon involvement in the feet of patients with gout: a dual-energy CT study. Ann Rheum Dis 2013;72(9):1545–8.

22. Pache G, Krauss B, Strohm P, et al. Dual-energy CT virtual noncalcium technique: detecting posttraumatic bone marrow lesions—feasibility study 1. Radiology 2010;256(2):617–24.

23. Reagan AC, Mallinson PI, O'Connell T, et al. Dual-energy computed tomographic virtual noncalcium algorithm for detection of bone marrow edema in acute fractures. J Comput Assist Tomogr 2014; 38(5):802–5.

24. Ai S, Qu M, Glazebrook KN, et al. Use of dual-energy CT and virtual non-calcium techniques to evaluate post-traumatic bone bruises in knees in the subacute setting. Skeletal Radiol 2014;43(9): 1289–95.

25. Pache G, Bulla S, Baumann T, et al. Dose reduction does not affect detection of bone marrow lesions with dual-energy CT virtual noncalcium technique. Acad Radiol 2012;19(12):1539–45.

26. Guggenberger R, Gnannt R, Hodler J, et al. Diagnostic performance of dual-energy CT for the detection of traumatic bone marrow lesions in the ankle: comparison with MR imaging. Radiology 2012; 264(1):164–73.

27. Wang CK, Tsai JM, Chuang MT, et al. Bone marrow edema in vertebral compression fractures: detection with dual-energy CT. Radiology 2013;269(2):525–33.

28. Bierry G, Venkatasamy A, Kremer S, et al. Dual-energy CT in vertebral compression fractures: performance of visual and quantitative analysis for bone marrow edema demonstration with comparison to MRI. Skeletal Radiol 2014;43(4):485–92.

29. Reddy T, McLaughlin PD, Mallinson PI, et al. Detection of occult, undisplaced hip fractures with a dual-energy CT algorithm targeted to detection of bone marrow edema. Emerg Radiol 2015;22(1):25–9.

30. Rajayogeswaran B, Chhaya N, McLaughlin PD, et al. "A touch of colour": DE bone marrow v virtual noncalcium application for the assessment of bone marrow oedema in acute hand fractures. archiversnaorg. Available at: http://archive.rsna.org/2014/14009000.html. Accessed January 25, 2015.

31. Deng K, Sun C, Liu C, et al. Initial experience with visualizing hand and foot tendons by dual-energy computed tomography. Clin Imaging 2009;33(5): 384–9.

32. Mallinson P, Antoniades G, McLaughlin P, et al. Dual-energy computed tomographic tendon algorithm in acute trauma. J Comput Assist Tomogr 2014;38(3): 348–51.

33. Mallinson PI, Stevens C, Reisinger C, et al. Diagnosis using dual-energy computed tomography collagen material decomposition application. J Comput Assist Tomogr 2013;37(3):475–7.

34. Stevens CJ, Murphy DT, Korzan JR, et al. Plantar plate tear diagnosis using dual-energy computed tomography collagen material decomposition application. J Comput Assist Tomogr 2013;37(3):478–80.

35. Fickert S, Niks M, Dinter DJ, et al. Assessment of the diagnostic value of dual-energy CT and MRI in the

detection of iatrogenically induced injuries of anterior cruciate ligament in a porcine model. Skeletal Radiol 2013;42(3):411–7.

36. Glazebrook KN, Brewerton LJ, Leng S, et al. Case–control study to estimate the performance of dual-energy computed tomography for anterior cruciate ligament tears in patients with history of knee trauma. Skeletal Radiol 2013;43(3):297–305.

37. Coe FL. Uric acid and calcium oxalate nephrolithiasis. Kidney Int 1983;24(3):392–403.

38. Pak CY, Sakhaee K, Fuller C. Successful management of uric acid nephrolithiasis with potassium citrate. Kidney Int 1986;30(3):422–8.

39. Trinchieri A, Esposito N, Castelnuovo C. Dissolution of radiolucent renal stones by oral alkalinization with potassium citrate/potassium bicarbonate. Arch Ital Urol Androl 2009;81(3):188–91.

40. Qu M, Jaramillo-Alvarez G, Ramirez-Giraldo JC, et al. Urinary stone differentiation in patients with large body size using dual-energy dual-source computed tomography. Eur Radiol 2013;23(5):1408–14.

41. Qu M, Ramirez-Giraldo JC, Leng S, et al. Dual-energy dual-source CT with additional spectral filtration can improve the differentiation of non-uric acid renal stones: an ex vivo phantom study. Am J Roentgenol 2011;196(6):1279–87.

42. Li X, Zhao R, Liu B, et al. Gemstone spectral imaging dual-energy computed tomography: a novel technique to determine urinary stone composition. Urology 2013;81(4):727–30.

43. Ho LM, Marin D, Neville AM, et al. Characterization of adrenal nodules with dual-energy CT: can virtual unenhanced attenuation values replace true unenhanced attenuation values? Am J Roentgenol 2012;198(4):840–5.

44. Kaza RK, Platt JF, Cohan RH, et al. Dual-energy CT with single- and dual-source scanners: current applications in evaluating the genitourinary tract. Radiographics 2012;32(2):353–69.

45. Mangold S, Thomas C, Fenchel M, et al. Virtual nonenhanced dual-energy CT urography with tin-filter technology: determinants of detection of urinary calculi in the renal collecting system. Radiology 2012;264(1):119–25.

46. Graser A, Johnson TR, Hecht EM, et al. Dual-energy CT in patients suspected of having renal masses: can virtual nonenhanced images replace true nonenhanced images? 1. Radiology 2009;252(2):433–40.

47. Nute JL, Le Roux L, Chandler AG, et al. Differentiation of low-attenuation intracranial hemorrhage and calcification using dual-energy computed tomography in a phantom system. Invest Radiol 2015;50(1):9–16.

48. Tran DN, Straka M, Roos JE, et al. Dual-energy CT discrimination of iodine and calcium. Acad Radiol 2009;16(2):160–71.

49. Kim SJ, Lim HK, Lee HY, et al. Dual-energy CT in the evaluation of intracerebral hemorrhage of unknown origin: differentiation between tumor bleeding and pure hemorrhage. AJNR Am J Neuroradiol 2012;33(5):865–72.

50. Thieme SF, Johnson TR, Lee C, et al. Dual-energy CT for the assessment of contrast material distribution in the pulmonary parenchyma. Am J Roentgenol 2009;193(1):144–9.

51. Schoepf UJ. Right ventricular enlargement on chest computed tomography: a predictor of early death in acute pulmonary embolism. Circulation 2004;110(20):3276–80.

52. Kerl JM, Bauer RW, Renker M, et al. Triphasic contrast injection improves evaluation of dual energy lung perfusion in pulmonary CT angiography. Eur J Radiol 2011;80(3):e483–7.

53. Arnoldi E, Lee YS, Ruzsics B, et al. CT detection of myocardial blood volume deficits: dual-energy CT compared with single-energy CT spectra. J Cardiovasc Comput Tomogr 2011;5(6):421–9.

54. Ruzsics B, Schwarz F, Schoepf UJ, et al. Comparison of dual-energy computed tomography of the heart with single photon emission computed tomography for assessment of coronary artery stenosis and of the myocardial blood supply. Am J Cardiol 2009;104(3):318–26.

55. Wang R, Yu W, Wang Y, et al. Incremental value of dual-energy CT to coronary CT angiography for the detection of significant coronary stenosis: comparison with quantitative coronary angiography and single photon emission computed tomography. Int J Cardiovasc Imaging 2011;27(5):647–56.

56. De Cecco CN, Harris BS, Schoepf UJ, et al. Incremental value of pharmacological stress cardiac dual-energy CT over coronary CT angiography alone for the assessment of coronary artery disease in a high-risk population. Am J Roentgenol 2014;203(1):W70–7.

57. Schoepf UJ, Bamberg F, Ruzsics B, et al, editors. CT imaging of myocardial perfusion and viability. Berlin: Springer; 2014.

58. Romero J, Husain SA, Kelesidis I, et al. Detection of left atrial appendage thrombus by cardiac computed tomography in patients with atrial fibrillation: a meta-analysis. Circ Cardiovasc Imaging 2013;6(2):185–94.

59. Hur J, Kim YJ, Lee HJ, et al. Cardioembolic stroke: dual-energy cardiac CT for differentiation of left atrial appendage thrombus and circulatory stasis. Radiology 2012;263(3):688–95.

60. Berland LL, Silverman SG, Gore RM, et al. Managing incidental findings on abdominal CT: white paper of the ACR incidental findings committee. J Am Coll Radiol 2010;7(10):754–73.

61. Botsikas D, Triponez F, Boudabbous S, et al. Incidental adrenal lesions detected on enhanced

abdominal dual-energy CT: can the diagnostic workup be shortened by the implementation of virtual unenhanced images? Eur J Radiol 2014; 83(10):1746–51.

62. Gnannt R, Fischer M, Goetti R, et al. Dual-energy CT for characterization of the incidental adrenal mass: preliminary observations. Am J Roentgenol 2012; 198(1):138–44.

63. Ascenti G, Mileto A, Krauss B, et al. Distinguishing enhancing from nonenhancing renal masses with dual-source dual-energy CT: iodine quantification versus standard enhancement measurements. Eur Radiol 2013;23(8):2288–95.

64. Mileto A, Marin D, Ramirez-Giraldo JC, et al. Accuracy of contrast-enhanced dual-energy MDCT for the assessment of iodine uptake in renal lesions. Am J Roentgenol 2014;202(5):W466–74.

65. Lv P, Lin XZ, Li J, et al. Differentiation of small hepatic hemangioma from small hepatocellular carcinoma: recently introduced spectral CT method. Radiology 2011;259(3):720–9.

66. Ascenti G, Mazziotti S, Lamberto S, et al. Dual-energy CT for detection of endoleaks after endovascular abdominal aneurysm repair: usefulness of colored iodine overlay. Am J Roentgenol 2011; 196(6):1408–14.

67. Mileto A, Mazziotti S, Gaeta M, et al. Pancreatic dual-source dual-energy CT: is it time to discard unenhanced imaging? Clin Radiol 2012;67(4): 334–9.

68. Grimm J, Wudy R, Ziegeler E, et al. Differentiation of heroin and cocaine using dual-energy CT—an experimental study. Int J Legal Med 2014;128(3): 475–82.

69. Pomerantz SR, Kamalian S, Zhang D, et al. Virtual monochromatic reconstruction of dual-energy unenhanced head CT at 65–75 kev maximizes image quality compared with conventional polychromatic CT. Radiology 2013;266(1):318–25.

70. Scheske JA, O'Brien JM, Earls JP, et al. Coronary artery imaging with single-source rapid kilovolt peak-switching dual-energy CT. Radiology 2013;268(3): 702–9.

71. Yuan R, Shuman WP, Earls JP, et al. Reduced iodine load at CT pulmonary angiography with dual-energy monochromatic imaging: comparison with standard CT pulmonary angiography—a prospective randomized trial. Radiology 2012;262(1):290–7.

72. Quiney B, Harris A, McLaughlin P, et al. Dual-energy CT increases reader confidence in the detection and diagnosis of hypoattenuating pancreatic lesions. Abdom Imaging 2014. [Epub ahead of print].

73. Patel BN, Thomas JV, Lockhart ME, et al. Single-source dual-energy spectral multidetector CT of pancreatic adenocarcinoma: optimization of energy level viewing significantly increases lesion contrast. Clin Radiol 2013;68(2):148–54.

74. Robinson E, Babb J, Chandarana H, et al. Dual source dual energy MDCT: comparison of 80 kVp and weighted average 120 kVp data for conspicuity of hypo-vascular liver metastases. Invest Radiol 2010;45(7):413–8.

75. Potretzke TA, Brace CL, Lubner MG, et al. Early small-bowel ischemia: dual-energy CT improves conspicuity compared with conventional ct in a swine model. Radiology 2014;140875. http://dx.doi.org/10.1148/radiol.14140875.

76. Bamberg F, Dierks A, Nikolaou K, et al. Metal artifact reduction by dual energy computed tomography using monoenergetic extrapolation. Eur Radiol 2011; 21(7):1424–9.

77. Lee YH, Park KK, Song HT, et al. Metal artefact reduction in gemstone spectral imaging dual-energy CT with and without metal artefact reduction software. Eur Radiol 2012;22(6):1331–40.

78. Glazebrook KN, Guimarães LS, Murthy NS, et al. Identification of intraarticular and periarticular uric acid crystals with dual-energy CT: initial evaluation. Radiology 2011;261(2):516–24.

79. Choi HK, Burns LC, Shojania K, et al. Dual energy CT in gout: a prospective validation study. Ann Rheum Dis 2012;71(9):1466–71.

Improving Outcomes in the Patient with Polytrauma
A Review of the Role of Whole-Body Computed Tomography

Martin L. Gunn, MBChB, FRANZCR[a],*, Digna R. Kool, MD[b],
Bruce E. Lehnert, MD[a]

KEYWORDS

- Trauma • Polytrauma • Panscan • CT • Whole-body CT • Mortality • Survival rate
- Injury severity score

KEY POINTS

- Whole-body computed tomography (WBCT) has become a widely used technique for the workup of the patient with blunt polytrauma.
- Current evidence suggests that WBCT is associated with improved or no change in patient survival and reduces the emergency department (ED) length of stay (LOS).
- However, randomized studies, at least one of which is underway, are needed to determine for certain whether early WBCT improves survival, to clarify which patients benefit the most and to model the costs of this technique compared with traditional workup.
- Advancements in modern multidetector computed tomography (MDCT) technology and an improved understanding of optimal protocols have enabled one to scan the entire body and achieve adequate image quality for a comprehensive trauma assessment in a short period.

INTRODUCTION

Trauma remains a major cause of death and health care expenditure worldwide, accounting for nearly 10% of all deaths.[1] In the United States, trauma is the leading cause of death in patients aged 1 to 44 years, the third most common cause in patients aged between 45 and 54 years, and the fifth most common cause overall.[2] In 2010, there were 41.0 million US ED visits for injuries and more than 120,000 deaths.[3,4] Worldwide, road traffic injuries, falls, and drowning are the top 3 causes of death from unintentional injury.[1] The Centers for Disease Control and Prevention estimated that in 2005 the total cost of injury in the United States was approximately 172 billion dollars.

Evidence during the last 2 decades has shown that rapid patient triage followed by transportation to a designated trauma center is associated with a significant reduction in mortality after severe injury compared with transport to a nontrauma center.[5,6] During initial evaluation, an accurate and timely diagnosis of bleeding and other important injuries is essential to plan and prioritize therapy. Unfortunately, significant injuries are overlooked at an unacceptably high rate in patients with major trauma.[7] In particular, physical examination is unreliable in patients with a reduced level of

[a] Department of Radiology, University of Washington, Box 359728, 325 9th Ave, Seattle, WA 98104, USA;
[b] Nijmegen, The Netherlands
* Corresponding author.
E-mail address: marting@uw.edu

Radiol Clin N Am 53 (2015) 639–656
http://dx.doi.org/10.1016/j.rcl.2015.02.006
0033-8389/15/$ – see front matter © 2015 Elsevier Inc. All rights reserved.

consciousness or distracting injuries, necessitating imaging evaluation.[8] Radiographic evaluation detects many important injuries in the chest and pelvis, but radiographs fail to show important injuries in the head, spine, chest, abdomen, and pelvis because of lack of sensitivity, misinterpretation, or inadequate technique.[7] Computed tomography (CT) is much more sensitive for the detection of head, spine, and torso injuries than radiography, and the dramatic decline in mortality rates from polytrauma in the past few decades is likely, in part, because of the increased use of CT in the ED. CT has also lead to a reduction in the number of nontherapeutic laparotomies and an increase in nonoperative management of solid-organ injuries, including those involving the liver and spleen, with or without angioembolization.[9] Several studies have demonstrated that WBCT is a sensitive and comprehensive tool for the diagnosis of a wide range of traumatic injuries, especially in the severely injured patient.[10–14] Accordingly, there has been increasing interest in the development and utilization of WBCT techniques. It was reported that about 60% of European trauma centers use WBCT.[15]

However, several unanswered questions persist about the role of WBCT in major trauma. These uncertainties surround appropriate patient selection, potentially excessive radiation exposure, management of incidental findings,[16] and potentially increased health care costs. The relative sensitivity, time, and radiation dose of various WBCT scan protocols have not yet been studied sufficiently. Furthermore, there are persistent doubts about the clinical significance of additional injuries detected by WBCT and the mortality benefit of WBCT when compared with selective CT.[15–23] This article provides a detailed overview of the current concepts surrounding WBCT in trauma.

DEFINITION OF WHOLE-BODY COMPUTED TOMOGRAPHY IN TRAUMA

The techniques used for WBCT (otherwise known as pan-scan or total-body CT) in trauma vary tremendously, but generally, WBCT is considered to include CT of the head, neck, chest, abdomen, and pelvis during a single visit to the CT scanner. Less commonly, CT has been used to refer specifically to thoracoabdominal CT for trauma. Usually, a WBCT scan comprises a CT of the head without intravenous contrast, CT of the cervical spine (acquired before, or following, intravenous contrast), and CT of the chest, abdomen, and pelvis following intravenous contrast. This procedure differs from selective CT, in which one or

more body regions are scanned based on physical examination, prior tests (laboratory and radiographic), and the suspected pattern of injury.

INDICATIONS FOR WHOLE-BODY COMPUTED TOMOGRAPHY IN TRAUMA

There is no consensus in the literature and no validated clinical prediction rule that defines clear criteria for WBCT following trauma or to define patients in whom WBCT can be safely omitted. In the published studies to date, a range of indications have been applied to select patients with trauma for WBCT rather than selective CT. Broadly, indications for WBCT have included the mechanism of injury, injury location or pattern, initial vital signs, or a combination of these.[17]

Mechanism of Injury

Only a few studies have evaluated mechanism of injury as a decision-making tool for the use of WBCT.

Salim and colleagues[11] performed a prospective observational study in which WBCT was performed in 1000 hemodynamically stable patients without definitive signs of major injury. Inclusion criteria for WBCT were based on mechanism of injury in 60% of patients (motor vehicle collisions [MVCs] at >35 mph [55 km/h], fall >15 ft [4.5 m], automobile vs pedestrian injury with the pedestrian thrown more than 10 feet, and assault). However, WBCT was performed because of a depressed level of consciousness in 40% of subjects, independent of mechanism. Overall, these investigators found clinically significant abnormalities in 3.5% of head CT scans, 5.1% of cervical spine CT scans, 19.6% of chest CT scans, and 7.1% of abdominal CT scans when WBCT was performed based on mechanism of injury alone. These abnormal CT scan findings resulted in a change in treatment in 18.9% of patients. The investigators noted a change in treatment in 120 (20.3%) patients based on the abdominal CT scan, resulting in 8 laparotomies in patients with normal findings on abdominal examinations. One potential flaw of this study was the broad definition of a change in treatment resulting from the CT scan, which included early discharge from the ED, further imaging of any kind, admission for serial examination, or operation.

A retrospective analysis by Hutter and colleagues[24] evaluated 608 patients undergoing WBCT based on a high-energy mechanism (MVC with death of other occupants or extrication, falls from height, pedestrian injuries, bicycle injuries, and patients with unknown mechanism of injury). Patients had to be hemodynamically stable after resuscitation (systolic blood pressure >90 mm Hg). The investigators found a significant survival benefit with the use of the WBCT protocol (odds ratio [OR] for mortality: 0.28; 95% confidence interval [CI], 0.19, 0.42).[24] However, simultaneous improvements in departmental equipment and processes may have contributed to the results.

Not all studies evaluating the use of WBCT based on mechanism of injury alone have come to the same conclusion. A retrospective study of 108 hemodynamically stable and clinically evaluable patients with blunt trauma who underwent a CT of the chest, abdomen, and pelvis found only 11 patients (10%; 95% CI, 4.4, 15.6) had acute injuries detected on CT and none of these patients required direct medical intervention or hospital admission.[22] Of the 11 patients with injuries detected at CT, 8 were intoxicated or had distracting injuries. Most of these injuries were orthopedic but included small pneumothoraces and a single small, contained liver laceration.

Location of Injury

Some studies have evaluated location of suspected injury as an indication for WBCT. Hemodynamically stable patients with polytrauma who presented to the ED at a single center with trauma to 2 or more body regions (head, neck, chest, abdomen, and pelvis) were retrospectively analyzed by Sampson and colleagues.[10] Of 296 WBCT examinations, only 41 (13.8%) showed no traumatic injury. A wide range of injuries was described with the most common being pneumothoraces, lung contusions, and rib fracture. Positive findings included several clinically unsuspected injuries, including 19 cervical spine fractures and 37% (36 of 97) of the pneumothoraces. As one would expect, the investigators found a strong likelihood of another injury if there were injuries to the head, chest, spine, and pelvis.

Combination of Physical Examination Findings, Injury Location, and Mechanism

Based on previous research, van Vugt and colleagues[25] developed a detailed list of criteria and an algorithm combining physical examination findings, injury location, and mechanism of injury that could be used to decide whether a patient underwent WBCT or selective CT. In a pilot study evaluating the use of this algorithm in the ED, the researchers reported that compliance with the protocol was excellent, unnecessary imaging was avoided, and no injuries were missed. For details of this algorithm readers are referred to their comprehensive description.

IMPACT OF WHOLE-BODY COMPUTED TOMOGRAPHY ON PATIENT MORTALITY

A recent Cochrane systematic review attempted to assess the effects of routine thoracoabdominal CT compared with selective CT on mortality in patients with high-energy blunt trauma.[20] This systematic review noted the absence of any randomized controlled trials meeting their inclusion criteria and concluded that "while the diagnostic value of WBCT seems clear, its benefits on mortality cannot be established."

Several prospective observational studies and retrospective cohort studies have been performed, and these have conflicting results (**Table 1**). A systematic review by Healy and colleagues[26] comprising 5 nonrandomized cohort studies (4 retrospective including 1 multicenter, 1 prospective multicenter) evaluated the impact of WBCT on mortality and time spent in the ED.[24,27–31] Most of the included studies reported a mortality benefit from WBCT in patients who were severely injured (based on an injury severity score [ISS] of >15) compared with selective CT. However, when the data were combined and WBCT was compared with selective CT in this meta-analysis, there was no significant reduction in mortality rate using the random effects model (OR, 0.68; 95% CI, 0.43, 1.09; $P = .11$), although the trend did suggest a potential mortality benefit.[26]

This meta-analysis included the most widely cited single study to examine the impact of WBCT, a retrospective multicenter study performed in Germany.[28] In this study, Huber-Wagner and colleagues[15] used data from the German Trauma Registry and compared mortality rates in 1494 patients who underwent WBCT (average ISS = 32.4, standard deviation [SD] = 13) with 3127 patients who did not (average ISS = 28.4 SD = 12, $P<.001$). Based on the trauma and injury severity score (TRISS) and revised injury severity classification (RISC), the investigators calculated the ratio of recorded to expected mortality in the 2 cohorts and found that WBCT was associated with a relative mortality reduction of 25% based on the TRISS and 13% based on the RISC and that WBCT was an independent predictor for survival. A further study by the same group using an expanded trauma registry including 216 trauma centers in predominantly German-speaking countries comparing 9233 patients who underwent WBCT with 7486 patients who did not also found a mortality benefit for patients undergoing WBCT. However, there were limitations in these studies: only patients with an ISS of 16 or more were included, the indications for WBCT were not

Table 1
Studies of WBCT mortality rate and ED length of stay

Author	Design	Description	Number of Subjects		Mortality Rate[a]			ED Length of Stay (min)		
			Selective CT	WBCT	Selective CT	WBCT	P Value	Selective CT	WBCT	P Value
Weninger et al,[27] 2007	Retrospective. Single center. Cohort	WBCT included patients who underwent on a new 16-channel scanner relocated in the center of the ED using a new protocol	185	185	0.16	0.17[b]	n.s.	70,104 ± 21	104 ± 21	.025
Wurmb et al,[31] 2011	Retrospective. Single center. Cohort	WBCT patients who underwent a new protocol on a sliding gantry 16-channel CT scanner in resuscitation room Selective CT group included radiography and portable ultrasonography for initial triage	155	163	0.09	0.09	n.s.	ISS 16–24: 125 ISS 25–75: 130	ISS 16–24: 110 ISS 25–75: 105	ISS 16–24: n.s. ISS 25–75: .022
Hutter et al,[24] 2011	Retrospective. Single center. Cohort	Selective CT group workup included radiography and portable ultrasonography before CT away from the trauma bay. WBCT group followed installation of a new 64-channel CT scanner by the trauma bay	313	608	0.23	0.08	.02	114.7 ± 115.8	83.5 ± 49.2	<.001
Yeguiayan et al,[30] 2012	Prospective. Nonrandomized. Multicenter. Cohort	Patients undergoing trial at 11 French hospitals to evaluate prehospital and hospital data about blunt trauma management	254	1696	0.22	0.16	.02	Not reported	Not reported	n/a

Study	Study design	Description								
Sierink et al,[32] 2014.	Retrospective. Nonrandomized. Single center. Case control	Selective CT group included standard workup with radiography, ultrasonography and selective CT on a 4-slice sliding gantry CT in the resuscitation room This historical cohort was case-matched by age, gender, and ISS to a WBCT cohort who were pilot subjects for a randomized controlled study of immediate WBCT using a 64-channled sliding gantry CT in the resuscitation room	152	152	0.13	0.13	n.s.	Not reported	Not reported	n/a
Huber-Wagner et al,[15] 2013	Retrospective. Multicenter. Cohort	Used data from German Trauma Society registry, for patients with blunt trauma with ISS>15 Compared patients who underwent WBCT with selective CT according to registry. Controlled for injury severity	7486	9233	0.21	0.17	<.001	Not reported	Not reported	n/a

Abbreviations: n/a, not applicable; n.s., not significant.
[a] Overall mortality rate (period not reported).
[b] In-hospital mortality rate.

described, differences between sites in the location of CT scanners relative to the resuscitation room were not detailed or analyzed, the preference for WBCT in more experienced centers was not controlled for, and intersite inconsistency for organ injury grading (which might influence the ISS) was not evaluated.

The reliance on the ISS as a means to compare WBCT with the non-WBCT cohorts is a limitation shared by several of the studies in Table 1, and as a result these findings should be interpreted with caution. The ISS can only be calculated retrospectively after comprehensive trauma assessment, often including injuries detected by CT. The ISS cannot be used as a prospective clinical decision tool in the trauma room to determine which patients are sent for WBCT and which ones should undergo limited imaging or selective CT. Furthermore, the ISS is likely to be higher in patients who undergo WBCT because WBCT is a more comprehensive examination, potentially revealing more injuries than more limited selective scans[24]; this means the apparent survival benefit in patients with higher ISS who undergo WBCT may be attributed to WBCT but may reflect, in part, the increased detection of less significant injuries that may not require treatment yet increase the ISS (eg, occult pulmonary contusions).

To control for these limitations, prospective randomized trials that examine the impact of WBCT on mortality, quality of life, health care costs, and radiation dose are necessary. A small prospective pilot study performed from 2009 to 2011 compared consecutive patients who underwent immediate WBCT with a case-matched historical cohort who underwent standard radiologic workup.[32] The investigators found that patients who underwent immediate WBCT had a similar mortality rate (13%) compared with those who did not. The WBCT group had a higher median Glasgow coma scale (GCS) (15 vs 10), but the study design matched the cases and controls by age, gender, and ISS category. After correction for differences in raw ISS and in-hospital GCS, there was a slight decrease in 30-day mortality in the WBCT group. This study was performed as a pilot for the Randomized Study of Early Assessment by CT Scanning in Trauma Patients (REACT)-2 study, a multicenter randomized controlled trial involving more than 1000 patients that is underway. The REACT-2 study focuses on several outcomes, including in-hospital, 30-day, and 1-year mortality; trauma workup time; radiation dose; general health; and cost-effectiveness.[33]

Impact of Whole-Body Computed Tomography on Emergency Department Length of Stay

For patients with blunt trauma, time to definitive surgery and ED LOS have been linked to mortality.[34,35] WBCT could improve survival by reducing the time from admission to definitive diagnosis and treatment.

Although no prospective study has been performed, several observational studies have examined the impact of WBCT on ED LOS and CT scan time.[27,29,31,35–40] Although ED LOS was reported in most of these studies, changes in CT scanner location, departmental redesign, or changes in trauma protocols often occurred during WBCT protocol implementation. A definitive link between the use of WBCT and ED LOS has not yet been demonstrated.

Weninger and colleagues[27] compared 185 consecutive patients who underwent whole-body fluoroscopy and selective CT with 185 consecutive patients who underwent WBCT following installation of a new 16-channel CT scanner and trauma management protocol. In the new protocol, patients were transported directly to the new CT scanner located in the emergency room. Using this new protocol, the ED LOS was reduced from 104 ± 21 to 70 ± 17 minutes. The researchers also noted a reduction in length of intensive care unit stay in patients who underwent the new algorithm with WBCT.

In a similar retrospective study, Wurmb and colleagues[29] compared 79 patients who underwent a conventional trauma protocol, including a radiographic trauma series, focused abdominal sonography for trauma, and selective CT on a single-detector row scanner located in the radiology department, with 82 patients who underwent a new diagnostic algorithm with WBCT on a new 16-channel CT scanner located in the trauma resuscitation room. The researchers found that completion of the imaging workup was reduced from 70 to 23 minutes in these patients. In a follow-up retrospective study of an expanded cohort, a reduction in time of arrival in the emergency room to the start of emergency surgery from 120 to 105 minutes was demonstrated, but the group did not find a mortality benefit from WBCT.[31]

Soon after the introduction of the 16-channel CT scanner technology, Fanucci and colleagues[40] compared 20 patients who underwent a segmented WBCT acquisition technique (where separate body segments are acquired in separate contrast phases) with 26 patients who underwent a single-pass technique. They found that the single-pass technique was associated with a reduction in CT scanner room time from 32 to 22 minutes.

A study by Sedlic and colleagues[37] examined the use of single-acquisition WBCT without patient repositioning compared with a segmented whole-body acquisition with repositioning between the chest and abdomen. Use of the new rapid protocol seems to have been nonrandomized and based on referrer choice. In this study, the CT scan time was reduced from 18 to 10 minutes. Moreover, much greater time reductions were achieved in the ED before and after the WBCT scan, confirming that protocol optimization can reduce scan time as well as ED LOS.

Hutter and colleagues[24] also found a reduction in ED LOS from 96 to 84 minutes following the implementation of a standard WBCT protocol, with accompanying stepwise improvements in CT equipment and co-location of CT close to the trauma resuscitation room.

In a pooled analysis of 4 studies comprising 2369 patients who underwent WBCT and 3704 patients who underwent selective CT, Healy and colleagues[26] demonstrated that performing WBCT saved an average of 32 minutes of ED time. Although this result is encouraging, the investigators note that simultaneous changes in ED processes, technology, and CT location may also have affected this ED time.

SCAN TECHNIQUE
Arm Positioning and Imaging Quality

There is no consensus regarding the best WBCT technique. Varying approaches categorized into 2 broad groups, multipass and single pass, have been described.

A multipass CT acquisition technique generally involves separate helical CT phases of different body regions. Typically, this approach involves noncontrast CT of the head and cervical spine, with the upper extremities resting beside the patient's torso. Following acquisition of the cervical spine, the upper extremities are raised beside the head and neck, and CT of the chest, abdomen, and pelvis is obtained as a single helical acquisition or as separate arterial and venous phases following intravenous contrast. Repositioning of the arms, intravenous lines, and ventilation tubing following acquisition of noncontrast CT of the head and cervical spine has been shown in one study to lengthen total scan time by an average of 4 to 8 minutes.[41,42]

The single-pass CT technique typically involves noncontrast CT of the head, followed by a single helical acquisition of the neck, chest, abdomen, and pelvis without repositioning the upper extremities. Single or multiple contrast-enhanced phases may be obtained.

For a single-pass technique, upper extremity positioning has an impact on radiology dose and image quality. The principal arm positioning techniques include (1) arms up, whereby the arms rest beside the head and neck; (2) the swimmer's position, whereby one arm rests beside the neck and the other is beside the torso; (3) the arms down position, whereby both arms are beside the torso; and (4) propping the arms anterior to the chest or abdomen (**Fig. 1**).

For torso CT (chest, abdomen, and pelvis) single-pass techniques that involve placing the arms beside the neck are associated with the highest image quality of the visceral organs and lowest overall radiation dose. Brink and colleagues[43] evaluated the effect of arm positioning on radiation dose and thoracoabdominal image quality using a 16-channel CT scanner with automated tube current modulation. They found that the arms-up technique was associated with the lowest radiation dose (18.6 mSv) and highest image quality of the thoracoabdominal organs. When the arms were placed in the swimmer's position the mean radiation dose was approximately 18% higher, and when the arms-down position was used, the mean radiation dose was 45% higher. In common with torso CT protocols on nearly all modern CT scanners, the CT scan protocol they used had automated exposure control, which modulates the tube current based on photon attenuation derived from the topograms and during the helical scan acquisition.[44] The additional attenuation caused by placing the arms in the scan field causes the scanner to upmodulate the tube current, resulting in an increase in radiation dose-length-product.

A novel technique was described by Karlo and colleagues,[45] in which subjects crossed their upper extremities and rested them on a pillow placed across the chest. The investigators compared this technique to the arms-up and arms-down positions. They confirmed that the arms-up position was associated with the lowest radiation dose (approximately 25% lower) and highest image quality but found that image quality was significantly improved when the arms were placed across the chest compared with the standard arms-down position. As this technique avoids the need to reposition the arms and life-support tubing between passes, this approach is used at the authors' institution (**Fig. 2**).

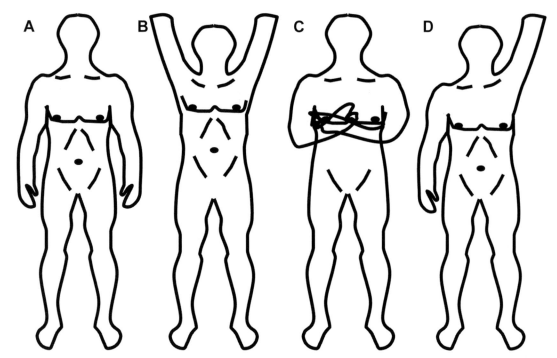

Fig. 1. Arm position for WBCT. (*A*) Arms down. (*B*) Arms up. (*C*) Arms crossed anterior to lower chest. (*D*) Swimmers. The lowest radiation dose and highest image quality can be achieved by scanning the head and neck without contrast with the patient in the arms-down position (*A*), then positioning the patient in the arms-up position (*B*) and scanning the chest, abdomen, and pelvis following intravenous contrast. The arms-up position can also be used for an arterial phase scan of the neck, chest, abdomen, and pelvis, achieving an adequate-quality CTA of the neck vessels and good-quality CT of the torso with low radiation dose. The position shown in (*C*), where the arms are crossed anterior to the lower chest, achieves excellent quality imaging of the neck, with fewer artifacts in the abdomen compared with CT of the abdomen and pelvis in the arms-down position. The compromise swimmers position (*D*) provides adequate image quality in multiple regions and avoids kinking of intravenous catheters when placed in the right antecubital fossa.

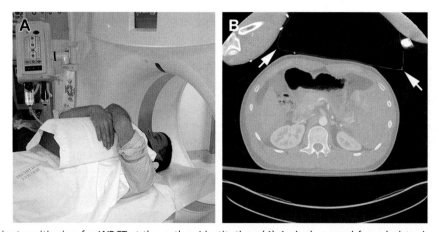

Fig. 2. Patient positioning for WBCT at the authors' institution. (*A*) A vinyl-covered foam bolster is placed over the chest and the arms are crossed anterior to the lower chest, taking a slightly oblique craniocaudal course. Conscious patients tolerate this position well. In unconscious patients, the wrists can be tied across the chest to a slider board using soft bandages to position them securely. Moving the arms away from the body reduces beam hardening artifacts through the liver and spleen. (*B*) Axial CT through the upper abdomen showing the position of the bolster. The radiolucent vinyl-coated bolster (*white arrows*) is placed on the patient's chest separating the arms from the abdomen.

Scanning the Cervical Spine Without Contrast Versus Computed Tomographic Angiography of the Carotid and Vertebral Arteries

Owing to recent advances in CT scanner technology, particularly the introduction of faster MDCT scanners and long tables, it is possible to perform computed tomographic angiography (CTA) of the whole body from the circle of Willis to the lower extremities (Fig. 3). One major difference in the WBCT protocols used at different centers involves the technique for evaluating the neck. At centers using a multipass technique, the cervical spine is scanned without contrast before repositioning of the arms, whereas at centers using a single-pass technique, CTA of the neck vessels to screen for blunt cerebrovascular injury (BCVI) is obtained at the same time as screening for cervical spine injury and torso injury. Patients with blunt polytrauma are at risk of BCVI, with a reported incidence of up to 3.3%.[46,47] Although clinical prediction rules based on defined risk factors have been extensively developed and investigated, approximately 20% to 37% of patients with polytrauma who have BCVI do not meet traditional BCVI screening criteria[46,48,49] Early BCVI detection and treatment has been shown to reduce the incidence of, and morbidity from, posttraumatic ischemic stroke.[50] With recent advances in MDCT technology and refinement of contrast injection techniques, it has become possible to perform CTA neck screening as part of WBCT acquisition using a single contrast bolus and helical acquisition. Evidence suggests that neck CTA performed as part of WBCT on 16+ channel MDCT is as good as dedicated neck CTA for the diagnosis of BCVI.[46,51,52] Consequently, the authors perform CTA of the neck vessels concurrent with CT of the cervical spine as part of the WBCT protocol (Table 2).

Radiation Dose

Valid concerns have been raised about the radiation exposure and the potential increase in the lifetime attributable risk of radiation-induced cancer resulting from WBCT.[17,18] A study that compared the impact of a new WBCT protocol on radiation dose found that the proportion of patients exposed to a radiation dose of greater than 20 mSv increased by 8% and the risk of receiving a higher dose scan occurred regardless of patient age or injury severity.[17] However,

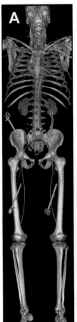
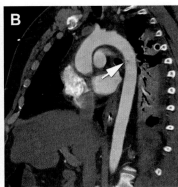
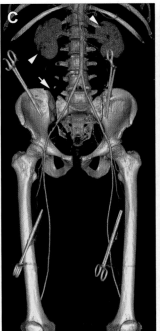
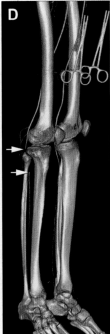

Fig. 3. WBCT in the arterial phase in a 44-year-old man who was riding a motorcycle when he was hit by a car. (A) Using modern fast scanners with scan long tables, it is possible to perform CTA of the whole body from the circle of Willis to the lower extremities. (B) Oblique sagittal reformat of the thoracic aorta shows a filling defect of the proximal descending thoracic aorta (arrow), consistent with a minimal aortic injury. (C). Volume-rendered view of the pelvis shows a right sacroiliac joint fracture dislocation (arrow) and transverse process fractures, as well as bilateral renal infarcts (arrowheads), presumed to result from embolization from the aortic injury. (D) As a result of a transient right knee dislocation, the patient also had a traumatic occlusion of the right popliteal artery (arrows).

Table 2
Parameters for CT scan acquisition following blunt polytrauma[a]

Head	
Parameter	**Setting**
Helical detector configuration	128 × 0.6 mm
kVp	120
Quality reference milliampere second (mAs) for automated tube current modulation	310
Pitch	1:0.6
Rotation time (s)	1.0
Contrast material	None
Superior range	Vertex
Inferior range	Foramen magnum If a maxillofacial CT is requested, the inferior scan range is extended to the angle of the mandible
Scan angulation	Intraorbital meatal line
Scan direction	Caudal to cranial
Axial reconstruction thickness (mm)	5
Axial reconstruction interval (mm)	5
Reconstruction kernel	Soft tissues: J45 Bone: H70
Multiplanar reformations	Coronal brain 2 mm at 2 mm intervals If a maxillofacial CT is requested, axial reconstructions at 0.6 mm (kernel: H70 and H41) are performed, and H41 coronal 1.5 mm thick at 1.5-mm interval images are generated
Neck, Chest, Abdomen, and Pelvis[b]	
Parameter	**Setting**
Helical detector configuration	128 × 0.6 mm
kVp	120
Quality reference mAs for automated tube current modulation	190 (for a reference of 120 kV)
Pitch	1:0.8
Rotation time (s)	0.5
Contrast material	Iohexol 350 mg/mL
Injection rate (mL/s)[c]	Contrast: 60 mL at 5 mL/s Contrast: 60 mL at 4 mL/s Saline: 30 mL at 4 mL/s

Scan delay (s)	Arterial phase
	  20 s (patient age <55 y)
	  25 s (patient age 55 + years)
	Venous phase
	  45 s after completion of arterial phase
	Delayed phase (optional)[d]
	  5–10 min after beginning of contrast

Helical scan direction	Cranial to caudal
Superior range (arterial phase)	1.5 cm above the sella turcica
Inferior range (arterial phase)	No pelvic ring disruption (5 cm above iliac crests) Pelvic ring disruption on radiograph: ischial tuberosities

(continued on next page)

Table 2
(continued)

Neck, Chest, Abdomen, and Pelvis[b]	
Parameter	**Setting**
Superior range (venous phase)	Dome of highest hemidiaphragm
Inferior range (venous phase)	Ischial tuberosities
Arm position	Bolstered anterior to lower chest
Oral/rectal contrast	Not used
Reconstruction section thickness (mm)	3
Reconstruction interval (mm)	3
Reconstruction kernel	Soft tissues: I31f. Sinogram affirmed iterative reconstruction (SAFIRE) strength of 2 Spine: b60f (separate limited FOV reconstructions)
Multiplanar reformation planes and thickness (torso)	3 mm thick at 3 mm intervals axial, sagittal, coronal reformations of all phases Dedicated axial (2 mm at 1 mm interval), sagittal (2 mm at 2 mm interval), and coronal (2 mm at 2 mm interval) reformations of spine 0.6 mm thick at 0.6 mm interval I31f (SAFIRE 2) images sent to 3D postprocessing workstation
Multiplanar reformation planes and thickness (CTA neck)[c]	Kernel: b45 Axial 1 mm thickness at 1 mm intervals Oblique sagittal 2 thickness at 2 mm intervals Coronal MIPs 5 mm at 2.5 mm intervals 6.6 mm axial images sent to 3D workstation

Abbreviations: FOV, field of view; kVp, peak tube kilovoltage; MIP, maximum intensity projection.

[a] This protocol is used only in adults 18 years or older who have not had prior outside imaging of one of the included scan range. A radiologist reviews images on the CT scanner before every patient is removed from the CT table and communicates urgent findings to the trauma team.

[b] Patient is not repositioned between CT of the head and CT of the remainder of the body.

[c] A dedicated CTA neck is not reconstructed unless one is required based on intuitional guidelines for BCVI or an injury is suspected on the standard arterial phase images of the neck.

[d] After review of the venous phase images on the CT table, radiologist may elect to do a low-radiation dose delayed phase through injured organs. This procedure uses a quality reference mAs of 150. If the patient has indications for a CT cystogram and the patient is hemodynamically stable, this can be performed as part of this acquisition.

some researchers have found that, although the emergency room radiation dose increased along with increased use of WBCT, the total radiation dose throughout the hospital stay did not change.[53]

Newer dose-saving techniques have the potential to considerably reduce absolute radiation dose from WBCT. A well-designed prospective study (Dose Reduction in Whole-Body Computed Tomography of Multiple Injuries [DoReMI]) of 1000 patients plans to compare a cohort of consecutive patients undergoing WBCT using regular radiation dose parameters with a subsequent cohort of consecutive patients undergoing WBCT with lower dose parameters accompanied by iterative image reconstruction.[54] In addition to radiation exposure, subjective and objective image quality, diagnostic accuracy, and the incidence of delayed diagnoses will be measured.

Contrast Injection Protocols

Several protocols for the use of intravenous iodinated contrast in major trauma have been reported.

Traditionally, trauma protocols used a noncontrast CT protocol followed by a contrast-enhanced protocol. A single-center retrospective study that evaluated 84 patients who underwent CT with and without intravenous contrast for abdominopelvic CT found that contrast-enhanced images were significantly more sensitive (77%–96%) than noncontrast CT (8%–54%) for the detection of solid-organ injuries (liver, spleen, adrenal gland, and kidneys).[55] The investigators also found that a precontrast phase before the contrast-enhanced phase did not significantly improve detection of solid-organ injuries and recommended omitting the precontrast phase through the abdomen and pelvis. In accordance with this finding, and to avoid the unnecessary additional radiation, most centers perform only postcontrast CT for the evaluation of solid-organ injuries.

Contrast phases

There is little doubt that contrast-enhanced CT is sensitive for the detection and exclusion of active vascular extravasation in both phantoms and patients with trauma when compared with catheter angiography, with sensitivities ranging from 87% to 95% and negative predictive values ranging from 93% to 98%.[56–59] However, there is considerable debate and diversity in the literature about the number of postcontrast phases, bolus timing, and bolus injection protocol for the optimal identification and characterization of injuries with the lowest radiation and contrast dose.

As described earlier, arterial phase WBCT including the carotid and vertebral arteries has adequate sensitivity for the detection of BCVI. An arterial phase of the thorax is also preferred for the detection and characterization of blunt thoracic great vessel injury (see **Fig. 3**; **Fig. 4**).[60]

Performing routine arterial phase CT of the upper abdomen for the detection and characterization of vascular injuries (pseudoaneurysms, arteriovenous fistula, and active arterial bleeding) of blunt splenic injury has been suggested.[61,62] Limited studies have shown that routine use of an arterial phase improves the sensitivity for the detection of splenic pseudoaneurysms compared with venous phase CT alone, and the highest sensitivity for detection of splenic vascular and parenchymal injury is achieved with dual-phase CT (**Fig. 5**).[61–63]

It is possible that dual-phase (arterial and venous) CT may be able to discriminate between arterial and venous hemorrhage in the pelvis and therefore determine the need for pelvic angioembolization. However, the studies to date contained small numbers and some patients with what seemed to be venous-only hemorrhage on CT who were found to have arterial hemorrhage on catheter angiography.[64,65] Therefore, an arterial phase CT may contribute to decision making for pelvic angioembolization in patients with pelvic trauma, although this is yet to be confirmed.

Accordingly, if WBCT is to be performed, arterial phase CT of the neck, chest, upper abdomen, and potentially the pelvis should be included. As venous phase CT is essential for the detection of solid-organ injuries in the upper abdomen, this is also recommended (**Fig. 6**). Based on local preference, some sites include arterial phase CT of the abdomen and pelvis with venous phase CT of the abdomen, whereas other sites, such as the authors', perform an arterial phase CT of the upper abdomen and venous phase CT of the abdomen and pelvis.

Split bolus injection protocols

As described earlier, dual- (arterial, venous) or triple- (arterial, venous, and delayed) phase helical CT passes are often used for optimal detection and characterization of injuries to the vasculature and parenchymal organs. However, scanning

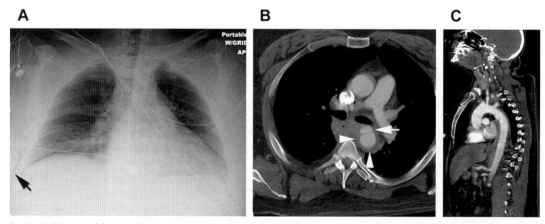

A   **B**   **C**

Fig. 4. A 47-year-old man who was an unrestrained driver during a motor vehicle collision. (*A*) Supine portable chest radiograph demonstrates a small quantity of extrapleural gas in the right chest wall (*arrow*). No rib fractures were visible on radiographs. Axial (*B*) and sagittal reformation (*C*) of an arterial phase component of a WBCT shows a pseudoaneurysm (*arrow*) at the site of a blunt traumatic aortic injury of the proximal descending thoracic aorta (*arrowheads*). A small right pneumothorax, rib fractures, and multiple abdominal injuries were also present.

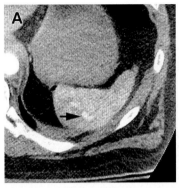
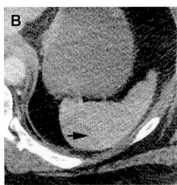
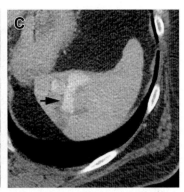

Fig. 5. (A) Arterial phase imaging of the upper abdomen shows a small pseudoaneurysm within the spleen (*arrow*) that was not visible on venous phase imaging. The splenic lesion had the appearance of a laceration on venous phase imaging and no pseudoaneurysm was visible (B). This condition was treated conservatively. Ten days later, the pseudoaneurysm had increased in size (C), and the patient underwent coil angioembolization.

regions of the body 2 or more times may substantially increase the radiation dose. To avoid this, the use of split bolus contrast infusion techniques has been proposed.[41,66–68] Split bolus techniques can include 2 or 3 sequential contrast boluses, with a delay period (or saline bolus) between each bolus, followed by a single scan pass through the torso, thus eliminating multiple acquisition phases and radiation exposures. The single helical acquisition may thus include arterial and venous or arterial, venous, and delayed (urinary excretory) contrast-enhanced phases in the 1 acquisition.

Beenen and colleagues[41] described the use of a double-split bolus technique on a 64-channel CT scanner. Their technique involved injecting a contrast bolus of 80 mL at 4 mL/s (20-second injection duration), not injecting contrast for 20 seconds, then injecting a contrast bolus of 40 mL at 5 mL/s

(8-second injection duration), and beginning their torso scan acquisition 12 seconds later. This method yields a prescan delay of 60 seconds from the beginning of the first bolus and 20 seconds from the beginning of the second bolus and uses 120 mL contrast in total. They used a saline flush after each contrast bolus (40 mL at 4 mL/s). The investigators found that quantitative (Hounsfield unit [HU]) and qualitative (reader scoring) measures of vascular and parenchymal enhancement were superior compared with a nonsplit bolus infusion of 100 mL of contrast, with scan acquisition in either the late-arterial or venous phases. Yaniv and colleagues[66] performed a similar study in which a conventional protocol was compared with a double-split bolus technique (80 mL contrast bolus at 3 mL/s, 13-second delay, 50 mL contrast bolus at 4 mL/s) with a 75-second interval between the

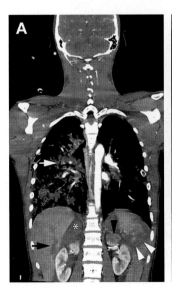
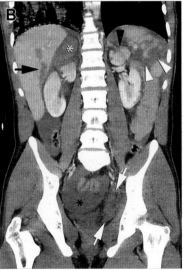

Fig. 6. Arterial phase CT of the chest and upper abdomen (A) and venous phase CT of the abdomen and pelvis (B) in a 19-year-old man who was riding a bicycle when hit by a truck demonstrates a large right pulmonary contusion (*white arrow*), liver laceration (*black arrows*), right adrenal hematoma (*white asterisk*), splenic laceration without pseudoaneurysm or active bleeding (*white arrowheads*), a left renal laceration (*black arrowheads*), hemoperitoneum (*black asterisk*), and left extraperitoneal hematoma in the pelvis. A right pulmonary contusion is also present.

beginning of the first contrast bolus and the final acquisition. These investigators reported improved enhancement and image quality in the abdomen but reduced vascular enhancement of the thoracic aorta, similar to a further study.[66,67]

Studies that have evaluated the use of the split bolus technique for the evaluation of torso trauma have used a noncontrast CT of the cervical spine, followed by a contrast-enhanced CT of the torso, excluding a CTA of the neck vessels (a potential limitation of the technique). Another possible limitation, not reported because of the small number of patients, is the potential for the combined arterial phase and parenchymal phase CT to mask vascular injuries of the liver and spleen, although this has yet to be described in the literature.

Single-bolus injection protocols
Several investigators have described single-bolus protocols that use varying flow rates during the bolus.[37,42,61,67] To maximize depiction of posttraumatic splenic pseudoaneurysms that are more apparent in the late arterial phase, Atluri and colleagues[61] described a biphasic injection protocol that used a high flow rate (6 mL/s) immediately followed by 4 mL/s, as well as late arterial and venous phase CT acquisitions of the upper abdomen. Others have described different protocols using a mixture of contrast and normal saline and other flow rates.[37,69]

Contrast timing
Nearly all published protocols for WBCT use a fixed scan delay from the beginning of the contrast bolus rather than using bolus tracking or a test

bolus of contrast. The advantage of this technique is that it takes less time for the technologist to prepare the CT; however, it carries the potential risk of mistiming the CT acquisition; this has not been a problem in the authors' experience.[70]

INCIDENTAL FINDINGS

Incidental radiologic findings are findings totally unrelated to the referring clinician's reason for obtaining the study, for which the term incidentaloma has been coined.[71] As the frequency and scope of medical imaging obtained on patients in the ED has increased, so too has the detection of unrelated but potentially clinically significant incidental findings. Some of the most common examples include small nodules in the lungs and adrenal gland. Several of these demonstrate imaging features that indicate benignity with a high level of confidence, such as calcified granulomas in the lung or lipid-rich adenomas in the adrenal glands. However, incidental lesions often lack the classic features of a benign entity and may therefore require further evaluation (**Fig. 7**).

The prevalence and significance of incidental findings on imaging obtained in the ED depends on the examination type and included anatomy and patient age. Incidental findings are most commonly identified on abdominopelvic CT scans, with prevalence ranging from 12% to 45%,[19,72–75] whereas the rate of incidental findings on head and neck scans is reportedly as low as 1% to 7%.[19,75,76] The prevalence of incidental findings increases with age, with a reported increase from

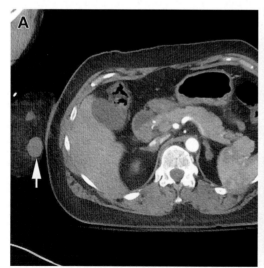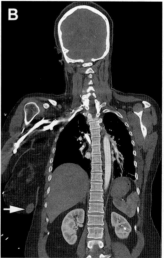

Fig. 7. Axial (*A*) and coronal (*B*) arterial phase postcontrast phase of a WBCT of a 44-year-old woman showing an incidental rounded mass in the right breast (*arrow*). She had a history of left mastectomy for breast cancer and recurrent masses in the right breast.

20% in patients younger than 40 years to 46% in those older than 40 years.[75]

The impact of WBCT in the ED on the rate of incidentaloma detection has not been extensively reported. The incidental finding rate on thoracoabdominal CT scans in the ED has been reported to be approximately 36%,[77] whereas total-body CT, from the vertex through the pelvis, has a reported incidental findings rate of 45%,[16] with most findings being located in the abdomen.

Although not typically immediately relevant to the visit of a patient with trauma to the ED, identification of incidental findings is a critical responsibility of the emergency radiologists. Ekeh and colleagues[72] found that a large majority (75%) of patients with trauma with incidental findings had no identified traumatic injury in the abdomen or pelvis. A higher probability of identifying an incidental abnormality than traumatic injury on CT in the ED was also demonstrated in a study by Munk and colleagues,[19] which reported an incidental findings rate of 30% in a population with an overall traumatic abnormality rate of 15% on all CT scans (head, chest, and abdomen/pelvis).

Many frequently encountered incidental findings, such as simple hepatic or renal cysts, are of little or no clinical importance and do not require follow-up. Incidental findings that have a high probability of being clinically significant, such as abdominal aortic aneurysm, lung mass, or breast mass, account for up to 15% of all incidental findings on trauma CT scans,[19] and it is the emergency radiologists responsibility to ensure these findings are communicated to the referring provider. With the reported documentation and follow-up rates for significant incidental findings on ED CT scans ranging from only 20% to 49%,[19,74,75] this represents an opportunity for emergency radiologists to significantly improve patient care in the ED.

SUMMARY

WBCT has become a widely used technique for the workup of the patient with blunt polytrauma. Evidence suggests that WBCT is associated with improved or no change in patient survival and reduces the ED LOS. However, randomized studies, at least one of which is underway, are needed to determine for certain whether early WBCT improves survival, to clarify which patients benefit the most, and to model the costs of this technique compared with traditional workup. Advancements in modern MDCT technology and an improved understanding of optimal protocols have enabled one to scan the entire body and achieve adequate image quality for a comprehensive trauma assessment in a short time period.

REFERENCES

1. World Health Organization. Injuries and violence: the facts. 2010. Available at: http://www.who.int/violence_injury_prevention/key_facts/en/. Accessed June 16, 2014.
2. Heron M. Deaths: leading causes for 2010. National vital statistics reports, vol. 62. no. 6. Hyattsville (MD): National Center for Health Statistics; 2013. p. 97.
3. Centers for Disease Control and Prevention. All injuries. 2013. Available at: http://www.cdc.gov/nchs/fastats/injury.htm. Accessed June 15, 2014.
4. Centers for Disease Control and Prevention. Accidents or unintentional injuries. Accidents or unintentional injuries. 2010. Available at: http://www.cdc.gov/nchs/data/ahcd/nhamcs_emergency/2010_ed_web_tables.pdf. Accessed January 5, 2013.
5. MacKenzie EJ, Rivara FP, Jurkovich GJ, et al. A national evaluation of the effect of trauma-center care on mortality. N Engl J Med 2006;354(4):366–78.
6. Haas B, Stukel TA, Gomez D, et al. The mortality benefit of direct trauma center transport in a regional trauma system: a population-based analysis. J Trauma Acute Care Surg 2012;72(6):1510–5 [discussion: 1515–7].
7. Pfeifer R, Pape HC. Missed injuries in trauma patients: a literature review. Patient Saf Surg 2008;2:20.
8. Schurink GW, Bode PJ, van Luijt PA, et al. The value of physical examination in the diagnosis of patients with blunt abdominal trauma: a retrospective study. Injury 1997;28(4):261–5.
9. Nicolaou S, Eftekhari A, Sedlic T, et al. The utilization of dual source CT in imaging of polytrauma. Eur J Radiol 2008;68(3):398–408.
10. Sampson MA, Colquhoun KB, Hennessy NL. Computed tomography whole body imaging in multi-trauma: 7 years experience. Clin Radiol 2006;61(4):365–9.
11. Salim A, Sangthong B, Martin M, et al. Whole body imaging in blunt multisystem trauma patients without obvious signs of injury: results of a prospective study. Arch Surg 2006;141(5):468–73 [discussion: 473–5].
12. Gupta M, Schriger DL, Hiatt JR, et al. Selective use of computed tomography compared with routine whole body imaging in patients with blunt trauma. Ann Emerg Med 2011;58(5):407–16.e15.
13. Stengel D, Ottersbach C, Matthes G, et al. Accuracy of single-pass whole-body computed tomography for detection of injuries in patients with major blunt trauma. CMAJ 2012;184(8):869–76.
14. Deunk J, Brink M, Dekker HM, et al. Routine versus selective multidetector-row computed tomography (MDCT) in blunt trauma patients: level of agreement

on the influence of additional findings on management. J Trauma 2009;67(5):1080–6.

15. Huber-Wagner S, Biberthaler P, Haberle S, et al. Whole-body CT in haemodynamically unstable severely injured patients–a retrospective, multicentre study. PLoS One 2013;8:e68880.

16. Sierink JC, Saltzherr TP, Russchen MJ, et al. Incidental findings on total-body CT scans in trauma patients. Injury 2014;45(5):840–4.

17. Asha S, Curtis KA, Grant N, et al. Comparison of radiation exposure of trauma patients from diagnostic radiology procedures before and after the introduction of a panscan protocol. Emerg Med Australas 2012;24(1):43–51.

18. Snyder GE. Whole-body imaging in blunt multisystem trauma patients who were never examined. Ann Emerg Med 2008;52(2):101–3.

19. Munk MD, Peitzman AB, Hostler DP, et al. Frequency and follow-up of incidental findings on trauma computed tomography scans: experience at a level one trauma center. J Emerg Med 2010;38(3):346–50.

20. Van Vugt R, Keus F, Kool D, et al. Selective computed tomography (CT) versus routine thoracoabdominal CT for high-energy blunt-trauma patients. Cochrane Database Syst Rev 2013;(12):CD009743.

21. van Vugt R, Kool DR, Deunk J, et al. Effects on mortality, treatment, and time management as a result of routine use of total body computed tomography in blunt high-energy trauma patients. J Trauma Acute Care Surg 2012;72(3):553–9.

22. Millo NZ, Plewes C, Rowe BH, et al. Appropriateness of CT of the chest, abdomen, and pelvis in motorized blunt force trauma patients without signs of significant injury. Am J Roentgenol 2011;197(6):1393–8.

23. Cowan I, Cresswell C, Liu H, et al. Selective versus mandatory whole-body computed tomography scanning in the multiply injured patient. Emerg Med Australas 2012;24(1):115–6.

24. Hutter M, Woltmann A, Hierholzer C, et al. Association between a single-pass whole-body computed tomography policy and survival after blunt major trauma: a retrospective cohort study. Scand J Trauma Resusc Emerg Med 2011;19:73.

25. van Vugt R, Kool DR, Lubeek SF, et al. An evidence based blunt trauma protocol. Emerg Med J 2013; 30:e23.

26. Healy DA, Hegarty A, Feeley I, et al. Systematic review and meta-analysis of routine total body CT compared with selective CT in trauma patients. Emerg Med J 2014;31(2):101–8.

27. Weninger P, Mauritz W, Fridrich P, et al. Emergency room management of patients with blunt major trauma: evaluation of the multislice computed tomography protocol exemplified by an urban trauma center. J Trauma 2007;62(3):584–91.

28. Huber-Wagner S, Lefering R, Qvick LM, et al. Effect of whole-body CT during trauma resuscitation on survival: a retrospective, multicentre study. Lancet 2009;373(9673):1455–61.

29. Wurmb TE, Fruhwald P, Hopfner W, et al. Whole-body multislice computed tomography as the first line diagnostic tool in patients with multiple injuries: the focus on time. J Trauma 2009;66(3):658–65.

30. Yeguiayan JM, Yap A, Freysz M, et al. Impact of whole-body computed tomography on mortality and surgical management of severe blunt trauma. Crit Care 2012;16(3):R101.

31. Wurmb TE, Quaisser C, Balling H, et al. Whole-body multislice computed tomography (MSCT) improves trauma care in patients requiring surgery after multiple trauma. Emerg Med J 2011;28(4):300–4.

32. Sierink JC, Saltzherr TP, Beenen LF, et al. A case-matched series of immediate total-body CT scanning versus the standard radiological work-up in trauma patients. World J Surg 2014;38(4):795–802.

33. Sierink JC, Saltzherr TP, Beenen LF, et al. A multicenter, randomized controlled trial of immediate total-body CT scanning in trauma patients (REACT-2). BMC Emerg Med 2012;12:4.

34. Clarke JR, Trooskin SZ, Doshi PJ, et al. Time to laparotomy for intra-abdominal bleeding from trauma does affect survival for delays up to 90 minutes. J Trauma 2002;52(3):420–5.

35. Mowery NT, Dougherty SD, Hildreth AN, et al. Emergency department length of stay is an independent predictor of hospital mortality in trauma activation patients. J Trauma 2011;70(6):1317–25.

36. Kanz KG, Paul AO, Lefering R, et al. Trauma management incorporating focused assessment with computed tomography in trauma (FACTT) - potential effect on survival. J Trauma Manag Outcomes 2010;4:4.

37. Sedlic A, Chingkoe CM, Tso DK, et al. Rapid imaging protocol in trauma: a whole-body dual-source CT scan. Emerg Radiol 2013;20(5):401–8.

38. Hudson S, Boyle A, Wiltshire S, et al. Plain radiography may be safely omitted for selected major trauma patients undergoing whole body CT: database study. Emerg Med Intern 2012;2012:432537.

39. Rieger M, Czermak B, El Attal R, et al. Initial clinical experience with a 64-MDCT whole-body scanner in an emergency department: better time management and diagnostic quality? J Trauma 2009;66(3):648–57.

40. Fanucci E, Fiaschetti V, Rotili A, et al. Whole body 16-row multislice CT in emergency room: effects of different protocols on scanning time, image quality and radiation exposure. Emerg Radiol 2007;13(5):251–7.

41. Beenen LF, Sierink JC, Kolkman S, et al. Split bolus technique in polytrauma: a prospective study on scan protocols for trauma analysis. Acta Radiol 2014. [Epub ahead of print].

42. Nguyen D, Platon A, Shanmuganathan K, et al. Evaluation of a single-pass continuous whole-body

16-MDCT protocol for patients with polytrauma. Am J Roentgenol 2009;192(1):3–10.

43. Brink M, de Lange F, Oostveen LJ, et al. Arm raising at exposure-controlled multidetector trauma CT of thoracoabdominal region: higher image quality, lower radiation dose. Radiology 2008;249(2):661–70.

44. Gunn ML, Kohr JR. State of the art: technologies for computed tomography dose reduction. Emerg Radiol 2010;17(3):209–18.

45. Karlo C, Gnannt R, Frauenfelder T, et al. Whole-body CT in polytrauma patients: effect of arm positioning on thoracic and abdominal image quality. Emerg Radiol 2011;18(4):285–93.

46. Bonatti M, Vezzali N, Ferro F, et al. Blunt cerebrovascular injury: diagnosis at whole-body MDCT for multi-trauma. Insights Imaging 2013;4(3):347–55.

47. Liang T, Plaa N, Tashakkor AY, et al. Imaging of blunt cerebrovascular injuries. Semin Roentgenol 2012;47(4):306–19.

48. Franz RW, Willette PA, Wood MJ, et al. A systematic review and meta-analysis of diagnostic screening criteria for blunt cerebrovascular injuries. J Am Coll Surg 2012;214(3):313–27.

49. Burlew CC, Biffl WL, Moore EE, et al. Blunt cerebrovascular injuries: redefining screening criteria in the era of noninvasive diagnosis. J Trauma Acute Care Surg 2012;72(2):330–5 [discussion: 336–7, quiz: 539].

50. Bromberg WJ, Collier BC, Diebel LN, et al. Blunt cerebrovascular injury practice management guidelines: the Eastern Association for the Surgery of Trauma. J Trauma 2010;68(2):471–7.

51. Sliker CW, Shanmuganathan K, Mirvis SE. Diagnosis of blunt cerebrovascular injuries with 16-MDCT: accuracy of whole-body MDCT compared with neck MDCT angiography. AJR Am J Roentgenol 2008;190(3):790–9.

52. Fleck SK, Langner S, Baldauf J, et al. Incidence of blunt craniocervical artery injuries: use of whole-body computed tomography trauma imaging with adapted computed tomography angiography. Neurosurgery 2011;69(3):615–23 [discussion: 623–4].

53. Sierink JC, Saltzherr TP, Wirtz MR, et al. Radiation exposure before and after the introduction of a dedicated total-body CT protocolin multitrauma patients. Emerg Radiol 2013;20(6):507–12.

54. Stengel D, Ottersbach C, Kahl T, et al. Dose reduction in whole-body computed tomography of multiple injuries (DoReMI): protocol for a prospective cohort study. Scand J Trauma Resusc Emerg Med 2014;22:15.

55. Naulet P, Wassel J, Gervaise A, et al. Evaluation of the value of abdominopelvic acquisition without contrast injection when performing a whole body CT scan in a patient who may have multiple trauma. Diagn Interv Imaging 2013;94(4):410–7.

56. Marmery H, Shanmuganathan K, Mirvis SE, et al. Correlation of multidetector CT findings with splenic arteriography and surgery: prospective study in 392 patients. J Am Coll Surg 2008;206(4):685–93.

57. Maturen KE, Adusumilli S, Blane CE, et al. Contrast-enhanced CT accurately detects hemorrhage in torso trauma: direct comparison with angiography. J Trauma 2007;62(3):740–5.

58. Hamilton JD, Kumaravel M, Censullo ML, et al. Multidetector CT evaluation of active extravasation in blunt abdominal and pelvic trauma patients. Radiographics 2008;28(6):1603–16.

59. Anderson SW, Lucey BC, Rhea JT, et al. 64 MDCT in multiple trauma patients: imaging manifestations and clinical implications of active extravasation. Emerg Radiol 2007;14(3):151–9.

60. Gunn ML. Imaging of aortic and branch vessel trauma. Radiol Clin North Am 2012;50(1):85–103.

61. Atluri S, Richard HM 3rd, Shanmuganathan K. Optimizing multidetector CT for visualization of splenic vascular injury. Validation by splenic arteriography in blunt abdominal trauma patients. Emerg Radiol 2011;18(4):307–12.

62. Boscak AR, Shanmuganathan K, Mirvis SE, et al. Optimizing trauma multidetector CT protocol for blunt splenic injury: need for arterial and portal venous phase scans. Radiology 2013;268(1):79–88.

63. Uyeda JW, LeBedis CA, Penn DR, et al. Active hemorrhage and vascular injuries in splenic trauma: utility of the arterial phase in multidetector CT. Radiology 2014;270(1):99–106.

64. Pinto A, Niola R, Tortora G, et al. Role of multidetector-row CT in assessing the source of arterial haemorrhage in patients with pelvic vascular trauma. Comparison with angiography. Radiol Med 2010;115(4):648–67.

65. Anderson SW, Soto JA, Lucey BC, et al. Blunt trauma: feasibility and clinical utility of pelvic CT angiography performed with 64–detector row CT. Radiology 2008;246(2):410–9.

66. Yaniv G, Portnoy O, Simon D, et al. Revised protocol for whole-body CT for multi-trauma patients applying triphasic injection followed by a single-pass scan on a 64-MDCT. Clin Radiol 2013;68(7):668–75.

67. Loupatatzis C, Schindera S, Gralla J, et al. Whole-body computed tomography for multiple traumas using a triphasic injection protocol. Eur Radiol 2008;18(6):1206–14.

68. Leung V, Jones H, Sastry A. Can split bolus CT protocols prevent excess radiation dose in trauma CT? Clin Radiol 69:S23.

69. Geyer LL, Koerner M, Wirth S, et al. Polytrauma: optimal imaging and evaluation algorithm. Semin Musculoskelet Radiol 2013;17(04):371–9.

70. Gunn ML, Lehnert BE, Cornea AM, et al. CTA in the ED: impact of contrast timing technique on scan duration. Radiological Society of North America

annual meeting. Chicago (IL), November 30 – December 5, 2014.

71. Berlin L. The incidentaloma: a medicolegal dilemma. Radiol Clin North Am 2011;49(2):245–55.

72. Ekeh AP, Walusimbi M, Brigham E, et al. The prevalence of incidental findings on abdominal computed tomography scans of trauma patients. J Emerg Med 2010;38(4):484–9.

73. Ahmad NA, Ather MH, Rees J. Incidental diagnosis of diseases on un-enhanced helical computed tomography performed for ureteric colic. BMC Urol 2003;3:2.

74. Messersmith WA, Brown DF, Barry MJ. The prevalence and implications of incidental findings on ED abdominal CT scans. Am J Emerg Med 2001; 19(6):479–81.

75. Paluska TR, Sise MJ, Sack DI, et al. Incidental CT findings in trauma patients: incidence and implications for care of the injured. J Trauma 2007;62(1): 157–61.

76. Eskandary H, Sabba M, Khajehpour F, et al. Incidental findings in brain computed tomography scans of 3000 head trauma patients. Surg Neurol 2005;63(6):550–3 [discussion: 553].

77. van Vugt R, Dekker HM, Deunk J, et al. Incidental findings on routine thoracoabdominal computed tomography in blunt trauma patients. J Trauma 2011;72(2):416–21.

Pearls for Interpreting Computed Tomography of the Cervical Spine in Trauma

CrossMark

Kathryn Darras, MD[a], Gordon T. Andrews, MD, FRCPC[b],
Patrick D. McLaughlin, MB BCh BAO, FFR RCSI, FRCPC[b],
Nivmand Khorrami-Arani, BSc, BMBS, FRANZCR, FRCPC[c],
Alexandra Roston, BA[d], Bruce B. Forster, MD, FRCPC[b],
Luck Louis, MD, FRCPC[b,*]

KEYWORDS

• Cervical spine • Trauma • Computed tomography • Polytrauma • Dose reduction

KEY POINTS

- Because computed tomography (CT) scan is the imaging modality of choice for all suspected cervical spine injuries, it is essential to incorporate dose-reduction techniques.
- Caution is recommended when applying the National Emergency X-Ray Utilization Study criteria and the Canadian C-Spine Rule to elderly patients and those with rigid spinal disease (eg, ankylosing spondylitis, diffuse idiopathic skeletal hyperostosis).
- If a reliable neurologic examination cannot be obtained within 48 hours postinjury, MR imaging should be performed to clear the cervical spine, even if the initial CT scan is unremarkable.
- Although there are classic patterns of cervical spine injury, in severe trauma these may be difficult or impossible to appreciate.
- In the trauma setting, it is important to have a systematic approach to evaluating the cervical spine, especially when the patient has multiple distracting injuries.

INTRODUCTION

Trauma to the cervical spine is a devastating injury with high morbidity and mortality. In the United States, most traumatic spinal injuries occur as a result of motor vehicle collisions (MVCs) (43%), followed by falls (27%).[1] An estimated 81% of all spinal injuries occur in men with an average age of 40 years.[1] In the trauma setting, there is immense pressure on radiologists to clear the cervical spine and missing even a subtle finding could have devastating consequences. In the polytrauma patient, this is especially true because attention is focused on detecting injuries that are an immediate threat to life, such as an aortic pathology. This article presents a systematic approach to evaluating the cervical spine in trauma using computed tomography (CT) scan. It also provides an update on the latest imaging techniques, reviews the anatomy and biomechanics of the cervical spine, and illustrates classic patterns of injury.

[a] University of British Columbia, 899 West 12th Avenue, Vancouver, British Columbia V5Z 1M9, Canada; [b] Department of Radiology, Vancouver General Hospital, University of British Columbia, 899 West 12th Avenue, Vancouver, British Columbia V5Z 1M9, Canada; [c] Department of Radiology, St Joseph's Hospital, 2137 Comox Avenue, Comox, British Columbia V9M 1P2, Canada; [d] Zanvyl Krieger School of Arts & Sciences, Johns Hopkins University, 1717 Massachusetts Avenue NW, Washington, DC 20036, USA
* Corresponding author.
E-mail address: lucklouis@gmail.com

Radiol Clin N Am 53 (2015) 657–674
http://dx.doi.org/10.1016/j.rcl.2015.02.015
0033-8389/15/$ – see front matter © 2015 Elsevier Inc. All rights reserved.

IMAGING RECOMMENDATIONS

According to the American College of Radiology (ACR) Appropriateness Criteria, only high-risk patients require imaging of the cervical spine.[2] Low-risk patients who do not require imaging can be identified using the National Emergency X-Ray Utilization Study (NEXUS) criteria or the Canadian C-spine Rule (Box 1).[2–4] It is controversial whether the NEXUS criteria or the Canadian C-Spine Rule is a better screening method; the choice depends on the referring clinician.[5–7] Caution, however, is recommended when applying these rules to the elderly population because there have been case reports of elderly patients who meet the low-risk criteria but who are subsequently found to have dens fractures.[8] When imaging is necessary, the ACR Appropriateness Criteria recommends that a noncontrast CT scan with both sagittal and coronal reconstructions and/or a noncontrast magnetic resonance (MR) imaging be performed.[2] A meta-analysis determined that the overall sensitivity of CT scan is 98%, whereas the pooled sensitivity of radiography is only 52%.[9] In the intubated patient, the sensitivity of the lateral cervical spine radiograph is only 39%.[9] In addition, CT scan is superior in assessing the craniocervical and cervicothoracic regions, which are relative blind spots on radiography. In the trauma setting, CT scanning is also faster than radiography, especially when the scanner is located within the emergency department.[2]

Currently, there is a very limited role for static radiography in the setting of cervical trauma. A single lateral projection can be a useful adjunct when the CT scan sagittal reconstruction is suboptimal.[2] Surgeons may also request cervical spine radiographs to assist in preoperative planning. Additionally, radiography remains the best modality to follow patients with stable injuries that are initially diagnosed and characterized completely by CT scan. There is essentially no role for dynamic flexion–extension radiography in the trauma setting. It is unreliable because of muscle spasm and may aggravate injury. Several studies have demonstrated that there is no benefit to these views compared with CT scan in the diagnosis of ligament and soft tissue injuries.[2] MR imaging is the modality of choice for suspected ligamentous injury.[2] For patients who warrant cervical spine imaging, CT scan is the best initial modality.[2] Adjunct imaging can also include a CT angiogram of the head and neck vessels to assess for vascular injury.[10] Most mechanisms of injury that warrant a CT scan also meet the criteria for angiography.[11] If vascular imaging is not included as part of the initial polytrauma CT scan protocol, it should be obtained if cervical abnormalities are detected. Upper cervical spine injuries and factures involving the skull base pose a particularly high risk for associated vascular injuries.[10]

Clearing the cervical spine in obtunded patients is controversial. A recent meta-analysis reported that the negative predictive value of a normal CT scan for ligamentous injury was 100% but other studies have demonstrated that CT scan alone is inadequate for clearing the cervical spine and should be used in combination with MR imaging.[12] The ACR Appropriateness Criteria recommends that, if a reliable neurologic examination cannot be obtained within 48 hours postinjury, MR imaging should be performed to clear the cervical spine.[2]

SCANNING TECHNIQUE

All CT scans of the cervical spine should be performed with thin slices (ie, in 1 mm or 0.75 mm axial sections) with coronal and sagittal reconstructions at 1 to 2 mm thick. At the corresponding author's institution, patients are scanned in a craniocaudal direction with a tube voltage of 140 or 120 kilovolt (peak), rotation time of 1 second, and pitch of 0.8, using a detector configuration of 64 × 0.6 mm. All images are reconstructed using

---

Box 1
NEXUS criteria and Canadian C-Spine Rule

NEXUS Criteria	Canadian C-Spine Rule
• No posterior midline cervical tenderness	• Age <65 y
	• No dangerous mechanism
• No intoxication	○ Fall from height >3 feet
• No focal neurologic deficit	○ Axial loading injury
	○ MVC at high-speed (>100 km/h), MVC with rollover or MVC with ejection
• No painful distracting injuries	○ Recreational motor vehicle accident
	• No paresthesia
	• Sitting position in emergency department
	• Ambulatory at any time
	• Neck rotation 45° to both right and left

both a standard bone deconvolution kernel, B75h very sharp, ASA (Siemens Healthcare, Forchheim, Germany) in the axial, sagittal, and coronal planes, as well as a soft tissue deconvolution kernel using hybrid iterative reconstruction, I30 strength 2, SAFFIRE (Siemens Healthcare, Forscheim, Germany) in both the axial and sagittal planes. Because trauma primarily affects younger patients, using dose-reduction strategies, such as tube current modulation, adaptive collimation, automated exposure control, and iterative reconstruction, is essential.[13,14] At the corresponding author's institution, the kilovolt (peak) is reduced from 140 to 120 for younger patients, which results in 40% dose reduction. Greater dose reduction can be achieved by reducing both kilovolt and quality milliamp seconds (mAs) reference values and using iterative reconstruction techniques to account for the increased noise.

CERVICAL SPINE ANATOMY AND BIOMECHANICS

To understand the biomechanics of the spine, it is important to understand its anatomy. The cervical spine can be thought of as 2 anatomically and functionally separate units.[15,16] The first unit includes the skull base (ie, the occipital condyles), first cervical vertebra (C1), and second cervical vertebra (C2). The second unit consists of the third through seventh vertebral bodies (C3–C7). This division, however, does not apply to patients with rigid spinal disease, such as ankylosing spondylitis or diffuse idiopathic skeletal hypertrophy (DISH), and their spine will respond differently to applied external forces.[16]

Most of the compressive forces through the cervical spine are transmitted through the vertebral bodies, which increase in strength from C1 through to C7. The facets carry approximately 30% of the load and contribute to 45% of the torsional strength of the cervical spine.[16] The C1 (atlas) and C2 (axis) vertebral bodies are anatomically unique to allow for the articulation with the skull base and permit a wide range of movements at the head (**Fig. 1**).[16] The C3 through C7 vertebral bodies have similar shape; however, the C7 vertebral body is slightly different, with a longer spinous process, to allow for the transition to the thoracic spine.

The craniocervical junction is the most anatomically intricate part of the cervical spine. It is defined by 3 key associations between joints and ligaments: the occipitoatlantal relationship, the occipitoaxial relationship and the atlantoaxial relationship (**Fig. 2**).[16–18] The atlantoocipital relationship, between the occipital condyles and

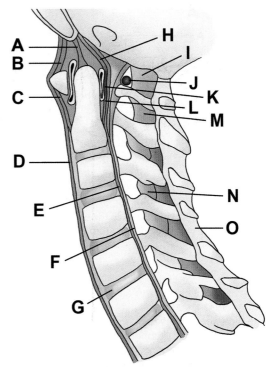

Fig. 1. Midsagittal anatomy of the cervical spine. A, apical ligament; B, anterior occipitoatlantal ligament; C, anterior atlantoaxial ligament; D, anterior longitudinal ligament; E, posterior longitudinal ligament; F, tectorial membrane; G, intervertebral disc; H, superior longitudinal band of the cruciate ligament; I, posterior occipitoatlantal ligament; J, vertebral artery; K, transverse ligament of atlas; L, inferior longitudinal band of the cruciate ligament; M, posterior atlantoaxial ligament; N, ligamentum flavum; O, interspinous ligament.

C1, consists of the anterior, posterior, and lateral atlantooccipital ligaments, as well as the paired atlantooccipital joints and anterior or posterior atlantodental joints. The occipitoaxial relationship, between the occipital condyles and C2, consists of the apical, occipitoaxial, and paired alar ligaments. The atlantoaxial relationship consists of 2 paired atlantoaxial joints as well as the cruciate ligament complex, which includes the transverse ligament and the superior and inferior longitudinal bands. The transverse ligament is responsible for holding the dens securely against C1. The tectorial membrane also helps stabilize the atlantoaxial association by covering the dens and other ligaments.

The lower cervical spine is primarily supported by long ligaments that extend from the C2 to the sacrum along the anterior and posterior aspects of the vertebral bodies, termed the anterior and

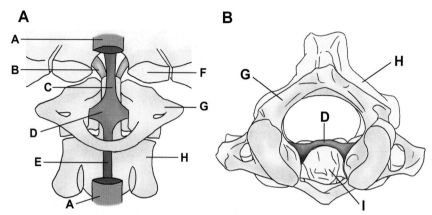

Fig. 2. Anatomic relationships of the upper cervical spine in the coronal (A) and axial (B) planes. A, tectorial membrane (cut); B, alar ligament (paired); C, superior longitudinal band of the cruciate ligament; D, transverse ligament of atlas; E, inferior longitudinal band of the cruciate ligament; F, occipital condyle; G, C1 (atlas); H, C2 (axis); I, dens.

posterior longitudinal ligaments, respectively.[16] The ligamentum flavum, interspinous ligament, and supraspinous ligament also provide support to the posterior elements. Additionally the intervertebral discs and the facets, which are synovial joints surrounded by thick capsules, confer additional integrity to the lower cervical spine (see **Fig. 1**).[16]

DETERMINING STABILITY OF CERVICAL SPINE INJURIES

When the cervical spine cannot maintain normal alignment and protect the spinal cord and exiting nerve roots under physiologic conditions, it is considered unstable.[16,19] Stability is determined by the integrity of the osseous and ligamentous structures, as well as the intervertebral discs and facet joints. Usually, if more than one of these structures is disrupted so as to allow motion at, above, or below the level of the injury, there is instability.[16,19] However, there is such a wide range of potential injuries as well as unique contributing patient factors that it can be challenging to predict stability on an individual patient basis, especially on CT scan.

The recently proposed Subaxial Cervical Spine Classification (SLIC) system incorporates the degree of osseous and ligamentous injury and the patient's neurologic status to assess the stability of injuries.[20] Points are awarded in each of the following categories: osseous morphology, disco-ligamentous complex, and neurologic status. An increased number of points denote a potentially more unstable injury. Although this system has been validated, it is not particularly helpful to the radiologist interpreting the initial CT imaging because information about the disco-ligamentous complex, which is determined by MR imaging as well as the neurologic status, is usually not available. In addition, this scale is unreliable in intubated or obtunded patients.

In the radiology literature, the definition of stability of the vertebral column has typically been assessed using the 3-column model.[19] The anterior column, which consists of the anterior longitudinal ligament, the anterior one-half of the vertebral body, and the intervertebral disc, is responsible for bearing the axial load and resisting extension. The middle column, which includes the posterior longitudinal ligament, the posterior one-half of the vertebral body, and the intervertebral disc, is responsible for bearing axial load and resisting flexion. The posterior column, which consists of the posterior bony elements and the facet joints, is also responsible for resisting flexion in addition to stabilizing the spine during rotation and lateral bending. An injury involving 2 or more columns is considered unstable and disruption of the middle column is synonymous with instability. Also, any injury of the craniocervical junction should be regarded as potentially unstable and MR imaging is required for further characterization.

EVALUATING THE CERVICAL SPINE

In the trauma setting, it is extremely important to have a systematic approach to interpreting studies because the emergency department is extremely busy and patients are often critically ill. At the corresponding author's institution, the first step is labeling the cervical spine using the annotation tool on the workstation; this will help correlate areas of concern across reconstructions. Using the sagittal reconstructions, the intervertebral discs and vertebral bodies are assessed for uniformity in height and shape. Next, evaluate the anterior vertebral, posterior vertebral, spinolaminar, and posterior spinous lines, similar to interpretation of the lateral radiograph. Subluxation of beyond 3 mm within the anterior and posterior vertebral lines is abnormal. It is important to scrutinize the interspinous distances because widening (or fanning) indicates ligamentous injury. Assessment of the prevertebral soft tissues is typically not reliable, especially in intubated patients. Use of the blood windows (width 135; length 72 Hounsfield units [HU]) to look for subtle epidural hematoma can be helpful.

Once the overall alignment has been assessed, divide the search pattern according to the upper and lower, or subaxial, cervical spine. Recall that the upper segment includes the occipital condyles, C1 and C2, and the lower segment consists of C3 through C7. Using this pattern, injuries occurring in these 2 biomechanically distinct units can be better evaluated and characterized.

Evaluation of the Craniocervical Junction

The craniocervical junction is a relative blind spot on CT scan, especially in severely injured patients. It is important to consider the occipital condyles as cervical vertebra zero (C0) to guarantee that they are individually assessed.[15] In the sagittal plane, ensure that there is perfect congruity between the occipital condyles and the C1 lateral masses (**Fig. 3A**). If the alignment is perfect, it is extremely unlikely that there is a pathology at this level (**Fig. 4A**). Evaluate the condyle-to-C1 interval and the condylar sum. The condyle-to-C1 interval should be less than or equal to 2 mm and, therefore, the condylar sum, which is the sum of the distance between each condyle and the condylar fossa of C1, should be less than 4 mm (see **Fig. 3B**).[21] Widening of the condyle-to-C1 interval or condylar sum may be associated with a fracture of the occipital condyle at the alar ligament insertion (ie, type 3 occipital condyle fracture) (see **Fig. 4B**).

Use all the reconstructions to assess the C1 and C2 vertebral bodies. The atlantooccipital relationship is best evaluated in the sagittal plane using the bone algorithm. The basion-dens interval (BDI), which is the distance from the basion to the dens, should be less than 9 mm on CT scan (**Fig. 5A**).[22] Values greater than 9 mm are in keeping with craniocervical dissociation, which is a rare injury, often immediately fatal (see **Fig. 5B**).[23,24] When assessing the atlantoaxial junction, ensure that there is not more than 2 mm of overhang of the lateral masses of C1 on C2 in the coronal plane (see **Fig. 3B**). If there is overhang of the lateral masses of C1 on C2, assess carefully for C1 fractures (see **Fig. 4B**). In the axial plane, the anterior atlantodental interval should be less than 2 mm (**Fig. 6A**).[24] Values greater than this are concerning for atlantoaxial dissociation (see **Fig. 6B**).[24]

Injuries at the Craniocervical Junction

Occipital condyle fractures

Occipital condylar fractures frequently occur in high-speed MVCs, especially with airbag deployment. They are associated with C1, C2, and basal skull fractures; 30% of affected patients will have cranial nerve abnormalities.[15,25] The most widely used classification system for occipital condyle

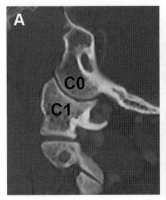
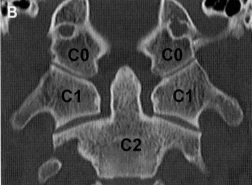

Fig. 3. Normal alignment of the upper cervical spine. (*A*) In the sagittal plane, the occipital condyles and C1 should be perfectly aligned. (*B*) In the coronal plane, the condylar sum (bilateral distance between the midpoint of the occipital condyle and the condylar fossa of C1) should be less than 4 mm. The lateral masses of C1 should overhang the C2 lateral masses by less than 2 mm.

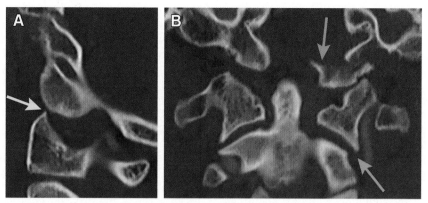

Fig. 4. Abnormal alignment of the upper cervical spine in a 25-year-old male cyclist involved in an MVC. (*A*) In the sagittal plane, there is abnormal alignment of the occipital condyle and the lateral mass of C1 (*yellow arrow*). (*B*) The coronal reconstruction of a left type 3 occipital condyle fracture (*blue arrow*) results in dislocation of both condyles on C1 (*red arrow*). There is 4 mm of overhang of the lateral mass of C1 on C2 (*green arrow*).

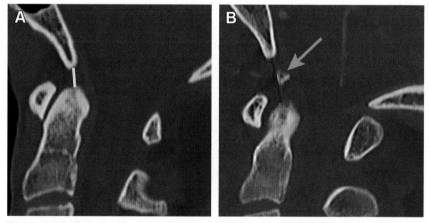

Fig. 5. Normal and abnormal BDI. (*A*) Normal BDI should be less than 9 mm (*yellow line*) on CT scan (*B*) A 56-year-old man involved in a motorcycle accident has craniocervical dissociation. The BDI measures 16 mm (*red line*). An occipital condyle fracture is only partially visible (*blue arrow*).

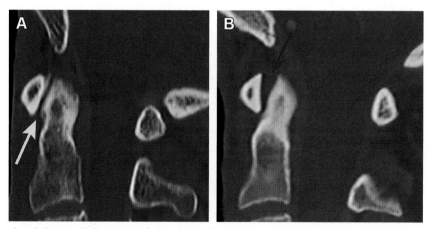

Fig. 6. Normal and abnormal alignment of the atlantodental interval. (*A*) Normal anterior atlantodental interval (*yellow arrow*) should be less than 2 mm. (*B*) A 23-year-old man involved in a cycling accident shows widening of the superior aspect of the atlantodental interval measuring 4 mm (*red arrow*), consistent with atlantoaxial dissociation.

fractures, developed by Anderson and Montesano in 1988, describes 3 types of occipital condyle fractures.[26] Type 1 fractures, due to loading of the occipital condyle, are a crush-type fracture with minimal comminution and impaction (**Fig. 7**). Type 2 fractures result from an extension of a basal skull fracture into the occipital condyle and may be unilateral or bilateral (**Fig. 8**). Type 3 fractures are due to an alar ligament avulsion fracture off the anterior aspect of the occipital condyle (**Fig. 9A, B**). These fractures are unstable due to the fracture fragment's location in the foramen magnum and avulsion of the alar ligament. It is important to measure the size of the fragment and displacement into the foramen magnum, which is easiest on the coronal reconstructions.[15] Also, if there are bilateral occipital condyle fractures of any type, these are considered unstable (see **Fig. 9C**).

Jefferson fracture

Jefferson, or C1 burst, fractures are due to sudden direct axial loading. There is compression of the C1 lateral masses between the occipital condyles and C2 superior facets, resulting in a fracture occurring through the weakest part of C1, which is at the junction of the anterior and posterior arches with the lateral masses.[15] By definition, this type of fracture requires only a fracture of the anterior arch although any combination may occur.[27] The classic Jefferson fracture has 4 parts (**Fig. 10**); however, a spectrum of atypical fractures can occur depending on the head position at the time of injury (**Fig. 11**). The number of fragments is best characterized on the axial source images

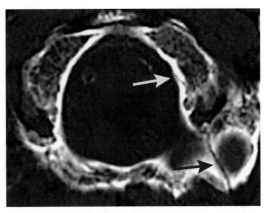

Fig. 8. Type 2 left occipital condyle fracture in a 48-year-old man involved in a motorcycle accident. The left occipital skull base fracture (*red arrow*) extends through the left occipital condyle (*yellow arrow*).

and the distance between fragments should be documented. Separation of fragments greater than 7 mm should be considered unstable.[28] Additionally, if the atlantoaxial distance is greater than 3 mm, the injury is considered unstable because of the concomitant rupture of the transverse ligament.[15] Other fractures may occur at C1 that do not fit the criteria for a Jefferson fracture. These typically involve the lateral masses and are considered unstable because of disruption of the transverse ligament.[28] Assess carefully for extension into the transverse foramen and potential vertebral artery injuries (**Fig. 12**).[10,29]

Dens fracture

Injury to the dens can result from a wide range of mechanisms and is commonly seen in elderly patients.[30] Anderson and D'Alonzo[5] classified dens fractures into 3 types. In Type 1 fractures, which are the least common, the fracture line is obliquely oriented at the superolateral aspect of the dens due to avulsion of the alar ligament (**Fig. 13A**). These fractures are unstable because of the ligamentous disruption. Type 2 fractures are the most common and are defined by horizontally oriented fracture at the base of the dens (see **Fig. 13B**).[30] Acute and/or nonunited Type 2 fractures may be unstable. Type 3 fractures are fractures that extend into the vertebral body (see **Fig. 13C**). On the sagittal reconstruction, assess for the degree and direction of angulation of the dens because this defines the integrity of the transverse ligaments (**Fig. 14**).[15] If there is a large degree of displacement, atlantoaxial dislocation should be considered.

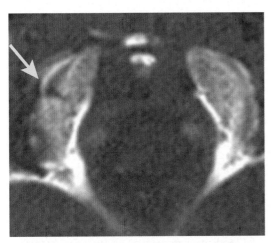

Fig. 7. Type 1 occipital condyle fracture (*yellow arrow*) in a 70-year-old woman who fell down the stairs. The anterior aspect of the occipital condyle is depressed and comminuted in keeping with a crush-type injury.

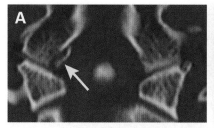
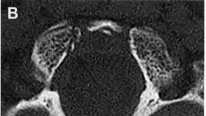
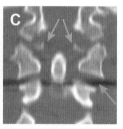

Fig. 9. Two patients with type 3 occipital right condyle fractures. (*A*) Type 3 occipital condyle fracture (*yellow arrow*) in a 24-year-old man involved in an MVC in the coronal plane. (*B*) The fracture (*red arrow*) on the axial source image. (*C*) Bilateral type 3 occipital condyle fractures (*green arrows*) in another patient also involved in an MVC. There is widening of the distance between the lateral masses of C1 and C2 in keeping with associated atlantoaxial instability (*blue arrow*).

Hangman's fracture

Hangman's, or C2, fractures are primarily due to hyperextension and distraction (**Fig. 15**). The classic Hangman's fracture, first described in hanging victims, is comprised of bilateral C2 pedicle fractures and complete distraction of C2 on C3. However, this classic description only describes 30% of fractures and the term Hangman's fracture is used to refer to a spectrum of C2 fractures described in a classification scheme by Levine and Edwards.[31] In general, there is typically extensive prevertebral soft tissue swelling and epidural hematoma. The axial source images provide the best assessment of the number of fracture fragments as well as the amount of distraction and angulation. When there is more than 3 mm between fragments or greater than 15° of angulation, the injury is considered unstable.[15] The fractures through the pars interarticularis are best evaluated on the sagittal reconstruction and there may be subtle anterior subluxation of C2 on C3, which is also a feature of instability. The posterior column, however, should remain aligned. In 33% of injuries, there will be a fracture in an adjacent vertebra and it is important to carefully scrutinize for a second site of fracture because concomitant C1 and C2 fractures are inherently unstable.[15] Also, if the fracture extends into the transverse foramen, a CT angiogram must be obtained.

EVALUATING THE LOWER CERVICAL SPINE

The facet joints are best assessed on the sagittal reconstruction and axial source images. Ensure that there is no overlap of facets or widening greater than 2 mm (**Fig. 16**). On the axial source images, normally aligned facet joints have a hamburger bun configuration. It may be helpful to link the axial bone and axial soft tissue algorithms and view them side by side to appreciate subtle soft tissue swelling and evaluate for epidural hematoma. It is important to use all 3 planes to assess for fractures, which are frequently subtle. Vertically oriented fractures are best appreciated on the coronal and axial planes, whereas horizontally oriented fractures are best appreciated on the coronal and sagittal planes. Having a detailed understanding of fracture patterns will help increase the sensitivity of individual search patterns.

Injuries to the Lower Cervical Spine

Hyperflexion injuries

Hyperflexion injures, usually occur in the middle or lower cervical spine, and are most commonly sustained in younger patient in MVCs. Injuries may be due to pure flexion, although they may occur with axial loading or distraction.[17] Typically, in hyperflexion injuries with axial loading the vector of force is directed through the anterior aspect of the spinal column with the anterior column being injured first, followed by the middle and posterior columns.[15] In

Fig. 10. Classic 4-part Jefferson fracture. Fracture lines extend through both anterior arches (*yellow arrows*) and posterior arches (*red arrows*) in a 25-year-old man involved in a snowmobile accident.

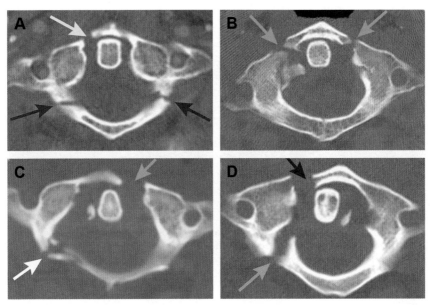

Fig. 11. Spectrum of atypical Jefferson fractures. (A) Three-part Jefferson fracture with a single fracture through the anterior arch (*yellow arrow*) and bilateral fractures through the posterior arch (*red arrows*). (B) Anterior one-half fracture through the anterior arch (*blue arrows*). (C) Contralateral hemiring with fractures through the left anterior arch (*green arrow*) and contralateral right posterior arch (*white arrow*). (D) Ipsilateral hemiring fracture through the right anterior arch (*blue arrow*) and ipsilateral right posterior arch (*orange arrow*).

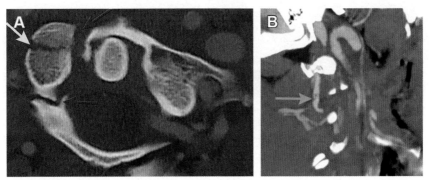

Fig. 12. Atypical Jefferson fracture with associated vertebral artery injury in a 25-year-old man involved in a snowmobile accident. (A) Axial source images of a right ipsilateral hemiring fracture (*red arrows*) with an associated right lateral mass fracture (*yellow arrow*). (B) CT angiogram of a dissection of the right vertebral artery (*blue arrow*) in the sagittal plane.

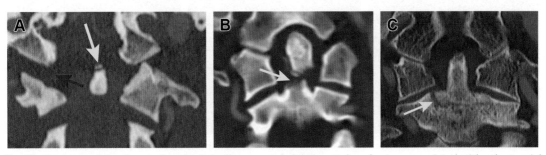

Fig. 13. Fractures of the dens in 3 patients (*yellow arrows*). (A) Type 1 dens fracture associated with atlantoaxial instability (*red arrow*). (B) Type 2 dens fracture. (C) Type 3 dens fracture.

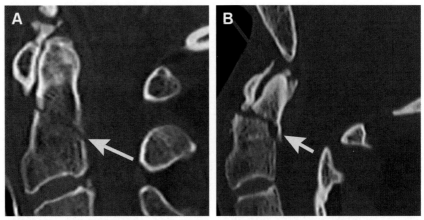

Fig. 14. Type 2 dens fractures in the sagittal plane in 2 patients. (*A*) Example of a nondisplaced dens fracture (*yellow arrow*). (*B*) Example of a displaced dens fracture with posterior angulation and migration (*yellow arrow*). The atlantodental interval is also minimally widened (*red arrow*).

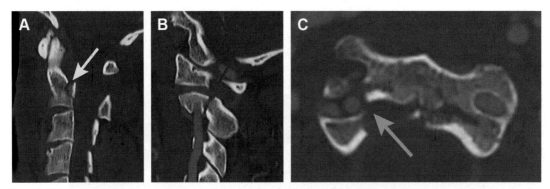

Fig. 15. Hangman's fracture in a 69-year-old woman involved in an MVC. (*A*) On the sagittal image, there is retropulsion of the fragment into the spinal canal (*yellow arrow*). (*B*) The fracture line extends into the right pars inticularis (*red arrow*). (*C*) The axial image shows extension into the right transverse foramen (*blue arrow*).

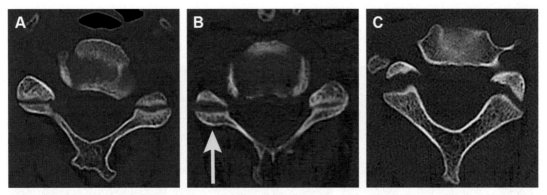

Fig. 16. Normal and abnormal facet alignment. (*A*) Normal facet alignment with the symmetric hamburger bun appearance. (*B*) Subtle widening of the right facet (*yellow arrow*). The left facet remains normal. (*C*) Bilateral facet widening with minimal distraction.

hyperflexion with distraction, the vector of force is superior and perpendicular to the spine and injury involves the posterior elements before the middle and anterior columns. Although it is important to have a general understanding of these mechanisms, these vectors have been shown to be unreliable predictors of fracture type, especially in complex injuries.

Anterior wedge compression fracture

Anterior wedge compression fractures are the result of both hyperflexion and compression.[17] In this injury, the anterior aspect of the vertebral body receives most of the impact and although the posterior ligaments stretch, they should not rupture. Anterior wedging greater than 3 mm is suggestive of a fracture; however, there should not be more than 25% vertebral body height loss (Fig. 17).[15] Prevertebral soft tissue swelling, focal kyphosis and narrowing of the intervertebral disc space at the level above the affected vertebral body are usually present. Although slight fanning

of the spinous processes may be present because of strain on the posterior ligaments, there should not be fracture extension into the middle or posterior columns. If there is, this connotes a more serious injury and is considered an unstable fracture.

Burst fracture

Burst fractures are due to extreme axial loading of the spine and typically occur in the lower cervical spine. In a true burst fracture, there are at least 2 fracture lines resulting in a multipart fracture (Fig. 18). Commonly, there is retropulsion of fragments into the central spinal canal, producing permanent neurologic damage. The degree of retropulsion and number of fragments is best appreciated on the axial source and sagittal images.[15]

Flexion teardrop fracture

Flexion teardrop fractures are due to extreme flexion and axial compression, which results in an obliquely-oriented fracture through the anteroinferior aspect of the vertebral body and complete disruption of the posterior ligaments (Fig. 19).[15,17,32] This is the most severe and most unstable injury of the cervical spine. The anteroinferior fracture of the vertebral body is best appreciated on the sagittal reconstructions, whereas the vertically oriented component of the fracture is best identified in the coronal plane. It is important to measure the distance of fragment migration into the canal. In severe cases, there may also be distraction of the facets.

Bilateral facet dislocation

In bilateral facet dislocation, there is extreme flexion and disruption, which results anterior subluxation of the vertebral body as well as subluxation of the inferior articular facets over the superior articular facets at the level below (Fig. 20).[15] As a result, there is uncovering of the facets immediately inferior to the affected level. This is an unstable injury due do the ligamentous disruption of the middle and posterior columns; however, there are usually no associated fractures. Prevertebral soft tissue swelling and focal kyphosis are present. There is often neurologic compromise due to cord injury and there is a strong association with vertebral artery injury. In bilateral facet dislocation injuries, there is also a high association with disc herniation.[33]

Unilateral facet dislocation

Unilateral facet dislocation typically occurs in the lower cervical spine due to asymmetric hyperflexion and/or rotation (Fig. 21).[15,17,34] During rotation, the superior facets slide over the inferior facets

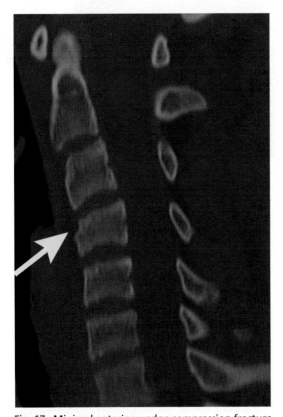

Fig. 17. Minimal anterior wedge compression fracture of C4 is identified with approximately 10% of vertebral body height loss (*yellow arrow*) in a 19-year-old woman involved in a diving accident. There is slight anterior cortical buckling.

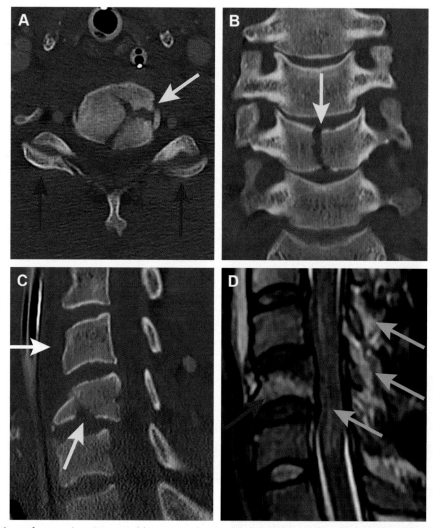

Fig. 18. C5 burst fracture in a 24-year-old woman who dove into shallow water. (*A*) Comminuted fracture of the vertebral body (*yellow arrow*) with bilateral facet widening (*red arrows*) in keeping with disruption of the posterior elements. (*B*) The vertical component of the fracture is best appreciated in the coronal plane (*yellow arrow*). There is loss of the vertebral body height. (*C*) Fracture through the anteroinferior corner of the C5 vertebral body (*yellow arrow*) with swelling of the prevertebral soft tissues (*white arrow*). (*D*) Sagittal T2-weighted MR imaging of edema in the posterior soft tissues (*blue arrows*) and edema of the spinal cord at this level (*green arrow*). There is bone marrow edema present within the fractured C5 vertebra (*red arrow*).

resulting in various degrees of facet displacement, including perched, locked, and complete dislocation. Diastasis of the contralateral facet is common and is best appreciated in the axial plane. In about 10% of cases, there will be a concomitant avulsion fracture of the posterior elements and 73% of patients will have associated fractures of the articular pillars.

Clay shoveler fracture

Clay shoveler fracture is a pure flexion injury in which there is a vertically or obliquely oriented avulsion fracture of the spinous process of C6, C7, or (occasionally) the first thoracic vertebra (**Fig. 22**).[35] Due to the avulsion fracture, the posterior ligaments remain intact. Typically, this type of fracture is limited to the spinous process, although it may extend into the lamina of the vertebral body, which is considered a more severe injury because of the potential for neurologic compromise.[15]

Hyperextension Injuries

Extension injuries account for less than 25% of cervical spine injuries.[15] However, they are much

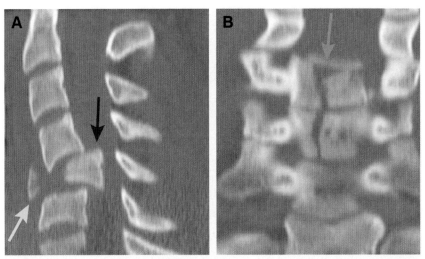

Fig. 19. Flexion teardrop injury in a 43-year-old woman involved in an MVC. (*A*) Midsagittal image demonstrates focal kyphosis with a fracture through the anterior inferior aspect of the C5 vertebral body (*yellow arrow*). There is retropulsion of the posterior fragment into the spinal canal (*red arrow*) resulting in neurologic compromise. (*B*) On the coronal image, the vertical component of this fracture extends through both the C4 and C5 vertebral bodies.

more common in the elderly and patients with rigid spinal disease.[36,37] These injuries result from hyperextension with axial compression or rotation. Typically, the direction of force is through the posterior column, which results in a range of injuries from a sprain, to ligamentous rupture, to fracture. Injuries are subtle and it is important to have a high index of suspicion. The history is usually misleading because patients often undergo relatively minor trauma (eg, fall).[38]

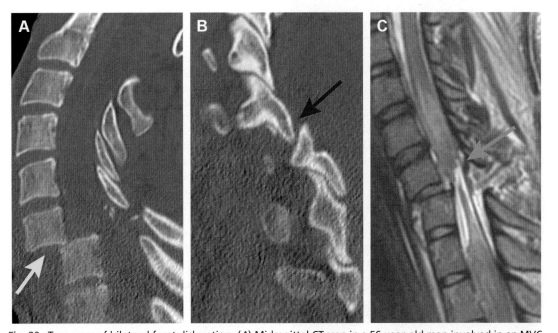

Fig. 20. Two cases of bilateral facet dislocation. (*A*) Midsagittal CT scan in a 56-year-old man involved in an MVC. There is greater than 50% subluxation of C6 on C7 (*yellow arrow*). (*B*) Sagittal image through the facets shows a dislocated facet (*red arrow*). (*C*) Midsagittal T2-weighted sequence in another patient who was involved in a rollover MVC, shows complete transection of the spinal cord (*blue arrow*). There was spontaneous reduction of the bilateral facet dislocation immediately following the injury.

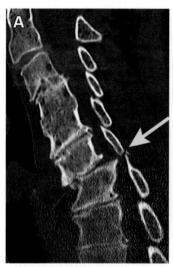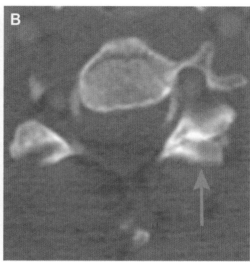

Fig. 21. Unilateral facet dislocation in 2 patients. (A) Unilateral facet dislocation (*yellow arrow*) in a 72-year-old woman involved in an MVC with degenerative ankylosis from C3 through C5. There is perched facet (*yellow arrow*) and focal kyphosis and anterior subluxation of C6 on C7 (*red arrow*). (B) Unilateral locked facet (*blue arrow*) in a 56-year-old man involved in a separate MVC. This left facet has the reverse hamburger sign.

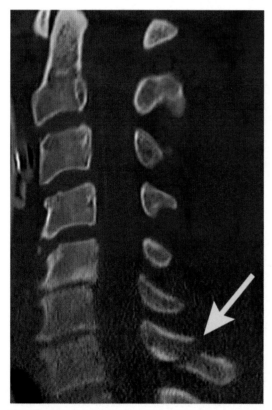

Fig. 22. Clay-shoveler's fracture. Obliquely oriented fracture through the spinous process of C7 (*yellow arrow*) in a 61-year-old man who fell down the stairs.

Hyperextension sprain dislocation

This injury occurs due to head trauma, commonly assault, which causes severe muscular and ligamentous injury of the cervical spine.[39] The anterior longitudinal ligament is disrupted, resulting in widening of the anterior disc space.[15] Depending on the force, the intervertebral disc and posterior ligaments may also rupture (**Fig. 23**). In severe hyperextension sprain injuries, there is posterior movement of the vertebral body, which strips of the superior aspect of the intervertebral disc off the undersurface of the vertebral body causing neurologic compromise.[17] Generally, the middle and posterior columns remain intact. However, in high velocity trauma, there may be ligamentous damage in the middle column, resulting in dislocation of the vertebral body directly above the level of injury. It is important to have a high index of suspicion because these injuries reduce within seconds and there may not be evidence of dislocation on initial CT scan. MR imaging will be the key to characterizing this injury.

Hyperextension fracture dislocation

Fractures from hyperextension injuries usually occur in elderly patients and in patients with ankylosing spondylitis and DISH.[15] In the elderly, the mechanism is similar to hyperextension sprain dislocation except there are associated fractures of the posterior column, including the pedicles and spinous process, as a result of decreased

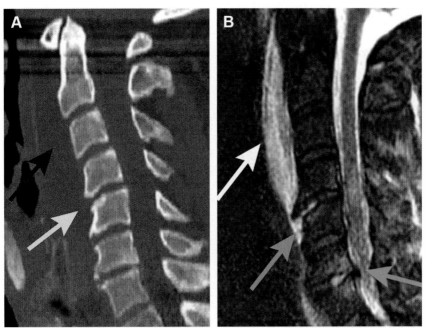

Fig. 23. Hyperextension sprain dislocation in a 65-year-old man involved in an MVC. (*A*) On the CT scan, there is loss of the normal curvature of the spine with disruption of the spinolamellar and anterior spinal lines (*yellow arrow*). There is extensive prevertebral soft tissue swelling (*red arrow*). (*B*) Sagittal T2-weighted MR imaging sequence confirms marked prevertebral soft tissue swelling (*white arrow*) and disruption of the anterior longitudinal ligament (*blue arrow*). Although there was immediate reduction of the dislocation, there is transection of the spinal cord (*green arrow*).

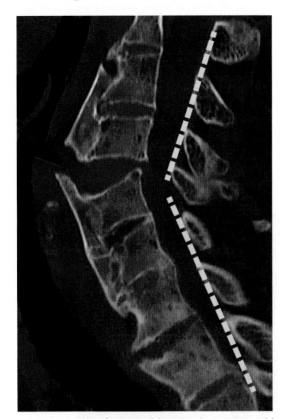

Fig. 24. Extension fracture dislocation in a 72-year-old man with DISH who presented 2 days after injury with left arm numbness. The fracture of the anterior flowing osteophyte (*red arrow*) and disruption of the spinolamellar line indicates extension into the posterior elements (*dotted yellow line*).

range of motion in the lower cervical spine (**Fig. 24**). In rigid spinal disease, there is a fracture through the flowing osteophytes or fusion anteriorly with the fracture line extending obliquely into the adjacent vertebrae and the posterior elements.[40] The anterior disc space is usually asymmetrically widened.

Extension teardrop fracture

With forced extension and rotation, there is compression and distraction of the posterior column and avulsion of the anteroinferior corner of the vertebral body (**Fig. 25**).[40] The anterior longitudinal ligament is disrupted, resulting in widening of the disc space at or below the level of the fracture. This fracture is considered unstable, especially in extension, and can be associated with spinal cord injury.[15] If rotational force is large, there may be widening of the facet joints. In elderly patients, extension teardrop fractures are more common in the upper cervical spine due to reduced mobility of the lower cervical spine (**Fig. 26**).[41]

BEYOND THE SPINE

In a patient with suspected cervical spine trauma, there is a high likelihood of other injuries.[42] Evaluation of the cervical spine should include assessment of edge-of-film findings, which may indicate more extensive injuries and the need for

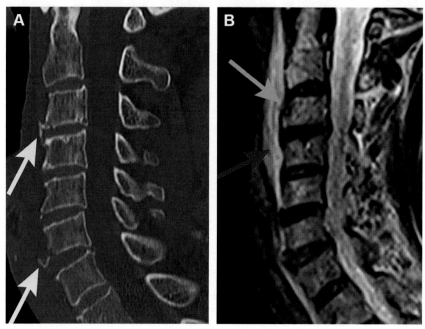

Fig. 25. Extension teardrop fracture in a 45-year-old woman involved in an MVC. (*A*) Sagittal CT scan of fractures at the anterior-inferior aspect of the C3 and C6 vertebral bodies (*yellow arrows*). (*B*) Sagittal T2-weighted MR imaging of extensive prevertebral soft tissue swelling (*red arrow*) and disruption of the anterior longitudinal ligament (*blue arrow*).

further imaging (**Fig. 27**). This includes evaluation of the mandible, which is typically only partially included in the field of view. This may be the only chance to assess the mandible because it is not routinely included in polytrauma scans. If dedicated images of the chest have not been acquired, look carefully at the clavicles, first ribs, and lung apices. Widen the soft tissue windows to assess for any organic foreign bodies that are not readily appreciated on standard windows.

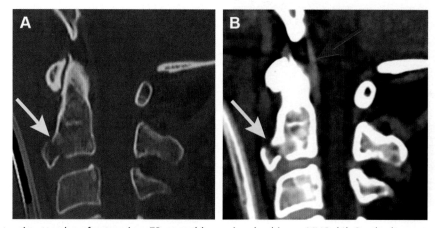

Fig. 26. Extension teardrop fracture in a 73-year-old man involved in an MVC. (*A*) On the bone sagittal reconstruction, the fracture line extends through the anteroinferior aspect of C2 (*yellow arrow*). (*B*) When the windows are narrowed on the soft tissue sagittal reconstruction, the fracture is still visible (*yellow arrow*) as well as the associated epidural hematoma (*red arrow*).

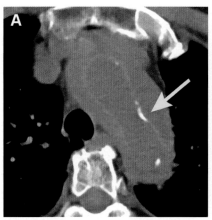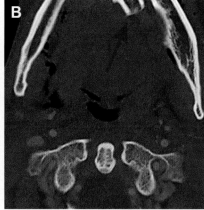

Fig. 27. Examples of edge-of-film findings on CT scans of the cervical spine. (*A*) Intramural hematoma (*yellow arrow*) discovered on a scan ordered in a 63-year-old woman who was found down, rule out fracture. (*B*) Displaced mandibular fracture (*red arrow*) identified in a 25-year-old man who was assaulted.

SUMMARY

Prompt identification and classification of cervical spine injuries is essential due to their high morbidity and mortality. In the trauma setting, it is important to have a systematic approach to evaluating the cervical spine, especially when the patient has multiple injuries. Although it can be useful to understand the classic patterns of cervical spine injury, it is important to realize that in severe trauma these patterns may be difficult or impossible to appreciate. In elderly patients and those with rigid spinal disease, injuries may be subtle and it is crucial to have a high index of suspicion even if the mechanism of injury is unimpressive.

CT scan is the imaging modality of choice for all suspected cervical spine injuries. At the corresponding author's institution, patients who meet the criteria for imaging receive a CT scan. Cervical spine radiographs are generally not obtained in the trauma setting. Because many trauma victims are young, it is essential to incorporate dose-saving CT scan protocols. In obtunded patients, an MR imaging is performed 48 hours postinjury if a meaningful neurologic examination cannot be obtained, even if the CT scan was unremarkable. If CT angiography is not performed as part of the initial polytrauma scan, it should be considered if there is cervical spine injury, especially fractures involving the transverse foramen.

REFERENCES

1. Looby S, Flanders A. Spine trauma. Radiol Clin North Am 2011;49(1):129–63.

2. Daffner RH, Hackney DB. ACR appropriateness criteria on suspected spine trauma. J Am Coll Radiol 2007;4(11):762–75.

3. Hoffman JR, Mower WR, Wolfson AB, et al. Validity of a set of clinical criteria to rule out injury to the cervical spine in patients with blunt trauma. National Emergency X-Radiography utilization study group. N Engl J Med 2000;343(2):94–9.

4. Stiell IG, Wells GA, Vandemheen KL, et al. The Canadian C-spine rule for radiography in alert and stable trauma patients. JAMA 2001;286(15):1841–8.

5. Anderson LD, D'Alonzo RT. Fractures of the odontoid process of the axis. J Bone Joint Surg Am 1974;56(8):1663–74.

6. Michaleff ZA, Maher CG, Verhagen AP, et al. Accuracy of the Canadian C-spine rule and NEXUS to screen for clinically important cervical spine injury in patients following blunt trauma: a systematic review. Can Med Assoc J 2012;184(16):E867–76.

7. Stiell IG, Clement CM, McKnight RD, et al. The Canadian C-spine rule versus the NEXUS low-risk criteria in patients with trauma. N Engl J Med 2003;349(26):2510–8.

8. Collins NC, McKenzie JV. The NEXUS criteria: do they stand the test of time? Eur J Emerg Med 2013;20(1):58–60.

9. Brohi K, Healy M, Fotheringham T, et al. Helical computed tomographic scanning for the evaluation of the cervical spine in the unconscious, intubated trauma patient. J Trauma 2005;58(5):897–901.

10. Hagedorn JC 2nd, Emery SE, France JC, et al. Does CT angiography matter for patients with cervical spine injuries? J Bone Joint Surg Am 2014;96(11):951–5.

11. Liang T, Tso DK, Chiu RY, et al. Imaging of blunt vascular neck injuries: a clinical perspective. AJR Am J Roentgenol 2013;201(4):893–901.

12. Stassen NA, Williams VA, Gestring ML, et al. Magnetic resonance imaging in combination with helical computed tomography provides a safe and efficient method of cervical spine clearance in the obtunded trauma patient. J Trauma 2006;60(1):171–7.

13. Becce F, Ben Salah Y, Verdun FR, et al. Computed tomography of the cervical spine: comparison of image quality between a standard-dose and a low-dose protocol using filtered back-projection and iterative reconstruction. Skeletal Radiol 2013;42(7): 937–45.

14. Mulkens TH, Marchal P, Daineffe S, et al. Comparison of low-dose with standard-dose multidetector CT in cervical spine trauma. AJNR Am J Neuroradiol 2007;28(8):1444–50.

15. Schwartz ED, Flanders AE. Spinal trauma: imaging, diagnosis, and management. Philadelphia: Lippincott Williams & Wilkins; 2007. p. xv, 419.

16. White AA, Panjabi MM. Clinical biomechanics of the spine. 2nd edition. Philadelphia: Lippincott; 1990. p. xxiii, 722.

17. Daffner RH, Deeb ZL, Rothfus WE. "Fingerprints" of vertebral trauma—a unifying concept based on mechanisms. Skeletal Radiol 1986;15(7):518–25.

18. Leone A, Cerase A, Colosimo C, et al. Occipital condylar fractures: a review. Radiology 2000; 216(3):635–44.

19. Denis F. Spinal instability as defined by the three-column spine concept in acute spinal trauma. Clin Orthop Relat Res 1984;(189):65–76.

20. Dvorak MF, Fisher CG, Fehlings MG, et al. The surgical approach to subaxial cervical spine injuries: an evidence-based algorithm based on the SLIC classification system. Spine 2007;32(23):2620–9.

21. Chang W, Alexander MT, Mirvis SE. Diagnostic determinants of craniocervical distraction injury in adults. AJR Am J Roentgenol 2009;192(1):52–8.

22. Rojas CA, Bertozzi JC, Martinez CR, et al. Reassessment of the craniocervical junction: normal values on CT. AJNR Am J Neuroradiol 2007;28(9):1819–23.

23. Green JD, Harle TS, Harris JH Jr. Anterior subluxation of the cervical spine: hyperflexion sprain. AJNR Am J Neuroradiol 1981;2(3):243–50.

24. Smoker WR. Craniovertebral junction: normal anatomy, craniometry, and congenital anomalies. Radiographics 1994;14(2):255–77.

25. Hanson JA, Deliganis AV, Baxter AB, et al. Radiologic and clinical spectrum of occipital condyle fractures: retrospective review of 107 consecutive fractures in 95 patients. AJR Am J Roentgenol 2002;178(5):1261–8.

26. Noble ER, Smoker WR. The forgotten condyle: the appearance, morphology, and classification of occipital condyle fractures. AJNR Am J Neuroradiol 1996;17(3):507–13.

27. Levine AM, Edwards CC. Fractures of the atlas. J Bone Joint Surg Am 1991;73(5):680–91.

28. Lee C, Woodring JH. Unstable Jefferson variant atlas fractures: an unrecognized cervical injury. AJNR Am J Neuroradiol 1991;12(6):1105–10.

29. Muratsu H, Doita M, Yanagi T, et al. Cerebellar infarction resulting from vertebral artery occlusion associated with a Jefferson fracture. J Spinal Disord Tech 2005;18(3):293–6.

30. Govender S, Maharaj JF, Haffajee MR. Fractures of the odontoid process. J Bone Joint Surg Br 2000; 82(8):1143–7.

31. Levine AM, Edwards CC. The management of traumatic spondylolisthesis of the axis. J Bone Joint Surg Am 1985;67(2):217–26.

32. Kim KS, Chen HH, Russell EJ, et al. Flexion teardrop fracture of the cervical spine: radiographic characteristics. AJR Am J Roentgenol 1989;152(2):319–26.

33. Doran SE, Papadopoulos SM, Ducker TB, et al. Magnetic resonance imaging documentation of coexistent traumatic locked facets of the cervical spine and disc herniation. J Neurosurg 1993;79(3): 341–5.

34. Crawford NR, Duggal N, Chamberlain RH, et al. Unilateral cervical facet dislocation: injury mechanism and biomechanical consequences. Spine 2002; 27(17):1858–64 [discussion: 64].

35. Cancelmo JJ Jr. Clay shoveler's fracture. A helpful diagnostic sign. Am J Roentgenol Radium Ther Nucl Med 1972;115(3):540–3.

36. Regenbogen VS, Rogers LF, Atlas SW, et al. Cervical spinal cord injuries in patients with cervical spondylosis. AJR Am J Roentgenol 1986;146(2):277–84.

37. Scher AT. Hyperextension trauma in the elderly: an easily overlooked spinal injury. J Trauma 1983; 23(12):1066–8.

38. Daffner RH, Goldberg AL, Evans TC, et al. Cervical vertebral injuries in the elderly: a 10-year study. Emerg Radiol 1998;5(1):38–42.

39. Edeiken-Monroe B, Wagner LK, Harris JH Jr. Hyperextension dislocation of the cervical spine. AJR Am J Roentgenol 1986;146(4):803–8.

40. Daffner RH, Daffner SD. Vertebral injuries: detection and implications. Eur J Radiol 2002;42(2):100–16.

41. Lomoschitz FM, Blackmore CC, Mirza SK, et al. Cervical spine injuries in patients 65 years old and older: epidemiologic analysis regarding the effects of age and injury mechanism on distribution, type, and stability of injuries. AJR Am J Roentgenol 2002;178(3):573–7.

42. Sinclair D, Schwartz M, Gruss J, et al. A retrospective review of the relationship between facial fractures, head injuries, and cervical spine injuries. J Emerg Med 1988;6(2):109–12.

Penetrating Thoracic Injury

Anthony M. Durso, MD[a], Kim Caban, MD[a], Felipe Munera, MD[b],*

KEYWORDS

- Penetrating chest trauma • Gunshot wounds • Transmediastinal injuries • Diaphragmatic injuries
- Multidetector CT • Pneumothorax • Lung injuries

KEY POINTS

- Penetrating thoracic trauma encompasses a wide variety of injuries.
- The role of imaging in evaluating these patients will be determined by hemodynamic stability, mechanism of injury, and location of injury.
- Although most injuries will be to the lungs and pleura and may only be evaluated with serial radiographs, multi-detector computed tomography is being used with increasing frequency in hemodynamically stable patients.
- With an understanding of injury mechanics and trajectory, the radiologist can play a vital role in diagnosing the extent of injury and guiding further diagnostic examinations or interventions.

INTRODUCTION

Trauma is a significant cause of morbidity and mortality, resulting in 100,000 deaths per year in the United States.[1] It is the leading cause of death for persons less than 44 years old.[1] Cardiovascular injury is the second leading cause of traumatic death, behind only central nervous system traumatic injuries.[2] Although blunt trauma accounts for approximately 70% of trauma cases,[1,3] penetrating trauma should not be overlooked as a cause of significant morbidity and mortality.

Penetrating trauma encompasses various mechanisms from stab and puncture wounds to gunshot wounds (GSW). GSW are the second leading cause of injury death after motor vehicle crashes.[4] From 2007 to 2011, there were 158,187 reported deaths caused by firearms in the United States.[5] In 2011 alone, there were just more than 32,000 deaths (approximately the US annual average) and nearly 74,000 nonfatal injuries from firearms in the United States.[5] Statistics on morbidity and mortality for stab wounds and other non-GSW penetrating trauma are more difficult to elucidate in the available national databases; although nonfatal cut/pierce injuries, of which they would be a subset, are more frequent, mortality is much lower than GSW.

MECHANISM

Penetrating trauma can be divided into ballistic and nonballistic injuries. The mechanism of injury from nonballistic injuries (ie, stab and puncture wounds) is more intuitive than the mechanism for injury from ballistic trauma. Nonballistic penetrating injuries are caused by tissue disruption and laceration along their trajectory; determining that trajectory on imaging can help identify the injuries it has caused.

The authors have nothing to disclose.
[a] Department of Radiology, Jackson Memorial Hospital/Ryder Trauma Center, University of Miami Miller School of Medicine, 1611 Northwest, 12th Avenue, WW-279, Miami, FL 33136, USA; [b] Department of Radiology, Jackson Memorial Hospital/Ryder Trauma Center, Radiology Services, University of Miami Hospitals, University of Miami Miller School of Medicine, 1611 Northwest, 12th Avenue, WW-279, Miami, FL 33136, USA
* Corresponding author.
E-mail address: Fmunera@med.miami.edu

Radiol Clin N Am 53 (2015) 675–693
http://dx.doi.org/10.1016/j.rcl.2015.02.010
0033-8389/15/$ – see front matter © 2015 Elsevier Inc. All rights reserved.

Ballistic trauma is a more complex topic; but in the least, a basic understanding of ballistics will be helpful in evaluating imaging of such wounds.

Ballistics is the science of the motion of projectiles. Ballistics as it relates to firearms can be divided into

- Internal ballistics, the study of projectiles within a firearm
- External ballistics, the study of projectiles in the air, from firearm to target
- Terminal ballistics, the study of projectiles within its target[6–8]

Wound ballistics is a subset of terminal ballistics that deals with the behavior of projectiles within living tissue and an analysis of the injuries they cause.[7,8] Although all 3 subcategories of ballistics will affect the wound potential of a projectile,[6] ballistics is a complex topic that cannot be covered in its entirety here. Wound ballistics is briefly discussed.

Although frequently divided into low-velocity and high-velocity projectiles (Box 1), a better classification for wound ballistics would be low-energy transfer and high-energy transfer injuries,[8] which emphasizes that the degree of injury will depend on how effectively the projectile transfers its kinetic energy into the target soft tissues.

This transfer of energy will be influenced by various factors:

- Velocity of the projectile
- Inherent characteristic of the projectile (bullet shape and design)
- Elasticity of the tissues it is penetrating (Lung, hollow viscus, and skeletal muscle are relatively more elastic than solid viscera like the liver and brain.)

Box 1
Projectile classification

Low velocity

- Typically handguns
- Muzzle velocity 250 m/s to 370 m/s

High velocity

- Typically rifles
- Muzzle velocity greater than 700 m/s

This loose classification of projectiles generally serves only as a differentiation of wounds caused by handguns or rifles.[8] An important consideration is that tissue damage is mainly related to the amount of energy dissipated in the target, which largely depends on projectile caliber and design.[13]

The exact mechanisms of energy transfer and the relative importance of each in wound potential remain controversial.[7–9] Mechanisms, as depicted in **Fig. 1**, include

- Direct tissue laceration and contusion will occur along the trajectory, referred to as the permanent cavity.
- An initial ballistic pressure wave, often referred to as a shockwave, will precede the bullet, although its capacity and contribution to injury is debated.[7–9]
- A second phase caused by pressure gradients results in tissue separation in a radial direction, forming a temporary cavity to develop along the trajectory.[7–9]

Of note, depending on bullet design and energy, the temporary cavity can be many times larger than the caliber of the projectile. Temporary cavitation becomes more significant at higher velocities. In one study, using computed tomography (CT) to measure the size of a temporary cavity formed in a ballistic soap block, a 0.357 Magnum hollow-point bullet caused a temporary cavity with a diameter up to 6.35 cm[10]; so a 9-mm diameter bullet can cause a temporary cavity approximately 7 times larger. The temporary cavity is caused by the shockwave as the projectile travels through tissue with resultant contusion around the bullet path. Therefore, the use of the term *temporary* as a descriptor of the concussion zone may be misleading.[11,12]

Wounding potential will also depend on the elasticity of the targeted soft tissues and how they can respond to these expansile forces. Lung is more elastic than solid organs like the liver, and can better absorb the cavitary forces. Vascular damage from temporary cavitation can be extensive, usually affecting capillary and small vessels with relative sparing of large vessels due to their elasticity, however endothelial injury and thrombosis still can occur in larger vessels (**Figs. 2 and 3**).[8]

IMAGING

Penetrating thoracic trauma encompasses a heterogeneous group of injuries with differing presentations. Most penetrating injuries involve only the chest wall and lung parenchyma[14,15] and may initially be imaged with chest radiography (CXR). Entry and exit wounds should be demarcated by radiopaque markers (a paper clip can be used) to help approximate the injury trajectory and its proximity to the mediastinum. Penetrating nonmediastinal thoracic trauma is historically treated

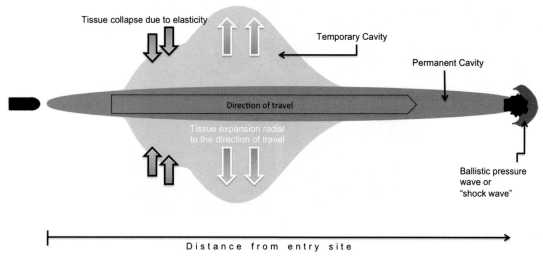

Fig. 1. Wound ballistics. A shock wave precedes the bullet; direct tissue laceration along the bullet path causes the permanent cavity; pressure gradients cause tissue separation radial to the bullet path with subsequent tissue recoil, the temporary cavity. The temporary cavity size and its distance from the entry site will depend on bullet design and velocity.

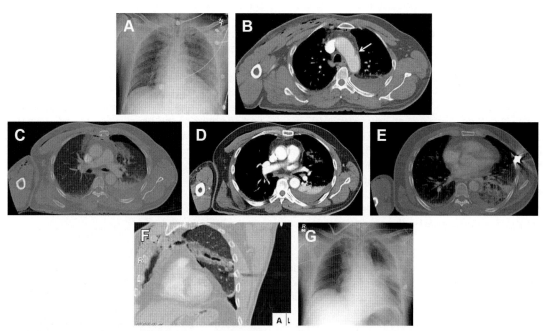

Fig. 2. Admission chest radiography (CXR) (*A*) of a 50-year-old man with a GSW to the right shoulder demonstrates a large bullet fragment in the left chest wall indicating a transmediastinal trajectory. Axial images from chest CT angiography (*B–E*, superior to inferior) with subcutaneous air in the right chest wall (*B–D*), pneumomediastinum (*B, C*), sternal fracture (*C*), left pneumothorax (*C*), left hemothorax (*B–D*), pulmonary contusion in the lingula of the left upper lobe (*C*), and main bullet mass in the left chest wall (*E*) indicating a transmediastinal GSW. Notice the intimal flap in the aortic arch (*white arrow* in *B*); the trajectory was anterior to the aortic arch and the injury likely was a result of cavitation. Oblique multiplanar reformatted image (*F*) was created by the radiologist to better demonstrate the trajectory. CXR after intervention (*G*) shows the aortic stent graft used to treat the aortic injury.

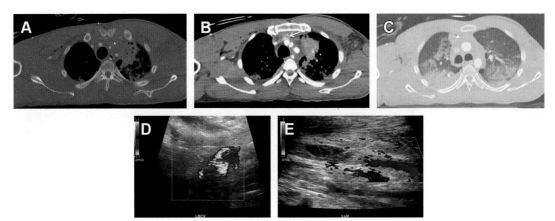

Fig. 3. A 31-year-old man who presented with transmediastinal injury through the superior mediastinum. Axial images from chest CT angiography (*A–C*, superior to inferior) demonstrate subcutaneous air in the right chest wall (*A–C*), bullet fragments in the anterior mediastinum (*A, C*), left upper lobe pulmonary contusion and laceration (*A, B*), and left pneumothorax (*C*). Notice the filling defect in the left brachiocephalic vein (*white arrow* in *B*) suspicious for brachiocephalic vein thrombus and injury. Color Doppler evaluation of the left brachiocephalic vein (*D*) confirmed intraluminal thrombus (*yellow arrow*) with extension into the left internal jugular vein (*E*).

conservatively with chest tube placement.[9,16–18] If these patients have a normal initial CXR, a short-term follow-up examination in 3 to 6 hours should be obtained to rule out development of a delayed pneumothorax,[14,15] though a recent series suggests that interval may be further decreased to 1 hour.[19]

Imaging evaluation of patients with suspected mediastinal or cardiac injury depends on the patient presentation. Most of these patients will be unstable and require emergent surgical intervention without any imaging at admission with the possible exception of an initial CXR or pericardial ultrasound (US) if time permits. Transmediastinal injury can be inferred from exit and entry wounds on opposite sides of the thorax, an entry site and main ballistic mass on opposite sides of the thorax, or a main ballistic mass projecting over the mediastinum. Any injury in the cardiac box should also raise concern for potential cardiac injury (**Fig. 4**).

The hemodynamically stable patient with mediastinal injury represents a small, select subset of penetrating thoracic trauma, that historically were evaluated by any combination of conventional angiography, bronchoscopy, esophagoscopy, esophagram, transthoracic or transesophageal echocardiography, pericardial window, or pericardiocentesis.[17,20–24] Currently, focused assessment by sonography in trauma (FAST) is used in the initial assessment of penetrating mediastinal injury to evaluate for pericardial fluid, an indication of pericardial or cardiac injury.[2,22–24] With the widespread availability of,

and improvements in CT, it has emerged as a more cost-effective technique for evaluating these patients.[2,17,20,23–26] In evaluating a series of 207 patients with penetrating mediastinal injury that presented over a 6-year period to a level 1 trauma center, Burack and colleagues[17] concluded that the combination of transesophageal echocardiography and contrasted-enhanced CT was an effective screening tool; patients with negative results can be safely observed, and patients with positive results are referred for further evaluation. This finding supports the conclusions of earlier smaller series that evaluated the use of CT in

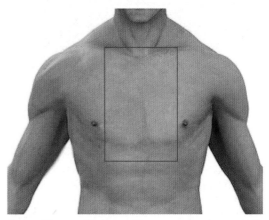

Fig. 4. The cardiac box. The rectangle denotes the boundaries of the cardiac box. Penetrating injuries within the rectangle should raise concern for potential injury to the heart. (*Courtesy of* Chris Granville, MD, Miami, FL)

hemodynamically stable patients with penetrating mediastinal injury.[24,25]

When evaluating penetrating thoracic injuries by chest CT angiography (CTA), depending on estimated bullet trajectory, a contiguous body part should also be included in the scan. For injuries in the supraclavicular region, CTA of the neck and chest can be obtained (**Fig. 5**); for injuries in the thoracoabdominal region, CTA of the chest and abdomen should be obtained for potential transdiaphragmatic injuries (**Fig. 6**). **Box 2** contains the multi-detector CT (MDCT) protocol used at the authors' institution for CTA of the chest in trauma patients.

CT has high sensitivity for pneumothorax, hemothorax, pneumopericardium, pericardial effusions, pericardial and myocardial injuries, and cardiac luxation and can be used to visualize ballistic or stab wound trajectory and retained foreign bodies.[27] MDCT demonstrates wound tract defects in the pericardium and myocardium.[15]

CT is useful in detecting the ballistic trajectory, the path of which can determine the need for additional evaluation (**Fig. 7**).[24,25,28] The bullet trajectory, or wound tract, is usually readily visible by MDCT; any combination of air, bullet, and bone fragments and hemorrhage can outline the wound tract (**Fig. 8**). These entities are usually more apparent with GSW, which are higher-energy injuries with ballistic fragments along the trajectory, as opposed to stab wounds whose full extent might not be readily apparent. To aid in determining the wound tract, radiopaque markers should be placed at entry and exit sites (again paper clips can be used). Pitfalls in determining wound tracts occur in cases of multiple penetrating injuries and when projectiles rebound off of bony structures causing a nonlinear trajectory. Mismatches in positioning resulting from differences in respiration and arm positioning between the time of trauma and the time of imaging can also potentially introduce sources of error but, in the authors' experience, usually do not prevent an accurate diagnosis.[1]

PENETRATING MEDIASTINAL INJURY

Most patients with thoracic trauma can be treated conservatively; the exception is the subset of patients with penetrating trauma to the mediastinum.[17] Transmediastinal penetrating injury is defined as penetrating injury that traverses any part of the mediastinum and by its nature can involve any of the sensitive structures it contains,

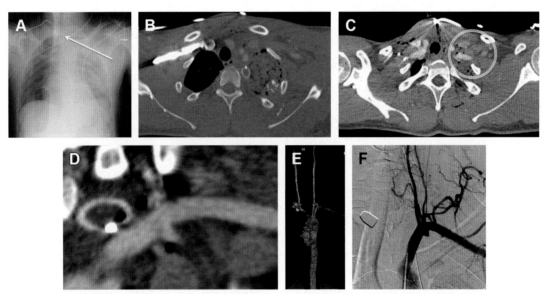

Fig. 5. A 21-year-old man status post GSW in the left chest wall. Portable CXR at presentation (*A*) paper clip demarcating entry site and bullet fragment to the right of the supraclavicular trachea indicating a transmediastinal trajectory (*white arrow* in *A*). Subsequent neck and chest CTA (*B*) in bone window demonstrates rib fracture fragments within the contused left upper lobe along the bullet trajectory. Axial image more superiorly (*C*) with the bullet anteriorly in the soft tissues of the lower neck and air along the trajectory; the trajectory is in close proximity to the left subclavian artery, which has an irregular contour and surrounding air bubbles (*white circle* in *C*). Curved multiplanar reformatted (*D*) and 3-dimensional volume-rendered (*E*) images generated from the CTA more clearly depict a small pseudoaneurysm of the left subclavian artery, a finding confirmed at conventional angiography (*F*).

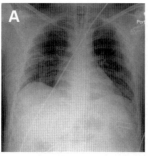 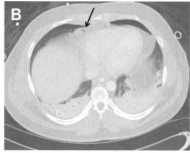 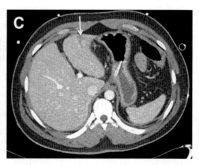

Fig. 6. A 27-year-old man presenting with multiple stab wounds to the lower thorax and upper abdomen as demarcated by paper clips on initial CXR (*A*); bilateral chest tubes had already been placed and the patient was intubated. Axial image from subsequent chest and abdomen CTA (*B*) in lung window demonstrates small bilateral pneumothoraces and bibasilar atelectasis. Notice the small amount of pneumomediastinum in close proximity to the right heart (*black arrow* in *B*). Axial image (*C*) in soft tissue window reveals a liver laceration in the left lobe (*white arrow* in *C*). Injuries above and below the diaphragm were suspicious for diaphragmatic injury. The patient was taken to the operating room and underwent repair of a right ventricular injury, right diaphragmatic injury, and liver laceration.

such as the heart, great vessels, trachea and bronchi, and the esophagus.

These patients have high operative and mortality rates.[2,14,17,20–23,27] They can be subdivided into hemodynamically unstable and stable patients at presentation. The unstable patients require emergent surgical intervention. Even though modern trauma systems have decreased prehospital times, and more patients arrive to the trauma center alive but in extremis, mortality remains high in hemodynamically unstable patients.[20]

Box 2
Protocol for MDCT (64 detector) chest CTA

Contrast: 100 mL iohexol, 350 mg Iodine/mL

Contrast bolus: 4 mL/sec × 20 sec, then 3.5 mL/sec × 20 sec, then normal saline 3.5 mL/sec × 14 sec

Scout: lower neck through abdomen

Scan mode: spiral

Kilovolts peak: 120

Effective milliampere seconds: 200

Dose modulation: on

Rotation time: 0.5 s

Pitch: 0.7

Arterial phase acquisition: 0.6-mm slice collimation, scan from lung apices to adrenals, reconstructed at 3-mm thickness in the axial, sagittal, and coronal planes; reconstructions at 1.5-mm slice thickness with 0.7-mm intervals in the axial plane

Postprocessing: maximum intensity projections and volume rendered images reconstructed from arterial phase acquisition

---

Hemodynamically stable patients are a select subset of these patients. As discussed previously, historically these patients underwent many expensive and invasive examinations; but the evaluation of these patients has shifted to contrast-enhanced CTA. The growing data suggest that a combination of echocardiography and MDCT can be used to effectively screen these patients and preclude the need for the more invasive work-up (**Fig. 9**).[6,17] CTA allows for better visualization of the ballistic path and determination of occult injury that can then be investigated by additional tests if indicated; if mediastinal injury can be excluded on CT, patients may be spared unnecessary and invasive procedures and tests (**Fig. 10**).[20] CT can also be useful in postoperative care of any survivors to evaluate for other occult injuries.[20]

Cardiac Injuries

Any penetrating wound to the chest or upper abdomen should raise the possibility of cardiac injury.[22] Most penetrating cardiac trauma is the result of stab wounds or GSW; the relative frequency largely depends on access to firearms.[22] Penetrating cardiac injury is associated with a prehospital mortality rate as high as 94%[2,22] and an in-hospital mortality rate of 50% among initial survivors.[2] The mechanism of injury also has prognostic value with a higher mortality rate for GSW than stab wounds.[2,22,23] Physiologic status on arrival is the other major predictor of outcome.[22]

Penetrating cardiac trauma accounts for only 0.1% of all trauma admissions.[22] Death results from cardiac tamponade or hemorrhage.[22]

Immediate surgical intervention is the only meaningful treatment of unstable patients with penetrating cardiac injury.[22] FAST is widely used

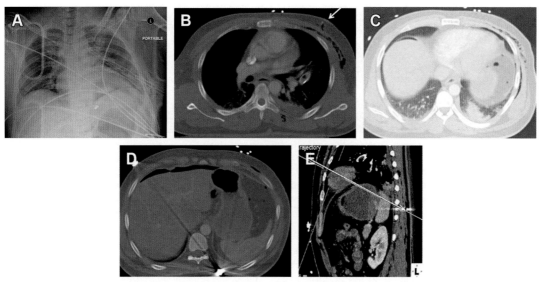

Fig. 7. Admission CXR (*A*) from a 27-year-old man status post GSW to the left chest wall with a paper clip denoting the entry site and the bullet projecting over the gastroesophageal junction. Axial images from the subsequent CTA (*B–D*) demonstrate the entry site in the anterior left chest wall (*arrow* in *B*), left pneumothorax and left lower lobe pulmonary contusion (*C*), pneumoperitoneum (*D*), and the bullet fragment in the posterior left chest wall (*D*). The trajectory above and below the diaphragm indicates diaphragmatic injury directing further management. Sagittal multiplanar reformatted image (*E*) created by the radiologist to better demonstrate the trajectory emphasizes the transdiaphragmatic bullet path and its proximity to the heart and stomach.

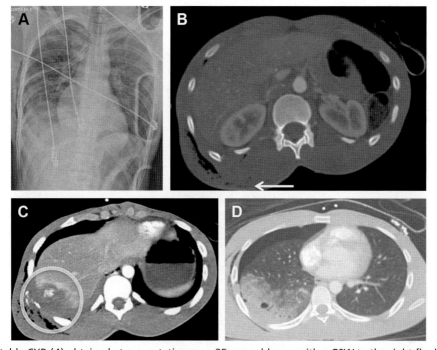

Fig. 8. Portable CXR (*A*) obtained at presentation on a 25-year-old man with a GSW to the right flank with subcutaneous emphysema along the right chest and abdominal wall. Axial images (*B–D*) from the subsequent chest and abdomen CTA at the level of the kidneys depict the entry site (*white arrow* in *B*). The bullet traveled superiorly and obliquely through the liver causing liver laceration with active extravasation (*white circle* in *C*), crossed the diaphragm, and caused a right lower lobe pulmonary laceration and right pneumothorax (*D*), before exiting the right chest wall.

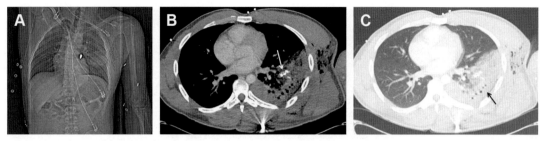

Fig. 9. Scout image (*A*) from a 23-year-old man who underwent chest CTA on presentation for a left chest GSW with left chest wall subcutaneous emphysema and a bullet fragment projecting over the left heart border. Axial image in soft tissue window (*B*) shows the bullet trajectory extending obliquely and posteriorly through the left hemithorax with the bullet path and fragment remote from the heart. Hyperdense foci in the left lower lobe pulmonary contusion (*white arrow* in *B*) represent active extravasation. Hemothorax is also seen. Axial image in lung window (*C*) better depict the concomitant left lower lobe pulmonary laceration (*black arrow* in *C*).

to evaluate for traumatic hemopericardium and has supplanted diagnostic pericardial window.[22,23] There is variability with the accuracy of FAST,[23] likely because of a combination of confounding factors from adjacent injury and operator experience.

The current evidence now supports the use of imaging in the smaller subset of hemodynamically stable patients with potential cardiac injury. CXR can be useful in initial triage to identify bullet fragments and potential ballistic trajectory. Emergent echocardiography can be performed to evaluate for hemopericardium; traumatic pericardial

effusions are an indicator of cardiac injury and can lead to emergent surgery.[2] CT has high sensitivity and specificity in detecting hemopericardium and pneumopericardium in the setting of penetrating injury.[2,23] CT will also better delineate the bullet trajectory than radiography.[24,25] A high negative predictive value (NPV) has been reported using a combination of CT and echocardiography in evaluating hemodynamically stable patients with suspected injury.[21] Plurad and colleagues[23] reported hemopericardium and/or pneumopericardium detected on CT had a sensitivity of 76.9%, specificity of 99.7%, positive predictive

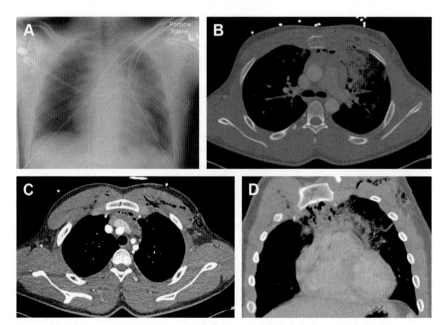

Fig. 10. A 16-year-old man status post GSW to the left chest wall. Admission CXR (*A*) with a paper clip demarcating the entry site and the bullet fragment projecting at the right shoulder. Axial images (*B, C*) from chest CTA demonstrate the transmediastinal trajectory with left lung contusion and laceration, pneumomediastinum, and anterior mediastinal hematoma. Vascular injury was not seen. Coronal multiplanar reformatted (*D*) from the CTA better depicts the trajectory and the absence of the hemopericardium.

> **Box 3**
> **Spectrum of cardiac injury**
>
> Myocardial contusion
>
> Myocardial rupture
>
> Pericardial injury[27]
>
> Can result in cardiac tamponade or cardiac herniation ± luxation, if pericardial defect is large enough
>
> Coronary arterial injury
>
> Less common injuries[22]
>
> Cardiac dysfunction from coronary arterial or valvular injury
>
> Septal defects
>
> Other complications[22]
>
> Ballistic fragment embolization
>
> Ventricular aneurysm
>
> Coronary arterial-cardiac chamber fistula
>
> Infection

value of 90.9%, and NPV of 99.1% for cardiac injuries.[23] **Box 3** lists the spectrum of cardiac injuries.

Indirect CT signs of cardiac injury include hemopericardium, pneumopericardium, mediastinal hemorrhage, retained foreign bodies or injury tract in close proximity to the heart (**Figs. 11** and **12**), mediastinal hematoma (**Fig. 13**), and traumatic injuries to the adjacent lung and pleura.

Multiple series report that the most commonly injured cardiac chamber was the right ventricle, followed by the left ventricle, right atrium, and left atrium.[22,27] Because of its anterior location, entry wounds are more common in the right ventricle, whereas mortality is increased with left ventricular injuries.[2] Left atrial and ventricular injuries have mortality rates as high as 80% compared with a 63% mortality rate for right atrial injury and a 49% mortality rate for right ventricular injury.[21] Patients presenting to the hospital with stab wounds more commonly have isolated right ventricular involvement (35%) than left ventricular involvement (25%) but have more than one chamber injured 30% of the time.[21] Ballistic injuries commonly have through-and-through injuries with concomitant hemorrhage, cardiac tamponade, and shock.[21]

The most important factor in determining survival is the nature of the penetrating injury (stab wound vs low-velocity GSW vs high-velocity GSW).[21] Mortality rates for ballistic injury are as high as 84% opposed to 35% for stab wounds.[21,23] Conflicting information exists regarding the prognostic significance of single chamber versus multiple chamber wounds, left ventricular versus right ventricular wounds, presence versus absence of tamponade, and isolated cardiac injury versus multi-organ injury.[22]

Vascular Injuries

In addition to cardiac injury, the great vessels and their branches, such as the internal mammary arteries, can be injured in penetrating mediastinal injury. The incidence of injury to the intrathoracic great vessels is low, but survival rates are poor.[14] CXR is not sensitive or specific in detecting

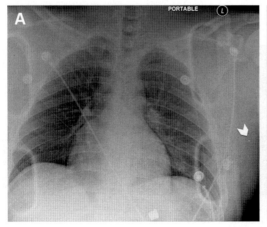 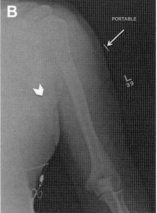

Fig. 11. A 20-year-old man status post single GSW to the left shoulder. Admission CXR (*A*) and left humeral radiograph (*B*) with a paper clip demarcating the entry site in the left shoulder (*white arrow* in *B*), ballistic fragments in the left lateral chest wall (*white arrowheads* in *A, B*), and the main bullet mass projecting over the cardiac apex and left upper quadrant.

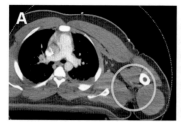
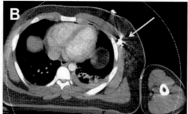
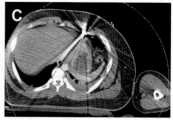

Fig. 12. Axial images (*A–C*, superior to inferior) from the chest CTA obtained at presentation from the same patient in **Fig. 11**. The bullet trajectory is demarcated by air in the left axilla (*white circle* in *A*), ballistic fragments in the left anterolateral chest wall (*white arrow* in *B*), and the main bullet mass resting along the left anterior cardiophrenic recess. Hemothorax and pulmonary laceration are also present at the left lung base. Injury to the heart was not demonstrated on CT, but the proximity of the main bullet mass and trajectory should prompt further diagnostic evaluation.

vascular injury; when the patients' condition allows for it, CTA is replacing conventional angiography for diagnosis. Direct signs of traumatic arterial injury are similar to other types of trauma (see **Fig. 2**). Indirect signs of vascular injury can be more subtle and include changes in the soft tissues around the vessel (**Box 4**). Of note, in the setting of ballistic penetrating injuries, streak artifact from adjacent bullet fragments can limit evaluation for direct signs of injury. In such cases, further evaluation may be indicated. Also the use of multiplanar reformatted (MPR) images and 3-dimensional (3D) images can help problem solve in such instances (see **Fig. 6**). MPRs are generally helpful in evaluating the vasculature, as not all vessels will be presented to full advantage on axial images.

Aerodigestive Injury

Penetrating trauma to the trachea and esophagus is rare,[9,14] but variable incidence rates have historically been reported ranging from 0% to 33%.[17]

However, Burack and colleagues[17] reported only a 1.4% incidence rate of aerodigestive tract injury in a series of 207 transmediastinal injuries. These injuries are more commonly seen in GSW than nonballistic penetrating injuries.[29]

The cervical trachea and right bronchus are most commonly injured (**Fig. 14**).[15] These injuries can be lethal if not detected expeditiously. Given their location in the mediastinum, isolated injuries of either structure are rare.[25]

Tears involving the mainstem bronchi or intrathoracic trachea place patients at an increased risk of death. Patients usually present with hemoptysis, neck or chest emphysema, pneumomediastinum, persistent large pneumothorax, or large air leak despite chest tube placement. CT is more sensitive in detecting pneumomediastinum (**Fig. 15**). With MDCT, one may identify the site of tracheal wall discontinuity, focal tracheal deformity, and tracheal ring fracture (see **Fig. 14**). An overdistended endotracheal balloon (>2.8 cm), a balloon that extends beyond the normal confines of the trachea, and a dumbbell or Mickey Mouse

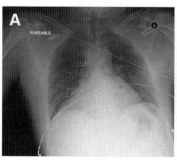
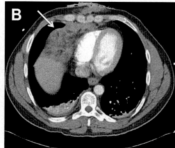
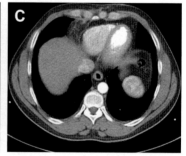

Fig. 13. A 36-year-old man presented with a puncture wound to the right parasternal chest from a large grilling utensil. Portable CXR (*A*) on presentation demonstrates an abnormal contour to the right lower mediastinal border and an obscured right heart border. The patient subsequently had a chest CTA (*B*) demonstrating a large mediastinal hematoma (*white arrow* in *B*) without active extravasation. Hemopericardium was not present on the initial CTA or subsequent echocardiogram. Chest CT 7 weeks later (*C*) shows marked resolution of the mediastinal hematoma.

Box 4	
Signs of vascular injury	
Direct Signs	**Indirect Signs**
• Abrupt caliber change can be a sign of dissection	• Indistinct perivascular fat planes
• Vessel occlusion	• Perivascular hematoma
• Contrast extravasation	• Proximity to ballistic fragment
• Intraluminal filling defects	• End organ infarcts (distal emboli from intraluminal thrombus)
○ Mural thrombi	
○ Intimal flaps	
• Abrupt change in vessel contour	
• Pseudoaneurysm	
• Arteriovenous fistulas	

ears–shaped trachea should arise suspicion for the presence of a tracheal injury.[30] Bronchoscopy is the gold standard in diagnosing a tracheobronchial injury. These injuries can lead to the development of tracheoesophageal fistulas, tracheal stenosis, mediastinitis, and empyemas.[31]

Esophageal injury mortality rates have remained fairly constant for the last 2 decades. Extraluminal mediastinal air adjacent to these structures is an indirect sign of injury, but air can be introduced into the mediastinum from penetrating trauma or as the result of a pneumothorax and can be a potential pitfall. A close proximity to the injury tract may be the most useful sign of aerodigestive trauma on CT (**Fig. 16**).[14]

MDCT is better than conventional radiography in diagnosing airway injuries, with a reported overall sensitivity of 85% for tracheal injuries, whereas its use in esophageal injuries has not yet been established.[15] Although a direct injury to the airways or esophagus may be difficult to detect on CT, if there is suspicion of injury based in injury trajectory or presence of air adjacent to these structures, that should prompt further investigation such as by endoscopy. In the case of esophageal injury, esophagram is another alternative.

PULMONARY INJURY
Pulmonary Contusion

Pulmonary contusions are frequently encountered after penetrating chest injuries. Histologically contusions are a result of disruption of the alveolar-capillary membrane and small blood vessels leading to the subsequent filling of the alveoli and interstitium with hemorrhage or fluid.[32] Contusions appear as fluffy air-space, nonsegmental opacities that do not respect the pleural boundaries. Typically they occur close to the chest wall in the periphery of the lung demonstrating a 2- to 3-mm area of subpleural sparing. Air bronchograms are often present. Most develop within

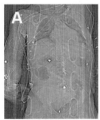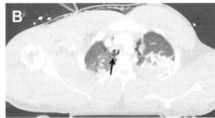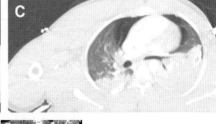

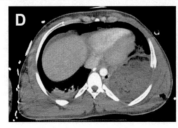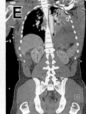

Fig. 14. A 30-year-old man status posts multiple GSW to the chest and abdomen who underwent CTA. Scout image (*A*) with multiple bullet fragments; determining trajectories is made more difficult with multiple GSW. Axial images in lung windows (*B, C*) with bilateral hemopneumothoraces, pneumomediastinum, and a small tracheal defect (*black arrow* in *B*). Axial image in soft tissue window (*D*), more inferior to (*B*) and (*C*), shows the stomach in the lower left hemithorax. Gastric herniation through a diaphragmatic defect is more easily seen on coronal MPR image (*E*).

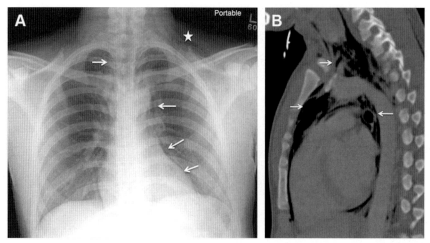

Fig. 15. Supine portable CXR (*A*) of a patient after sustaining a stab wound to the neck demonstrating pneumo-mediastinum (*white arrows*) and left neck supraclavicular subcutaneous emphysema (*white star*). Sagittal refor-matted CT image (*B*) of the chest demonstrating pneumomediastinum (*white arrows*).

several hours of injury and tend to resolve within a few days (48–72 hours). Some contusions may persist for more than a week. Volume resuscitation may cause contusions to increase in size. It may be difficult to visualize contusions on CXR. They are, however, readily apparent on CT within minutes after the injury (**Fig. 17**). A contused lung can result in respiratory compromise and serve as a nidus for development of infection.[33] Presumed contusions that persist should be further assessed for superimposed processes, such as acute respiratory distress syndrome (ARDS) and pneumonia.

Pulmonary Laceration

Lacerations are also a common occurrence with penetrating chest trauma and are usually located along the wound trajectory. They are characterized as a disruption of the alveolar spaces typically leading to formation of a round or oval-shaped cavity filled with blood and/or air. The inherent natural recoil of the lung tissue accounts for their shape. Initially pulmonary lacerations may be obscured on CXR by surrounding lung contusions but become more apparent as the contusions begin to clear. Pulmonary lacerations typically resolve in 3 to 5 weeks. However, in patients with ARDS or on positive pressure ventilation, they make take months to resolve.[33] Positive airway pressure ventilation can result in their expansion and subsequent mass effect on the surrounding lung leading to respiratory compromise. Lacerations also serve as a nidus for infection and abscess formation.

On CT, lacerations are seen as linear, round, or oval spaces filled with air and/or blood frequently surrounded by contusions (see **Fig. 9***C*; **Fig. 18**).

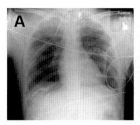
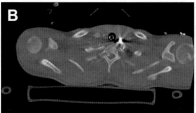
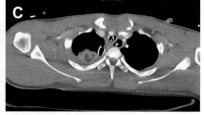

Fig. 16. A 17-year-old male patient who suffered multiple gunshot wounds to the chest and abdomen and was emergently operated on for abdominal injuries. Postoperative CXR (*A*) demonstrates a bullet fragment projecting just to the left of the endotracheal tube and nasogastric tube, a finding raising the possibility of tracheal and/or esophageal injury. Subsequent chest CTA in bone window (*B*) demonstrates fracture of the right second rib and T2 vertebral body with the bullet fragment directly adjacent to the esophagus; axial image in soft tissue window (*C*) slightly more inferiorly demonstrates injury to the right lung apex. The constellation of findings indicate a transmediastinal injury from left to right; though artifact from the bullet limits evaluation of the esophagus at this level, injury should be suspected and direct further diagnostic examinations.

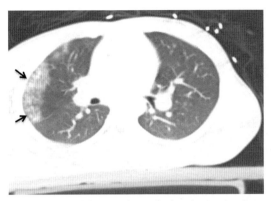

Fig. 17. Axial CT image through the chest using lung windows demonstrates the typical appearance of lung contusions. Fluffy air-space opacities with subpleural sparing (*black arrows*) are demonstrated in the right upper lobe.

If they are solely filled with air, they are referred to as *pneumatoceles*. When they are completely filled with fluid or hemorrhage (also known as *pulmonary hematoma*), they will appear nodular or masslike. The varying appearances of lacerations lend them to be mistaken for pneumonia, abscess, nodule, mass, or loculated pneumothorax. Lacerations involving the visceral pleura may lead to the development of a pneumothorax. If they involve both the visceral pleura and the airway, a bronchopleural fistula forms resulting in a persistent air leak.

Lung Herniation

A portion of the lung may herniate through a chest wall defect at sites of penetrating injuries, displaced rib fractures, or chest tube insertions. Lung herniations commonly occur within the anterior thorax because of a lack of muscular support.[34] On CXR, the herniated lung appears as a well-delineated locule of subcutaneous gas. They are seen to better advantage on CT and usually do not resolve on their own. Narrow necked hernias may result in incarceration and strangulation of the lung resulting in respiratory compromise and possibly necrosis. The risk of incarceration is greater in mechanically ventilated patients.

PLEURAL INJURY
Pneumothorax

Another common sequela of penetrating trauma is the formation of a pneumothorax. Pneumothoraces can form directly from the penetrating trauma itself or from a leak in the airway. On both CXR and CT, a pneumothorax appears as an air-filled pleural space, devoid of lung markings, surrounding the thin visceral pleura of the lung (**Fig. 19**). On an erect or semierect CXR, a pneumothorax will most commonly be seen along the apicolateral aspect of the hemithorax.[35] They can be overlooked on the initial supine or semierect portable CXR, as air tends to collect in the anterior and inferior pleural space. In one study,[36] supine CXR missed almost 40% of pneumothoraces that were subsequently diagnosed via CT. Small pneumothoraces may not demonstrate the classic features on standard radiography. An expiratory, decubitus, or lateral CXR may accentuate a pneumothorax. Visualization of subcutaneous

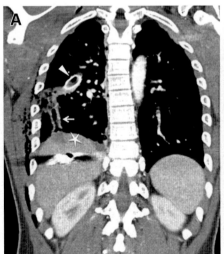
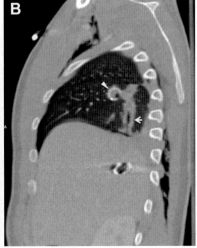

Fig. 18. Coronal (*A*) and sagittal (*B*) reformatted CTA images through the thorax after a GSW to the chest and placement of a chest tube (*white arrowhead*). The bullet trajectory is demonstrated by the lung laceration (*white arrows*) with resultant penetration of the right hemidiaphragm and subsequent laceration of the liver (*white star*). Bullet shrapnel retained within the liver parenchyma can also be seen. Artifact by the bullet limits evaluation of the surrounding hepatic parenchyma.

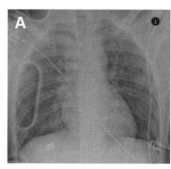
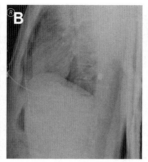
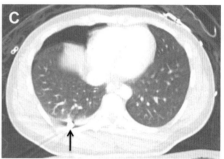

Fig. 19. A 32-year-old man status post GSW to the right chest wall. Posteroanterior and lateral views of the chest (*A, B*) demonstrate a bullet fragment residing in the posterior right hemithorax. Axial image in lung window from CTA (*C*) performed at presentation with a right pneumothorax, right middle lobe contusion, and the bullet fragment residing in a small right hemothorax (*black arrow* in *C*).

emphysema should prompt a closer investigation for a pneumothorax, although subcutaneous air may be introduced by the penetrating trauma itself. If the initial CXR is negative, a repeat should be done in 3 to 6 hours to exclude the formation of a delayed pneumothorax.[14] A few signs exist that may help one recognize the presence of a pneumothorax (**Box 5**). A persistent pneumothorax is usually the result of a malpositioned or kinked chest tube or airway leak from a direct injury or fistula. When a pneumothorax resolves, the ipsilateral lung may immediately develop reexpansion pulmonary edema (**Fig. 20**). The development of reexpansion pulmonary edema is associated with the size of the pneumothorax and how quickly it resolved.

The diagnosis of a pneumothorax regardless of size is critical to the management of patients on positive pressure ventilation or those undergoing general anesthesia as they are at increased risk of developing a tension pneumothorax. In these patients chest tube thoracotomy

is performed despite the size of a pneumothorax.[33] A tension pneumothorax occurs when the air trapped in the pleural space is under pressure resulting in mass effect on the mediastinal structures and contralateral lung (**Fig. 21**). A tension pneumothorax can easily be recognized on CXR (**Box 6**).

US can also be used to diagnose a pneumothorax and was shown to be more sensitive (98%) than a supine CXR (76%).[37] With US, in the absence of a pneumothorax, one should be able to visualize the visceral and parietal pleura of the lung slide against each other. If there is an absent sliding lung sign, one should suspect a pneumothorax. Subcutaneous emphysema, lung emphysema, lung contusions, and pleural adhesions may lead to a false positive diagnosis of a pneumothorax on US.

Box 5
Classic features of a pneumothorax on CXR

- Visualization of the thin visceral pleura of the lung with surrounding lucency devoid of lung markings
- Deep costophrenic sulcus sign-air collects in the deep lateral costophrenic sulcus
- Visualization of the anterior costophrenic sulcus
- Upper quadrant lucency
- Double diaphragm sign-air outlines the dome and anteroinferior insertion of the diaphragm
- Sharp cardiac silhouette

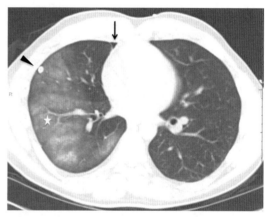

Fig. 20. Axial CT image through the chest obtained after placement of a chest tube (*black arrowhead*) for tension pneumothorax. A small residual anterior right-sided pneumothorax (*black arrow*) can be seen along with reexpansion pulmonary edema (*white star*).

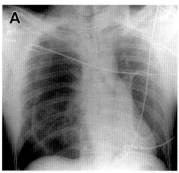
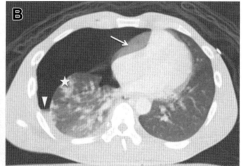

Fig. 21. Teenage boy sustained a stab wound to the right hemithorax. Anteroposterior CXR (*A*) demonstrates a large tension pneumothorax. Leftward mediastinal shift is seen. Axial CTA image (*B*) through the chest demonstrates a hydropneumothorax (*white arrowhead*) under tension (*white arrow*) and lung contusions (*white star*).

Pleural Collections

Fluid of varying types will frequently accumulate in the pleural space in the setting of penetrating thoracic injury. They can be detected by CXR, CT, and US.

A supine CXR may underestimate the degree of pleural fluid. A lateral decubitus CXR can detect as little as 5 mL of pleural fluid.[38] Various signs can be detected on CXR to indicate the presence of pleural fluid (**Box 7**).

CT is highly sensitive in detecting the presence of a pleural collection and its type. US is also sensitive in detecting pleural fluid and can be done at the bedside in unstable patients. Commonly the presence of a pneumothorax coexists with a pleural collection especially in the setting of trauma producing an air fluid level, aka hydropneumothorax. Hemothorax is a collection of blood within the pleural space and is considered massive when more that 1500 mL of blood accumulates.[31] Hemothorax may result from lung, rib, pleural, diaphragmatic, mediastinal, or vascular injuries. Hematocrit levels may be seen in these collections as clotted blood layers. Arterial sources of hemothorax often are large and rapidly accumulate, resulting in mass effect and displacement of the mediastinum and lung. Active extravasation on

CTA would also indicate an arterial source of hemothorax. Venous sources are usually self-limited. Serous pleural effusions can be seen in patients with splenic, pancreatic, or hepatic injuries.[39] There are other sources of pleural collections, and evaluating their attenuation values on CT may help characterize the source (**Table 1**).

Pleural collections are routinely treated with chest tube thoracotomy. If they go untreated, patients are at risk for developing infection, adhesions, and calcifications.[33] CXRs are unreliable in determining the amount of residual clot in the thoracic cavity; therefore, CT is preferred to evaluate their evolution.[31]

CHEST WALL

The initial CXR may not accurately demonstrate the extent of trauma to the chest wall. The bones of the thorax are frequently injured with penetrating injuries. Rib fractures can injure intercostal vessels, bleed themselves, or tear the chest wall musculature.[40] Fractures of the first 3 ribs may be associated with neurovascular and tracheobronchial injuries. Fractures of the lower 3 ribs are associated with diaphragmatic and abdominal organ injuries (particularly liver, spleen, and

---

Box 6
CXR signs of a tension pneumothorax

- Contralateral shift of the mediastinum
- Depressed or inverted ipsilateral diaphragm
- Intercostal space widening as a result of rib cage expansion
- Lucency of the hemithorax with the lung collapsed at its hilum

---

Box 7
Signs of pleural collection on CXR

- Obscured costophrenic angle
- Blunted costophrenic angle
- Meniscus sign at costophrenic angle
- Thickened fissures
- Increased density of the thorax
- Lateralization of the diaphragmatic apex, seen with subpulmonic collections (**Fig. 22**)

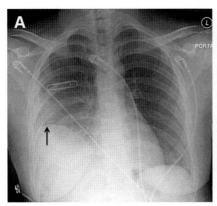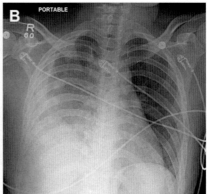

Fig. 22. Middle-aged woman status post stab wound to the chest. Initial supine anteroposterior (AP) portable CXR (*A*) demonstrates lateralization of the diaphragmatic apex (*black arrow*) indicating a subpulmonic effusion (hemothorax). A trace right apical pneumothorax can also be seen. Paper clip denotes the site of penetrating trauma. Four-hour follow-up supine AP portable CXR (*B*) demonstrates interval enlargement of the hemothorax. The right apical pneumothorax is not as conspicuous.

kidneys). Fracture of at least 4 consecutive ribs in 2 or more places constitutes a flail chest. Sternal fractures may be associated with vascular, cardiac, and mediastinal injuries. The presence of a presternal or retrosternal hematoma should prompt a search for a sternal fracture.[33]

Hemorrhage may occur in the extrapleural space. Extrapleural hematomas typically remain contained, do not migrate, or change in configuration. They are commonly associated with rib fractures. Extrapleural hematomas appear as a peripheral convex-shaped opacity demonstrating an apex that points toward the lung parenchyma. An expanding extrapleural hematoma should be further evaluated with CTA to evaluate for an arterial source, particularly when apical.

DIAPHRAGMATIC INJURIES

Diaphragmatic injuries (DI) are often subtle on imaging. The missed diagnosis of a DI can lead to herniation and subsequent strangulation of the herniated viscus even years after the initial injury. In cases of penetrating thoracoabdominal trauma, one must maintain a heightened awareness to the possibility of a DI. Penetrating injuries to the diaphragm usually result in a short defect, 1 to 2 cm in length, and without evisceration.[12,41,42] One should look closely for small fat-containing hernias as the only sign of a DI. These small diaphragmatic

---

Table 1
CT characteristics of pleural collections

Types of Pleural Fluid	Attenuation Values (HU)
Sympathetic	<15
Hemorrhagic	30–70
IV contrast extravasation with active bleeding	>90
Urogenic	<15
Bilious	<0
Chylous	<0
Enteric	≥15

Abbreviations: HU, Hounsfield unit; IV, intravenous.
From Mirvis SE, Shanmuganathan K. Imaging in trauma and critical care. Second edition. Philadelphia: Elsevier Science; 2003. p. 326; with permission.

Box 8
CXR findings of diaphragmatic injuries

Specific
- Nasogastric tube within the stomach above the diaphragm
- Collar sign, a waistlike constriction of the herniated viscera localizing the diaphragmatic defect

Nonspecific
- Ill-defined hemidiaphragm
- Elevated hemidiaphragm, 4 cm or greater above the contralateral diaphragm[45]
- Mediastinal shift to the contralateral side of the DI
- Pleural accumulation
- Air fluid level within the lower thorax
- Displaced lower thoracic rib fractures

Box 9
MDCT findings of DI in penetrating trauma

- *Contiguous injury,* juxtaposed injuries on both sides of the diaphragm
  - Most sensitive sign but decreased specificity with multiple wounds (see **Figs. 6** and **8**)
- *Discontinuous diaphragm sign*
- *Transdiaphragmatic trajectory sign,* focal defect along the wound track
  - Most specific sign even with multiple wounds (see **Fig. 7**)
- *Thickened diaphragm,*[31,46] nonspecific and may simply represent a contusion, hematoma, or contraction of the diaphragm without an associated defect
- *Collar sign,* waistlike constriction of the herniated viscera localizing the diaphragmatic defect (see **Figs. 14**; **Fig. 23**)
- *Dependent viscera sign* (see **Fig. 23**), loss of the diaphragmatic support and subsequent dependent positioning of an organ against the posterior thoracic wall in supine patients
- *Segmental diaphragmatic defect sign, a focal diaphragmatic defect*
- *Sinus cutoff sign,* herniated organs conform to dependent viscera sign interrupting pleural fluid in costophrenic sinus[47]
- *Dangling diaphragm sign,* torn free edge of diaphragm hangs and conforms to comma shape[45]
- *Visualization of contrast media extravasation from the diaphragm*
- *Elevated diaphragm and abdominal organs*
- *Pneumothorax associated with pneumoperitoneum*
- *Hemothorax associated with hemoperitoneum*

Box 10
Mimickers of diaphragmatic injuries

- Air-space opacities
- Lung collapse
- Diaphragmatic eventration
- Paralyzed diaphragm
- Subpulmonic effusion
- Congenital diaphragmatic hernia
- High apex of the right hemidiaphragm

defects are associated with an increased risk of viscus herniation and subsequent strangulation.[1]

Stab wounds have a predilection for the left hemidiaphragm that is attributed to the higher incidence of right-handedness in the general population (assailants) and assaults occurring when facing the victim. GSW affect both hemidiaphragms with equal frequency. GSW can create a blast effect that may result in a DI without formation of a defect.[12]

CXR are the most commonly performed initial imaging study for evaluating DI and may aid in the acute and late diagnosis of DI. However, the sensitivity of diagnosing a DI on CXR is only 24% to 50%.[43,44] There are multiple specific and nonspecific signs of DI on CXR (**Box 8**).

Recent studies show the sensitivity of MDCT in diagnosing DI is anywhere from 71% to 90% with a specificity of 98% to 100%.[42] The higher-quality MDCT images allow for generation of MPR and 3D images that aid in the diagnosis of DI (see **Figs. 7, 14,** and **18**). Many signs on MDCT have also been described to aid the diagnosis of DI (**Box 9**). One must keep in mind the imaging pitfalls that mimic DI, particularly on CXR (**Box 10**).

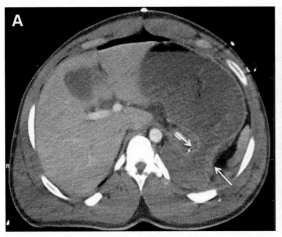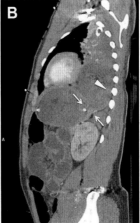

Fig. 23. Right-sided diaphragmatic injuries from a GSW. Axial (*A*) and sagittal (*B*) reformatted contrast-enhanced CT images demonstrate both a collar sign (*arrows*) and dependent viscera sign (*arrowhead*) with herniation of the stomach. Small bullet shrapnel can be seen adjacent to the diaphragmatic defect.

SUMMARY

Penetrating thoracic trauma encompasses a wide variety of injuries. The role of imaging in evaluating these patients will be determined by hemodynamic stability, mechanism of injury, and location of injury. Although most injuries will be to the lungs and pleura and may only be evaluated with serial radiographs, MDCT is being used with increasing frequency in hemodynamically stable patients. With an understanding of injury mechanics and trajectory, the radiologist can play a vital role in diagnosing the extent of injury and guiding further diagnostic examinations or interventions.

REFERENCES

1. Dreizin D, Munera F. Blunt polytrauma: evaluation with 64-section whole-body CT angiography. Radio-Graphics 2012;32:609–31.

2. Restrepo CS, Gutierrez FR, Marmol-Velz JA, et al. Imaging patients with cardiac trauma. Radio-Graphics 2012;32:633–49.

3. Steenburg SD, Ravenel JG, Ikonomidis JS, et al. Acute traumatic aortic injury: imaging evaluation and management. Radiology 2008;248(3):748–62.

4. Centers for Disease Control and Prevention, National Center for Health Statistics. Compressed mortality file 1999-2011 on CDC wonder online database. 2014. Available at: http://wonder.cdc.gov/cmf-icd10.html. Accessed August 21, 2014.

5. US Centers for Disease Control and Prevention WISQARS database. Available at: http://www.cdc.gov/ncipc/wisqars/. Accessed August 15, 2014.

6. Bastos R, Baisden CE, Harker L, et al. Penetrating thoracic trauma. Semin Thorac Cardiovasc Surg 2008;20:19–25.

7. Maiden N. Historical overview of wound ballistics research. Forensic Sci Med Pathol 2009;5:85–9.

8. Stefanopoulos PK, Filippakis K, Soupiou OT, et al. Wound ballistics of firearm-related injuries—part 1: missile characteristics and mechanisms of soft tissue wounding. Int J Oral Maxillofac Surg 2014;43:1445–58.

9. Garner J. The early hospital management of gunshot wounds. Part 1: head, neck, and thorax. Trauma 2005;7:143–54.

10. Rutty GN, Boyce P, Robinson E, et al. The role of computed tomography in terminal ballistic analysis. Int J Legal Med 2008;122:1–5.

11. Alonso RC, Nacenta SB, Martinez PD, et al. Kidney in danger: CT findings of blunt and penetrating renal trauma. RadioGraphics 2009;29(7):2033–53.

12. Lozano JD, Munera F, Anderson SW, et al. Penetrating wounds to the torso: evaluation with triple-contrast multidetector CT. RadioGraphics 2013;33(2):341–59.

13. Lichte P, Oberbeck R, Binnebösel M, et al. A civilian perspective on ballistic trauma and gunshot injuries. Scand J Trauma Resusc Emerg Med 2010;18:35.

14. LeBlang SD, Dolich MO. Imaging of penetrating thoracic trauma. J Thorac Imaging 2000;15:128–35.

15. DeVries CS, Africa M, Gebremariam FA, et al. The imaging of stab wounds. Acta Radiol 2010;1:92–106.

16. Kong VY, Sartorius B, Clarke DL, et al. The selective conservative management of penetrating thoracic trauma is still appropriate in the current era. Injury 2015;46:49–53.

17. Burack JH, Emad K, Sawas A, et al. Triage and outcome of patients with mediastinal penetrating trauma. Ann Thorac Surg 2007;83:377–82.

18. Loogna P, Bonanno F, Bowley DM, et al. Emergency thoracic surgery for penetrating, non-mediastinal trauma. ANZ J Surg 2007;77(3):142–5.

19. Berg RJ, Inaba K, Recinos G, et al. Prospective evaluation of early follow-up chest radiography after penetrating thoracic injury. World J Surg 2013;37(6):1286–90.

20. Okoye OT, Talving P, Teixeira PG, et al. Transmediastinal gunshot wounds in a mature trauma centre: changing perspectives. Injury 2013;44:1198–203.

21. Navid F, Gleason TG. Great vessel and cardiac trauma: diagnostic and management strategies. Semin Thorac Cardiovasc Surg 2008;20:31–8.

22. Kang N, Hsee L, Rizoli S, et al. Penetrating cardiac injury: overcoming the limits set by nature. Injury 2009;40:919–27.

23. Plurad DS, Bricker S, Van Natta TL, et al. Penetrating cardiac injury and the significance of chest computed tomography findings. Emerg Radiol 2013;20:279–84.

24. Stassen NA, Lukan JK, Spain DA, et al. Reevaluation of diagnostic procedures for transmediastinal gunshot wounds. J Trauma 2002;53(4):635–8.

25. Hanpeter DE, Demetriades D, Asensio JA, et al. Helical computed tomographic scan in the evaluation of mediastinal gunshot wounds. J Trauma 2000;49(4):689–94.

26. Ibiroga S, Nicol A, Navsaria PH. Screening helical computed tomographic scanning in haemodynamic stable patients with transmediastinal gunshot wounds. Injury 2007;38:48–52.

27. Co SJ, Yong-Hing CJ, Galea-Soler S, et al. Role of imaging in penetrating and blunt traumatic injury to the heart. Radiographics 2011;31:E101–15.

28. von See C, Stuehmer A, Gellrich NC, et al. Wound ballistics of injuries caused by handguns with different types of projectiles. Mil Med 2009;174(7):757–61.

29. Johnson SB. Esophageal trauma. Semin Thorac Cardiovasc Surg 2008;20(1):46–51.

30. Chen J, Shanmuganathan K, Mirvis SE, et al. Using CT to diagnose tracheal rupture. AJR Am J Roentgenol 2001;176:1273–80.

31. Shanmuganathan K, Killeen K, Mirvis SE, et al. Imaging of diaphragmatic injuries. J Thorac Imaging 2000;15(2):104–11.

32. Greene R. Lung Alterations in thoracic trauma. J Thorac Imaging 1987;2(3):1–11.

33. Kaewli R. Multidetector-row computed tomography of thoracic trauma. Int J Clin Pract 2011;65(Suppl 171):3–16.

34. Allen GS, Fischer RP. Traumatic lung herniation. Ann Thorac Surg 1997;63:1455.

35. Shanmuganathan K, Matsumoto J. Imaging of penetrating chest trauma. Radiol Clin North Am 2006;44:225–38.

36. Bridges KG, Welch G, Silver M, et al. CT detection of occult pneumothorax in multiple trauma patients. J Emerg Med 1993;11:179–86.

37. Blaivas M, Lyon M, Duggal S. A prospective comparison of supine chest radiography and bedside ultrasound for the diagnosis of traumatic pneumothorax. Acad Emerg Med 2005;12(9):844–9.

38. McCloud T. The pleura. In: McCloud T, editor. Thoracic radiology: the requisites. St Louis (MO): Mosby, Inc; 1998. p. 483–513.

39. Miller LA. Chest wall, lung, and pleural space trauma. Radiol Clin North Am 2006;44:213–24.

40. Mayberry JC. Imaging in thoracic trauma: the trauma surgeon's perspective. J Thorac Imaging 2000;15(2):76–86.

41. Madden MR, Paull DE, Finkelstein JL, et al. Occult diaphragmatic injury from stab wounds to the lower chest and abdomen. J Trauma 1989;29(3):292–8.

42. Murray JA, Demetriades D, Cornwell EE 3rd, et al. Penetrating left thoracoabdominal trauma: the incidence and clinical presentation of diaphragm injuries. J Trauma 1997;43(4):624–6.

43. Rodriguez-Morales G, Rodriguez A, Shatney CH. Acute rupture of the diaphragm in blunt trauma: analysis of 60 patients. J Trauma 1986;26(5):438–44.

44. Reber PU, Schmied B, Seiler CA, et al. Missed diaphragmatic injuries and their long-term sequelae. J Trauma 1998;44(1):183–8.

45. Desir A, Ghaye B. CT of Blunt Diaphragmatic Rupture. RadioGraphics 2012;32:477–98.

46. Leung JC, Nance ML, Schwab CW, et al. Thickening of the diaphragm: a new computed tomography sign of diaphragm injury. J Thorac Imaging 1999;14(2):126–9.

47. Kaya SO, Karabulut N, Yuncu G, et al. Sinus cut-off sign: a helpful sign in the CT diagnosis of diaphragmatic rupture associated with pleural effusion. Eur J Radiol 2006;59(2):253–6.

Imaging of Traumatic Brain Injury

Uttam K. Bodanapally, MBBS, Chandler Sours, PhD, Jiachen Zhuo, PhD,
Kathirkamanathan Shanmuganathan, MD*

KEYWORDS

- Trauma • Brain injury • Computed tomography • MR imaging

KEY POINTS

- Most patients with traumatic brain injury (TBI) have mild TBI (mTBI) and typically have no abnormalities on computed tomography (CT) and conventional MR imaging.
- Advanced MR imaging techniques including diffusion weighting, functional imaging, and spectroscopy are potential biomarkers for mTBI.
- CT is the initial diagnostic test in TBI. Conventional MR imaging in the acute phase is used as a problem solver when CT does not explain the neurologic deficit.

INTRODUCTION

Traumatic brain injury (TBI) is a major health and socioeconomic concern throughout the world[1,2] and is the leading cause of mortality and morbidity among young people.[3] The incidence of TBI is increasing in the developing countries, because of the increase in the number of motor vehicle accidents.[3] In advanced nations, the incidence of TBI caused by falls among the aging population is increasing[4] and is changing the occurrence of different forms of TBI, specifically increasing the incidence of focal brain injuries in the form of contusions. Meanwhile the incidence of diffuse axonal injury (DAI) caused by high-velocity traffic accidents is decreasing in developed nations.[4]

In the United States, an estimated 1.1 million emergency department visits and 235,000 hospital admissions occur yearly because of TBI.[5] Although most of these injuries are categorized as mild TBI (mTBI), a considerable number of these patients nevertheless experience permanent deficits.[6] Approximately 52,000 deaths are attributed to TBI per year in the United States.[7–9] TBI principally affects young men, resulting in lost productivity because of disability and lost years because of death. The financial burden to society is estimated to be more than $60 billion per year in the United States alone.[10] This article discusses the role of imaging in diagnosis and the spectrum of findings seen in patients with mild, moderate, and severe TBI.

CLASSIFICATION

TBI is usually classified by clinical severity using the Glasgow Coma Scale (GCS).[11] The mortality from TBI is related to the severity of injury as determined by GCS score.[12,13] GCS (range, 3–15) consists of the sum of the 3 component scores (eye, motor, and verbal scales): mTBI, greater than 12 to less than or equal to 15; moderate TBI, greater than 8 to less than or equal to 12; severe TBI, less than or equal to 8. TBI has also been classified according to the severity of structural damage based on neuroimaging.[14] However, the classification systems based on neuroimaging have limitations, because of severe underestimation of the extent of DAI by imaging modalities.

Funding support: None.

Disclosures/Conflicts of interest: None.

Department of Diagnostic Radiology & Nuclear Medicine, University of Maryland Medical Center, 22 South Greene Street, Baltimore, MD 21201, USA

* Corresponding author.

E-mail address: ksahnmuganathan@umm.edu

Radiol Clin N Am 53 (2015) 695–715

http://dx.doi.org/10.1016/j.rcl.2015.02.011

Also, the systems broadly place injuries into diffuse and focal categories and fail to account for the specific type of mass lesions (eg, epidural vs subdural). The lack of specification fails to correctly classify patients with combined DAI and focal injuries.[4,15]

TYPES OF BRAIN INJURY

TBI is divided into primary and secondary injuries.[4,5,16] Primary injuries occur as a direct result of traumatic impact. Secondary injuries result from a complex biochemical cascade of events that exacerbates the primary injury by resulting in cerebral edema and herniation.[17] The primary parenchymal lesions contain an epicenter with axons, glial cells, and vascular structures that sustain irreversible damage.[16] Primary injury can result in either focal or diffuse lesions. Primary injuries at the macroscopic level are calvarial fractures, extra-axial hemorrhage (epidural hematoma [EDH], subdural hematoma [SDH], subarachnoid hemorrhage [SAH], and intraventricular hemorrhage [IVH]), and intra-axial injuries (contusions, DAI, and brain stem injury).[16] At the cellular level, the initial events include microporation of membranes, leaky ion channels, and changes in the intracellular proteins that occur minutes to hours after initial injury.[4]

Surrounding the epicenter is traumatic penumbra with cells that have sustained reversible damage.[16] Penumbra is the site where most of the deleterious secondary biochemical changes occur. The extent of various physiologic changes that occur during the early or late posttraumatic period, such as hypoxia, hypotension, pyrexia, and coagulopathy, may exacerbate the secondary events and determine the evolution of penumbra either into irreversible lesions or complete resolution.[4] The evolutionary changes in penumbra explain the appearance of new lesions not apparent on initial scans.[18]

Secondary injury is initiated by various pathophysiologic cascades of events that follow the initial injury at both cellular and macroscopic levels to manifest as secondary lesions on neuroimaging. The cellular reactions that develop over hours and days include neurotransmitter release, free-radical generation, calcium-mediated damage, gene activation, mitochondrial dysfunction, and inflammatory responses.[4] The release of neurotransmitters exacerbates the already leaky ion channels that cause primary injury and results in astrocytic swelling and cerebral edema. Cell necrosis is mainly caused by free-radical generation and calcium-mediated injury. Gene activation and expression of proapoptotic protein factors cause apoptotic astrocytic and oligodendrocytic cell death. Mitochondrial dysfunction can decrease adenosine triphosphate production and oxygen consumption, which can further lead to axonal necrosis and apoptosis.[19]

The differentiation of TBI into primary and secondary injuries is important, because secondary injuries are often preventable, whereas primary injuries are not.[16]

MILD TRAUMATIC BRAIN INJURY

Most patients with TBI (up to 75%) are considered to have mTBI.[20,21] Computed tomography (CT) and conventional MR imaging examinations are typically normal and advanced neuroimaging techniques are required. Diffusion-weighted imaging (DWI), functional MR (fMR), arterial spin labeling (ASL), and spectroscopy show structural and functional abnormalities (Fig. 1).[22–29] Studies also indicate that these techniques can be used as biomarkers to diagnose and monitor recovery.

Blunt force from contact sports and blast injuries is a common mechanism for mTBI. The angular or rotational force that produces this injury results in widespread, diffuse effect on the entire brain parenchyma. Early diagnosis of mTBI and careful follow-up imaging to monitor healing holds the potential to prevent long-term neurodegenerative processes, such as chronic traumatic encephalopathy, that occur as a long-term complication of repetitive mTBI.[22,30]

The criteria to diagnose the 2 types of mTBI are shown in Table 1.[31] Unlike mTBI, patients with complicated mTBI have minor structural abnormality on CT or conventional MR imaging.

POSTCONCUSSIVE SYMPTOMS

Although most patients with mTBI are discharged quickly from the trauma center, a significant portion (∼40%) of patients with mTBI remain impaired for at least 3 months, and a substantial number of these patients show deficits up to 1 year after injury.[20,21,32] One year following injury, 82% of patients with mTBI reported the presence of at least 1 postconcussive symptom.[33] The resulting lost productivity has socioeconomic consequences. Postconcussive symptoms include neuropsychological (difficulty with socializing, depression, anxiety), cognitive (attention, executive function, working memory, reduced information processing speed), and somatic symptoms (headaches, chronic pain, sensory perception disorders, language difficulty).[34–38] These symptoms may also be present in patients with mTBI who lack evidence of intracranial injury on conventional

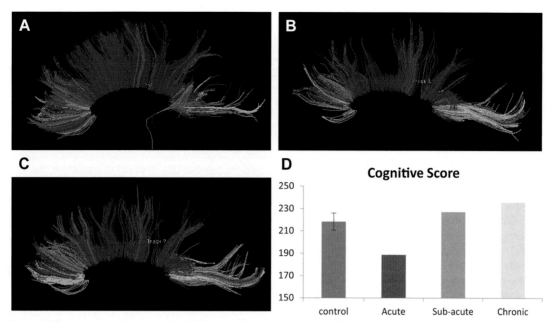

Fig. 1. Diffusion tensor imaging (DTI) fiber tracks and cognitive performance in a patient with mTBI admitted following a fall with no finding on CT or conventional MR imaging examinations. (*A*) Normal subject, (*B*) acute (7 days), and (*C*) subacute (1 month) stages show that disrupted fiber tracks from the corpus callosum partially recover in the subacute phase. (*D*) The decline in cognitive performance also shows corresponding recovery longitudinally.

CT or MR imaging, suggesting that more advanced MR imaging techniques are needed to fully characterize this supposedly mild injury.

MILD TRAUMATIC BRAIN INJURY
Diffusion-Weighted Imaging (Diffusion Tensor Imaging and Diffusion Kurtosis Imaging)

Diffusion MR imaging is an effective tool to study various neurologic disorders because it provides

Table 1
Definition of mTBI

Uncomplicated mTBI	Complicated mTBI
GCS 13–15	GCS 13–15
Loss of consciousness 0–30 min	Loss of consciousness 0–30 min
Alteration in consciousness or mental state for a moment up to 24 h	Alteration in consciousness or mental state for a moment up to 24 h
Posttraumatic amnesia 0–1 d	Posttraumatic amnesia 0–1 d
Normal structural imaging (CT or conventional MR imaging)	Minor structural changes on CT or conventional MR imaging

an in vivo measurement of changes in tissue microstructure. Diffusion tensor imaging (DTI) measures water diffusion in at least 6 directions to obtain an appropriate representation of a diffusion tensor, describing the preferential diffusion direction and an ellipsoidal diffusivity profile. Measurements such as mean diffusivity (MD), often referred to as apparent diffusion coefficient (ADC), and fractional anisotropy (FA) can be measured from such an acquisition; MD or ADC measures the overall diffusivity in the tissue, and FA measures the degree of diffusion anisotropy. Intact axons have high FA, because diffusion is greater along the axons (axial diffusivity) than perpendicular to it (radial diffusivity). Damaged axons have reduced FA, because of either reduced axial diffusivity (typically a result of axonal injury) or increased radial diffusivity (typically a result of myelin damage). Damaged axons may be visible when reconstructing white matter axons using diffusion tractography, a technique that provides axonal structure by measuring the principal diffusion direction within each voxel (see **Fig. 1**).[39] The disrupted fiber tracks observed at the acute stage tend to recover at the subacute stage, corresponding with the patient's cognitive function decline and symptoms followed by recovery.

As a result of secondary injuries, patients experience varied recovery paths, some enduring to chronic stages. In the chronic stages of TBI, commonly damaged regions as indicated by DTI include the corpus callosum,[32,40–42] internal capsule,[32,43] and cingulum bundles.[23] Furthermore, whole-brain analysis reveals more widely spread white matter abnormalities, including the superior and inferior longitudinal fasciculus, corona radiate, and frontal and temporal lobes, which are consistent with the diffuse nature of the injury.[44,45] Although reduced FA and increased MD are consistent findings in the chronic stages of injury thought to represent cell death and axonal damage, results in the acute and subacute stages of TBI are more heterogeneous. TBI is a dynamically evolving injury in the weeks following the initial impact, with multiple primary and secondary injury mechanisms occurring simultaneously. Nevertheless, in mTBI populations at very early stages postinjury, researchers have noted an increased FA and reduced MD. This finding has been hypothesized to indicate an inflammatory response including cytotoxic edema and axonal swelling.[32,46,47]

Diffusion Kurtosis Imaging

DTI is a sensitive tool to assess damage in white matter regions because of the sensitivity of FA to diffusion anisotropy changes; however, it has limited ability to assess alterations in gray matter regions because diffusion there is largely isotropic. Diffusion kurtosis imaging (DKI) has become the vanguard technique to probe the heterogeneity of the microenvironment of both gray and white matter. This technique overcomes a limitation of DTI by introducing a nongaussian term to the diffusion estimation model.[48,49] In addition to the diffusion tensor parameters measurable by the DKI model, the extra kurtosis parameter, the mean kurtosis (MK), captures the nongaussian diffusion property arising from the tissue microstructure heterogeneity. In a recent animal model of TBI, DKI measurements were sensitive to reactive astrogliosis caused by mild inflammation.[29] An increased MK was found in regions with reduced cerebral blood flow (CBF) measured by ASL (discussed later), without accompanying MD and fluid-attenuated inversion recovery (FLAIR) signal changes (Fig. 2). Regions may be affected by ischemia and inflammation following injury. In human studies of chronic mTBI, reduced MK was found in the thalamus and internal capsule, indicating a reduction of diffusion heterogeneity, which may suggest degenerative processes leading to neuronal shrinkage and changes in axonal and myelin density.[50] Furthermore, in the mTBI population, longitudinal changes in MK from the subacute to

chronic stages of injury have been shown to correlate with changes in cognitive functioning.[27]

Functional MR Imaging

fMR imaging is a valuable tool that can be used to noninvasively identify alterations in the communication within and between various neural networks. fMR imaging indirectly measures which regions of the brain are recruited to perform certain cognitive tasks or processes and interprets sensory inputs. This method is based on the MR signal differences between deoxygenated blood and oxygenated blood. When specific neurons for a given task are recruited or activated, there is an increase in freshly oxygenated blood to the local tissue to keep up with the increased neuronal activity. This change from deoxygenated blood to oxygenated blood in the activated region causes a change in the tissue signal as the local tissue changes from a predominantly paramagnetic state to diamagnetic state. This measured change is called the blood oxygen level–dependent (BOLD) signal. At present, fMR imaging data are acquired in one of 2 ways: using either a task-based fMR imaging paradigm or resting state fMR imaging paradigm.

Task-Based Functional MR Imaging

Using a task-based paradigm, participants are instructed to perform a specific task while in the scanner. Researchers are able to indirectly measure which regions of the brain are recruited to perform that task based on the regions that show increased BOLD signal compared with resting conditions.

Because of the susceptibility of the frontal lobe to the mechanical forces of TBI, task-based fMR imaging studies have focused primarily on attention and executive functioning deficits. Studies using task-based fMR imaging to investigate alterations in neural recruitment in patients with TBI have shown altered BOLD responses to tasks involving working memory,[51–54] executive function,[55] sustained attention,[56] and inhibitory control.[57] However, there is disparity with regard to increased[52,53,58] or reduced[59–61] task-induced activations in TBI populations because research groups have reported both. This discrepancy is likely related to differences in task and study design as well as inconsistencies in time since injury and the wide range in difficulty of tasks chosen in various studies.[62] Many of these inconsistencies can be addressed through the use of resting state fMR imaging, which can be administered at all stages of injury and is not influenced by task difficulty, study design, or patient participation.

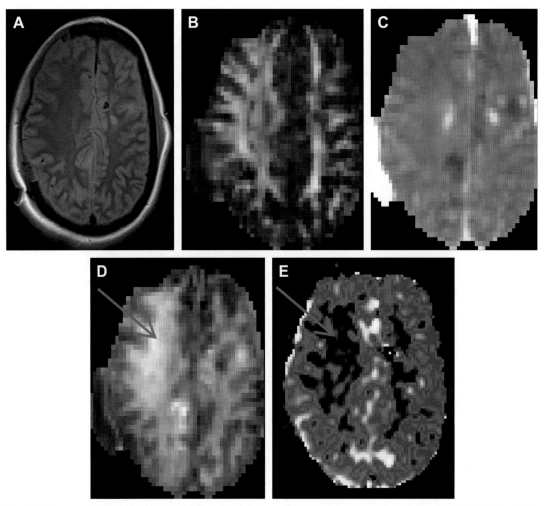

Fig. 2. A 22-year-old woman admitted following a motor vehicle collision, with a GCS of 6. Axial (*A*) FLAIR, (*B*) FA, (*C*) MD, (*D*) MK, and (*E*) CBF maps show decreased CBF (*arrow* in *E*) and increased MK (*arrow* in *D*) without accompanying MD or FLAIR abnormality. These findings may be caused by ischemia and inflammation caused by reduced blood flow and tissue heterogeneity.

Resting State Functional MR Imaging

Using a resting state paradigm, researchers are able to examine functional brain networks by measuring the interaction between brain regions. In this method, participants are not required to perform a task during the scan. Referred to as intrinsic functional connectivity or resting state functional connectivity (rs-FC), this method determines the strength of functional interactions between brain regions by measuring the correlations between small fluctuations in the BOLD signal across the brain.[63–65] Biswal and colleagues[63] discovered that regions recruited to perform a specific task display similar temporal patterns of fluctuations during resting conditions. At present, analysis can be conducted using a data-driven independent component analysis[66]

or a hypothesis-driven seed-based method. Resting state networks that are consistently replicated across both methods include networks that are associated with sensory systems (auditory, visual, somatosensory, and motor) and networks associated with cognitive processes.[67] Through understanding the difference in neural network communication among patients with TBI, researchers will gain a greater insight into the pathophysiology of postconcussive symptoms.

Both severe TBI and mTBI populations have shown reduced interhemispheric rs-FC,[25,60,68] which is likely caused by the compromised integrity of the corpus callosum. TBI also has been shown to reduce rs-FC in neural networks that are not directly linked through the corpus callosum, including the motor network,[69,70] thalamic network,[24,71] task-positive network,[25,72,73] and the default mode network.[29,72,74] It is hypothesized that the loss of structural integrity of the axonal tracts caused by both primary and secondary injury mechanisms contributes to the reduced rs-FC noted in many of these studies. However, some groups have provided evidence for increased rs-FC in the left frontoparietal network in patents with mTBI [75] and default mode network in patients with severe TBI.[75] Furthermore, increased rs-FC has been found in mTBI populations between 2 networks that are generally found to be anticorrelated: the default mode network and task-positive network.[72,74] An increased functional connectivity was observed between the thalamus and the motor cortex in patients with mTBI as opposed to controls, indicating a disturbed functional network (**Fig. 3**).

Longitudinal studies examining resting state fMR imaging over the time course of injury are still needed for a more complete understanding of these alterations and the subsequent effects on recovery from injury. Altered rs-FC within these networks as a result of TBI is an active area of research that has the potential for providing valuable information on the cognitive condition of patients, especially during the acute stage when they are unable to perform tasks or if they are in a vegetative state.

Arterial Spin Labeling

The MR imaging technique ASL is able to measure CBF using endogenous blood contrast by MR imaging. ASL has only recently been applied to TBI in the chronic stages. Using ASL during resting state conditions, patients with severe TBI show a global hypoperfusion,[76] whereas patients with mTBI show reduced CBF specific to the thalamus. Recently, investigators took the novel approach to collect perfusion measures during task-based conditions in order to tease apart the contribution of altered perfusion patterns to changes noted in task-based fMR imaging studies. For example, a severe TBI population showed hypoperfusion of the frontal lobe during a working memory task, suggesting cerebrovascular dysregulation of the cortical regions that modulate cognitive processes.[76] As shown in **Fig. 2**, ASL measured reduced CBF in a patient with severe TBI with otherwise normal FLAIR signal. It is likely that ASL will become widely used in the near future because it has great promise as a prognostic tool in determining patient outcomes.

Spectroscopy

MR spectroscopy (MRS) is unique in its ability to noninvasively measure cellular metabolites in vivo. Metabolites such as N-acetylaspartate (NAA), a neuronal and axonal marker; choline, a product of myelin breakdown products; lactate, a marker of anaerobic metabolism; and creatine (Cre) can be measured to evaluate metabolic changes in the brain following injury.

A common finding following TBI is reduced NAA, which is suggestive of neuronal injury through DAI.[77,78] Recent work in mild and moderate TBI found widespread reductions in NAA and increased choline, which correlated with neuropsychological assessments (**Fig. 4**).[79] In addition, strong correlations have been observed between metabolite concentrations and neuropsychological performance, suggesting that MRS provides novel information that can be used to determine the long-term outcome of patients with TBI (see **Fig. 4**).[26,80–83]

MRS is able to determine biochemical changes within brain tissue that appears healthy based on conventional structural imaging techniques. MRS may be able to detect abnormalities long before

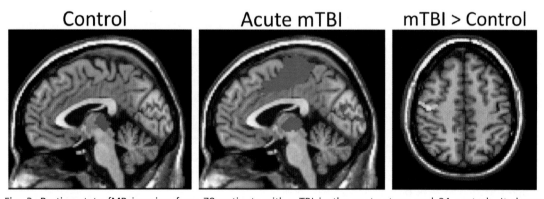

Fig. 3. Resting state fMR imaging from 78 patients with mTBI in the acute stage and 34 controls. It shows increased resting state functional connectivity between the thalamus and the primary motor cortex in the mTBI group compared with the control group. The contrast is shown at a voxelwise threshold of P<.005 (uncorrected) and a cluster threshold of P<.05 FWE corrected.

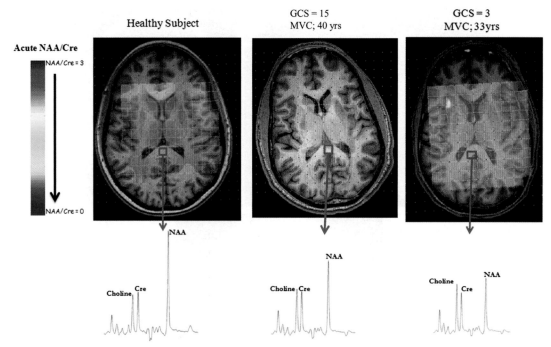

Fig. 4. MRS of a healthy individual, a 40-year-old man with mTBI (GCS, 15), and a 33-year-old man with severe TBI (GCS, 3 at acute stage). Both patients were admitted following a motor vehicle collision. Metabolite maps indicate reduced NAA/Cre in both patients compared with the healthy subject. MRS in the normal-appearing splenium showed reduced NAA and increased choline in patients, more severely in the patient with severe TBI compared with the patient with mTBI. On follow-up, both patients had poor GOSE and high PCS rating. GOSE, Extended Glasgow Outcome Scale; PCS, post concussive symptoms.

morphologic changes are seen using conventional MR imaging, which makes it especially helpful in the assessment of patients with mTBI who have normal structural scans but persistent symptoms. Although MRS is rarely conducted in clinical settings because of the long scan time, recent advances in scan parameters have reduced the length of scan time, making MRS collection in an acute setting increasingly feasible.

MODERATE AND SEVERE TRAUMATIC BRAIN INJURY
Diagnosis

CT is the initial diagnostic method used to assess patients with TBI. The wide availability, quick imaging, and rapid evaluation of patients with TBI support its use as the primary imaging modality. CT determines the presence of life-threatening structural lesions caused by primary injury and provides an opportunity for early treatment before secondary neurologic damage occurs.[14,84–86] Noncontrast CT readily identifies both extra-axial and intra-axial hemorrhages (detailed later).[4,87–89] CT shows intracranial lesions only in 15% of patients with mTBI with GCS of 14.[90] Hence, the current

guidelines support CT in all patients with TBI with a GCS of 14 or lower and in patients with a GCS of 15 in the presence of at least 1 risk factor.[91–93] The identified risk factors for intracranial lesions are severe headache, nausea, vomiting, age (<4 years; >65 years), amnesia, injury mechanism, neurologic deficits, and anticoagulant therapy.[94–96]

TBI is a dynamic process with evolving pathologic changes. Hence, presence of structural lesions on the initial CT or clinical deterioration requires follow-up studies.[96] Approximately 25% to 45% of contusions enlarge in size and 15% of diffuse injuries manifest with new lesions on CT.[97,98] Studies have shown that CT progression usually occurs within 6 to 9 hours after injury.[99] Follow-up CT imaging also allows the detection of evolving secondary lesions such as cerebral edema, ischemia/infarctions, and herniation that are relevant to the management of patients with TBI.[18,100–102]

MR imaging is seldom performed in the acute phase of TBI because of its complex logistics and the lengthy scan time.[4] However, MR imaging has a better sensitivity in identifying certain types of acute injuries that include nonhemorrhagic contusions and DAI lesions that are either

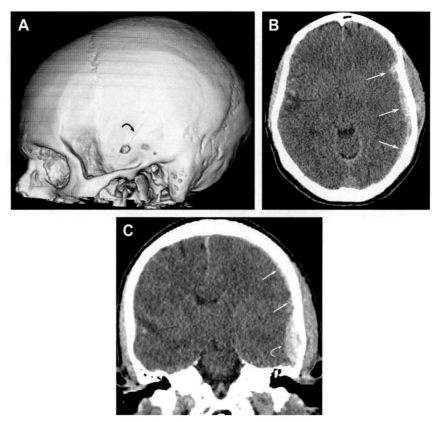

Fig. 5. Combined subdural and EDH in a 29-year-old man following an assault. (*A*) Three-dimensional (3D) volume rendered, (*B*) axial, and (*C*) coronal reformatted noncontrast axial CT images show squamous temporal bone fracture (*curved black arrow*), left convexity SDH (*white arrows*), and EDH (*curved white arrow*) in the lower middle cranial fossa. A contrecoup right temporal parenchymal bleed (*red arrows*) is also seen.

hemorrhagic or nonhemorrhagic.[103] Presently the role of conventional MR imaging is to evaluate patients with acute phase TBI for whom CT fails to explain neurologic status.[104] The role of advanced MR imaging techniques is yet to be determined in the management and diagnosis (see **Figs. 2** and **4**). However, in subacute and chronic phases of TBI, MR imaging is more informative than CT, with better detection of primary and secondary lesions, and also provides a better prediction of neurocognitive outcome.[105,106]

Skull Fractures

CT with bone-window setting is adequate to show skull fractures. Three-dimensional reconstruction with volume rendering provides a far superior ability to show both displaced and nondisplaced fractures and also provides insight into the nature of complex fractures (**Figs. 5A, 6A, 7A**). Although the presence of skull fracture is not correlated with the severity of brain injury, the incidence of intracranial hemorrhage in patients with skull fractures is much higher than in those without fractures. At the same time, approximately 25% of patients with fatal injuries do not show a skull fracture.[107] Skull fractures are commonly seen in patients after falls.[108] The most common types of fractures are linear fractures (see **Fig. 1A**), which are associated with the lowest incidence of intracranial injuries. Depressed skull fractures are usually associated with contusions and dural tears (see **Fig. 7**). Basilar fractures are divided into 4 major patterns: anterior transverse, posterior transverse, lateral frontal diagonal (**Fig. 8**), and mastoid diagonal (**Fig. 9**). Patient mortality caused by severe cerebral injury is more likely with diagonal fracture patterns than with transverse fractures. Complications associated with skull base fractures include blindness, cranial nerve injury, cerebrospinal fluid (CSF) leaks, and hearing loss.[109] Basilar skull fractures through the carotid canal may be associated with petrous carotid artery injuries, hence it is worthwhile performing CT angiography in these high-risk patients (see **Figs. 8** and **9**).[110]

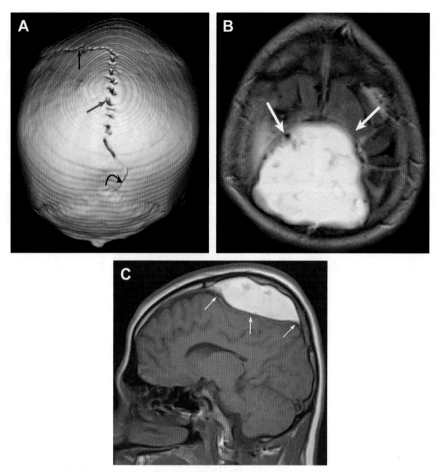

Fig. 6. Postseizure fall. (*A*) 3D volume rendered, (*B*) axial, and (*C*) sagittal reformatted MR images show fracture left parietal bone (*curved arrow*), diastasis of the coronal (*black arrow*) and sagittal (*red arrow*) sutures with a large parietal vertex EDH crossing the midline and limited by the inner dura (*white arrows*) striped from the calvarium. Mass effect is seen on the underlying parenchyma.

Extra-axial Hemorrhage

There are 3 types of extracerebral hemorrhage: EDH, SDH, and SAH or IVH.

Epidural Hematoma

EDH usually occurs at the site of impact (coup). EDH can cross the dural attachments but not the cranial sutures, because the hematoma exists in the potential space between the dura and the inner table of the skull (see **Fig. 6**). The most common locations are the temporal and parietal regions, and usually result from arterial disruption associated with a skull fracture (**Fig. 10**). The middle meningeal artery or one of its branches is the common source of hematoma (see **Fig. 10**).[111–113] EDH is common in young adults. Children, because of a compliant skull, and older people, because of a firm dural attachment to the skull, have lower incidences of EDH.

EDH can be caused by disruption of venous sinuses and often is associated with occipital or greater wing of sphenoid fractures.[114] Disruption of transverse or sigmoid venous sinuses, associated with occipital bone fracture, results in EDH in the posterior cranial fossa. Fracture of the greater wing of sphenoid results in disruption of the sphenoparietal sinus with EDH occurring in the middle cranial fossa. EDH arising from the sphenoparietal sinus is the most common EDH of venous origin.

EDH manifests as well-defined, biconvex, hyperdense, extra-axial blood on CT. The biconvex shape results from firm attachment of dura to the skull. Because EDHs can cross the dural attachments, they can be seen extending above and below the tentorium or extending across the midline (see **Fig. 6**B). Occasionally, an acute EDH can appear heterogeneous in density with foci of irregular areas of low attenuation (see

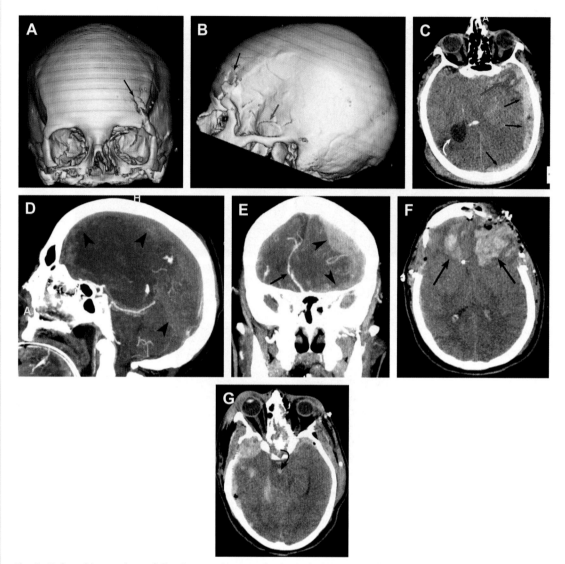

Fig. 7. Delayed hemorrhage following craniectomy for brain herniation and depressed skull fracture in 40-year-old man admitted following a motor vehicle collision. (*A* and *B*) 3D volume rendered images show a depressed left frontal bone (*black arrows*) and a nondepressed greater wing (*red arrow*) of sphenoid bone fractures. (*C*) Admission noncontrast axial CT image of the head shows a left temporal lobe contusion (*red arrow*), a large left acute SDH (*black arrows*) with dilatation of the occipital horn (*curved arrow*) caused by trapping of the right lateral ventricle. There is diffuse cerebral edema and loss of visualization of the basal cisterns. Contrast-enhanced (*D*) sagittal and (*E*) coronal maximum intensity projection images show a large left acute SDH (*arrowheads*) tracking up to the falx and tentorium causing mass effect with displacement of the anterior cerebral arteries (*black arrow*) to the right side and posterior cerebral arteries (*red arrow*) inferiorly caused by transfalcine and transtentorial herniation respectively. (*F* and *G*) Noncontrast axial CT shows bilateral new delayed parenchymal bleeds (*black arrows*), a right venous EDH (*red arrow*), and Duret hemorrhage (*curved arrow*) in the brain stem. The left frontal lobe bleed represents a hematoma.

Fig. 10A). The low density in the hematoma indicates active extravasation of fresh unclotted blood (swirl sign) and warrants immediate surgical attention.[115,116] Because of the high attenuation of EDH, they are well seen on CT, which also shows the associated skull fractures. MR imaging identifies EDHs, but the associated skull fractures are unlikely to be visualized. On MR imaging EDH can be easily differentiated from SDH by identifying the low-signal outer dura (see **Fig 7**C). Approximately one-fourth of EDHs enlarge on follow-up head CT scans.[117] Large EDHs causing mass effect and actively bleeding EDHs usually require surgical attention and evacuation.

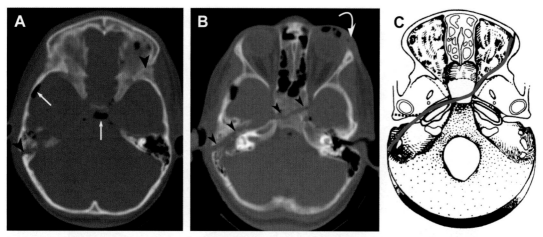

Fig. 8. Left frontodiagonal skull base fracture in 19-year-old man admitted following a motor vehicle collision. (*A* and *B*) Noncontrast axial CT images in bone windows. (*C*) Line diagram of the skull base shows a skull base fracture extending from the left lateral via the pituitary fossa region crossing the midline into right petrous temporal bone (*arrowheads, redline*). Impact site soft tissue swelling (*curved arrow*) and pneumocephalus (*arrows*) is also seen. (*From* West OC, Mirvis SE, Shanmuganathan K. Transsphenoid basilar skull fracture: CT patterns. Radiology 1993;188(2):334; with permission.)

Subdural Hematoma

SDH is located in the potential space between the dura and arachnoid and is usually venous in origin, resulting from the stretching and disruption of cortical veins.[118] Bridging veins can be stretched up to 30% to 35% before they tear and bleed.[24] SDH may be located at the point of impact (coup) (see **Fig. 5**B, C) or opposite to the point of impact (countercoup), the latter being more common. The loose connection between the dura and the arachnoid allows the SDH to spread over a large surface area of the brain and usually creates a crescentic configuration over the cerebral convexity (see **Fig. 7**C). SDH may continue to increase in size as progressive disruption of the already stretched and preloaded veins occurs as hematoma size increases. The phenomenon of lower intensity stretch below the threshold of rupture is called preloading of veins and results

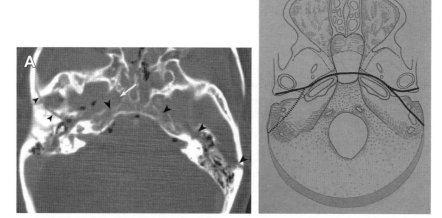

Fig. 9. Posterior transverse pattern skull base fracture. (*A*) Contrast-enhanced axial CT image and (*B*) line diagram show a skull base fracture (*arrowheads*) extending from the right to the left petrous temporal bone through the posterior petrous portion of the right and left carotid canals and pituitary fossa. No contrast material is seen within the lumen of right carotid artery (*arrow*) because it is a grade IV blunt carotid artery injury. ([*B*] *From* West OC, Mirvis SE, Shanmuganathan K. Transsphenoid basilar skull fracture: CT patterns. Radiology 1993;188(2):334; with permission.)

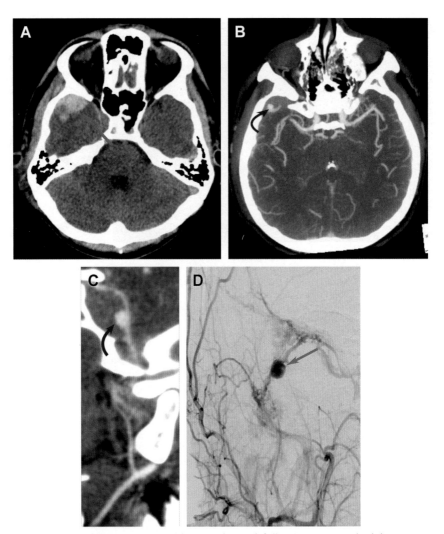

Fig. 10. Actively bleeding EDH in a 19-year-old man admitted following an assault. (*A*) Noncontrast axial CT image shows a mixed-attenuation right middle cranial fossa EDH (*arrow*). (*B*) Contrast-enhanced axial maximum intensity projection and (*C*) multiplanar images show a middle meningeal artery pseudoaneurysm (*curved arrow*). (*D*) Cerebral angiogram confirms the pseudoaneurysm (*arrow*), which was embolized (not shown).

in increased stiffness producing venospasm of varying degrees, which is prone to rupture with trivial force.[119] The same phenomenon explains the high incidence of SDH in patients with diffuse cerebral volume loss that result in preloading of veins that are susceptible to rupture with minimal force (eg, old age, chronic alcoholism). SDHs are also frequently seen along the dural reflections, namely falx (see **Fig. 7**C–E) and tentorium. Most of the SDHs are supratentorial and have uniform high attenuation on CT in the acute phase. Small SDHs may be subtle on CT, hence close scrutiny under proper window settings and multiplanar reformatted images are important (see **Fig 5**B, C). Approximately 40% of SDHs have heterogenous attenuation and the foci of

low attenuation are caused by unclotted blood products or a CSF leak into subdural space caused by associated arachnoid tears (see **Fig. 7**C).[120] In contrast with the EDHs, SDHs can cross cranial sutures but do not cross dural attachments (see **Fig. 7**C–E).

SDH manifests as well-defined, crescentic, hyperattenuated, extra-axial blood on CT. In the acute stage (first week), a traumatic SDH is typically hyperattenuating on CT (see **Fig. 7**C; **Fig. 11**). During the subacute phase (second and third weeks), the hematoma gradually decreases in attenuation, transforming into an isoattenuating collection with density similar to brain parenchyma (see **Fig. 11**).[121] Such isoattenuating SDHs are sometimes difficult to identify on CT; therefore, a

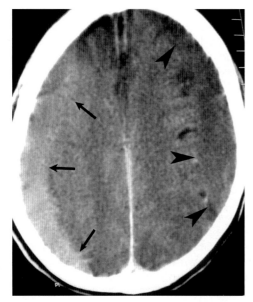

Fig. 11. Bilateral SDHs. Noncontrast axial CT image shows acute right (*arrows*) and isodense left (*arrowheads*) large SDHs causing mass effect leading to displacement of the cortical margins medially. Both extra-axial collections were surgically evacuated.

careful inspection should be performed for the following signs: medial displacement of gray-white matter junction, effacement of cortical sulci, and failure of surface sulci to reach the inner table of the calvarium.

SDHs in the chronic phase have a low attenuation on CT and signal intensities similar to CSF on all MR sequences. MR imaging can identify all phases of SDHs by identifying hematomas at varying stages of evolution by showing changing signal intensities of blood products depending on the oxidation state of blood.

Brain parenchymal injury is commonly associated with SDH (see **Fig. 7**C). Cerebral edema increases the parenchymal fluid, manifesting as decreased attenuation on CT images with a loss of gray-white matter differentiation. The degree of associated cerebral edema and cerebral injury determines the prognosis of patients with SDH.[122]

Rebleeding is frequently seen during the evolution of SDH, resulting in heterogeneous attenuation from the mixture of fresh blood and partially liquefied hematoma. Hematocrit effect results from sedimentation of blood products and is usually seen in patients after rebleeding or in patients with coagulopathy.

Subarachnoid Hemorrhage

SAH is commonly associated with moderate to severe TBI, and is seen in approximately 40% of patients.[123] Small SAHs result from laceration of small subarachnoid vessels and large hemorrhages result from direct extension of hemorrhagic contusions or hematomas into the subarachnoid space. Compared with aneurysmal SAH, posttraumatic SAH is peripheral in distribution, usually over the cerebral hemispheres. Intraventricular hemorrhage results from shearing force sustained by the subependymal veins along the surface of ventricles or by direct extension of parenchymal hematoma or SAH into the ventricular system. On CT, SAH appears as linear areas of increased attenuation along the sulci of cerebral hemispheres, sylvian fissures, or basilar cisterns. FLAIR MR imaging sequences are reliable in detecting SAH.[124]

INTRA-AXIAL LESIONS
Contusions

Contusions are typically focal or multifocal and located in cortical or subcortical regions, depending on the severity of impact. Focal contusions are the most common type of lesions, usually seen in older patients following falls. Cortical contusions are bruises and lacerations of the brain parenchyma. Contusions can occur in coup or counter-coup sites; the lesions at the latter sites are usually larger. Coup lesions that occur at the site of a depressed skull fracture are frequently associated with dural tears. Countercoup lesions occur as the brain, floating in CSF, is displaced in the opposite direction and bounces against the posterior skull. They also result from the cavitation effect of high negative pressures (see **Fig. 5**B, C).[125] The inferior frontal lobes and temporal lobes are especially at risk of such an injury as the brain glides over the irregular surface of the anterior and middle cranial fossa. In mild injuries, contusions are localized to the cortex and, in severe injuries, the lesions usually extend into subcortical white matter.

On imaging, approximately half of contusions are hemorrhagic at initial presentation.[88] Intracerebral hematomas and hemorrhagic contusions represent the same spectrum of injuries, rather than distinct entities. At greater severity of injury, microhemorrhages associated with contusions can coalesce into a larger intracerebral hematoma.

Cortical contusions, especially nonhemorrhagic contusions, are underestimated by CT. MR imaging has far superior sensitivity in the detection of nonhemorrhagic contusions.[88,126] Most hemorrhagic contusions are identified on CT and MR imaging. They appear as small hemorrhages in the cortex with or without surrounding edema (see **Figs. 5** and **7**). Approximately, 25% to 45% of contusions evolve and manifest, with hemorrhages increasing in size over time; this is known as hemorrhagic progression of contusion.[127] Approximately 15% of patients experience delayed microhemorrhages or hematomas in areas of the brain that were previously nonhemorrhagic, which is referred to as delayed traumatic intracerebral hemorrhage (see Fig. 7F).[128] Most progression of lesions occurs within 6 to 9 hours after injury,[99] so follow-up CT imaging should be timed accordingly.

Compared with CT, MR imaging with susceptibility-weighted imaging (SWI) or gradient recalled echo (GRE) sequences has a far superior sensitivity in detecting small hemorrhagic contusions.[105] Acute nonhemorrhagic contusions can be identified on DWI as bright lesions and on ADC maps as dark lesions because of restricted diffusion that results from cell necrosis.[129,130] In the nonacute setting, the lesions can manifest on FLAIR and T2-weighted sequences as hyperintense lesions because of vasogenic edema that develops around the neuronal disruption in the subacute phase and gliosis in the chronic phase. Contusions can lead to regional ischemia caused by the release of excitotoxic amino acids. Regional ischemia further exacerbates cytotoxic edema, vasogenic edema, and increased intracranial pressure associated with injury.[131] Cerebral edema that results from primary and secondary injuries may increase for approximately 72 hours and begins to heal after the first week of initial injury. Over the next few weeks to months, the lesions shrink because of gliosis. By 4 to 6 months after trauma, the lesions transform into cystic spaces called encephalomalacia and manifest as hypoattenuated areas on CT.[14,15]

Diffuse Axonal Injury

DAI is an indirect injury caused by impact or nonimpact trauma and usually results from shear strain at the gray-white matter junction caused by rotational acceleration.[132] DAI is one of the most common types of primary neuronal injuries in patients involved in high-velocity traffic accidents and is characterized by multiple small hemorrhagic and nonhemorrhagic lesions at the gray-white matter junction. The injury results in axonal stretching, and eventual disruption in severe shear injury. There can also be perforation of blood vessels resulting in microhemorrhages caused by shear injury. The deleterious cascade of biochemical events results in secondary injury over hours, days, weeks, and even years. The severity of DAI is proportionate to the magnitude of angular acceleration. With milder injury (grade I), lesions are localized to the gray-white matter

junction (Fig. 12F) of the subcortical white matter. Moderate injury (grade II) results in lesions in the corpus callosum (see Fig. 12E) in addition to subcortical white matter. With severe injury (grade III), the lesions are found in dorsolateral brain stem (Fig. 13), in addition to the subcortical white matter and corpus callosum. The grading of progressively deeper structural injury that occurs with increasing rotational acceleration is in accordance with the centripetal theory of shear injury. Patients with severe DAI usually manifest with profound coma, but not with high intracranial pressure, and frequently have a poor outcome compared with focal injury. The primary factor that generates coma in the immediate posttraumatic period is the axonal injury in the brain stem.[133] Coma that results from focal brain injuries is initiated by secondary injury resulting from increased intracranial pressure causing herniation and brain stem compression,[134] which is why the coma does not occur immediately after injury.

DAI lesions tend to be small (range, 1–15 mm), ovoid with long axis parallel to the axonal tracts, hemorrhagic or nonhemorrhagic, and multiple (15–20 lesions in severely injured patients) (see Fig. 12).[16,135] The distribution of lesions occurs along the corpus callosum complex, gray-white matter junction, parasagittal cortex, and deep periventricular white matter, especially in the frontal corner of the lateral ventricles, basal ganglia, internal capsule, hippocampal and parahippocampal regions, brain stem, and cerebellum (see Fig. 12D). Parasagittal cortical lesions are distinct and result from tearing of long perforating veins that are attached to the sagittal sinus.[16]

CT is notorious for underdiagnosing DAI, with only a minority of lesions appearing on CT (see Fig. 12). For the CT to be positive, the lesions usually are hemorrhagic and macroscopic and seen at the gray-white matter junction (Fig. 14).[88,89] The sensitivity of CT decreases following acute injury as the hemorrhages degrade and become isoattenuating within the brain parenchyma.[5]

Because CT has a low sensitivity in detecting DAI lesions, MR imaging is indicated in all patients with depressed consciousness and normal CT findings (see Fig 12).[88,89,130] MR imaging usually identifies lesions in these patients corresponding with their neurologic status.[88,89,132] The role of MR imaging, especially in patients with nonhemorrhagic lesions, cannot be understated. In acute stages of nonhemorrhagic DAI, DWI sequence is the most sensitive, with lesions manifesting as foci of restricted diffusion because of cytotoxic edema that results from axonal necrosis.[129,130] These lesions appear as bright foci on DWI sequence and dark lesions on ADC maps.

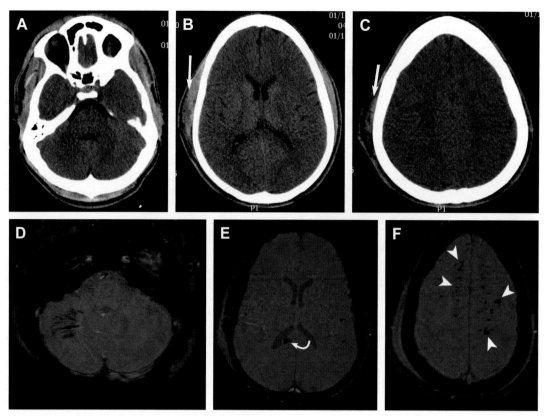

Fig. 12. Diffuse axonal shear injury only seen on MR images in a patient admitted with a GCS of 10. (*A–C*) Non-contrast axial CT of the head shows no intracranial bleed scalp contusion (*arrows* in *B* and *C*). (*D–F*) SWI images at corresponding anatomic regions show punctate bleeds in both hemispheres (*arrowheads*) at the gray-white junction and splenium of corpus callosum (*curved arrow*).

In the nonacute setting, the nonhemorrhagic lesions can manifest on FLAIR and T2-weighted sequences.[87–89] The vasogenic edema around the areas of neuronal disruption in the subacute phase results in FLAIR and T2-weighted

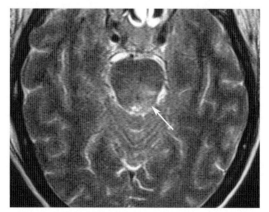

Fig. 13. Dorsolateral brain stem contusion. Axial T2-weighted image in the region of the brain stem shows a dorsolateral nonhemorrhagic contusion (*arrow*) caused by diffuse axonal shear injury.

hyperintensities. Acute hemorrhagic DAI lesions are identified on GRE and SWI sequences as focal susceptibility artifacts and signal loss caused by the paramagnetic effects of deoxyhemoglobin (see **Fig. 12**). SWI sequence is a high-resolution MR technique that contains images with phase information.[136] The sensitivity of these sequences further increases because of magnification of susceptibility artifacts with increase in the field strength of the MR imaging; 3-T MR imaging detects twice the number of lesions compared with 1.5 T.[137] SWI was found to detect approximately 4 times as many lesions as GRE sequences.[138]

Brain stem lesions are a frequent component of DAI caused by rotational acceleration impact forces, especially to the frontal and vertex regions.[16] Brain stem lesions occur because of a downward shift of the brain or impulsive rotational force. Such lesions usually involve the dorsolateral aspect of brain stem (see **Fig. 13**). In addition, note that DAI with vasogenic edema, cytotoxic edema, and microhemorrhages mimics cerebral fat embolism syndrome on MR imaging. Knowledge of the subtle differences on conventional MR imaging

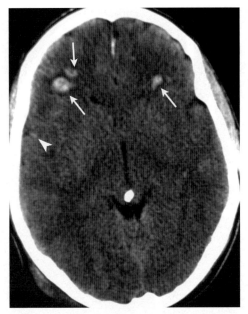

Fig. 14. Hemorrhagic diffuse axonal shear injury. Non-contrast axial CT image shows punctate hemorrhagic lesion (*arrows*) at the gray-white junction and small subarachnoid hemorrhage (*arrowhead*) typical for diffuse axonal shear injury.

and the differences in DTI parameters between the two conditions aids correct diagnosis.[139,140]

Brain Stem Injury

Brain stem injury can be caused either by primary injury or secondary injury. Primary injury may be caused by rotational acceleration with impact especially to the frontal and vertex regions resulting in a downward shift of the brain and direct injury to the dorsolateral aspect of the brain stem caused by contact with the free edge of the tentorium.[87] However, the most common form of primary brain stem injury is from DAI complex, with similar dorsolateral brain stem lesion distribution. Because brain stem DAI is observed in severe trauma (grade III DAI), these injuries are almost always associated with lesions in other typical locations, including subcortical white matter and the corpus callosum.[87]

Secondary lesions are also common in the brain stem and are a result of a delayed downward displacement of the cerebrum caused by the supratentorial mass effect, caused by cerebral edema intra-axial hemorrhage, or extra-axial hemorrhage. Secondary brain stem hemorrhages, called Duret hemorrhages, result from stretching and distortion of blood vessels in the interpeduncular cistern caused by transtentorial herniation from any cause that increases the supratentorial

intracranial pressure (see **Fig. 7**G). In contrast with primary lesions, secondary lesions usually involve the ventral or ventrolateral aspect of the brain stem, as opposed to dorsolateral distribution in primary injury.

On CT or MR imaging, special attention should be paid to analyzing the brain stem for traumatic lesions. Brain stem lesions are difficult to detect on CT because of the bone artifacts within the posterior fossa. MR imaging is the method of choice in brain stem injury analysis.[141–143] On imaging, the primary lesions follow a similar course and have similar appearance to the DAI lesions in other regions of the brain.

Brain Herniations and Infarctions

Cerebral herniations result from mechanical displacement of brain parenchyma from one cranial compartment to another. The recognized types of brain herniations are subfalcine herniation (see **Fig. 7**E), descending transtentorial herniation (see **Fig. 7**D), ascending herniation caused by upward herniation of the cerebellum, and tonsillar herniation caused by downward displacement of cerebellar tonsils through the foramen magnum. Subfalcine herniation manifests as midline shift and is caused by herniation of cingulate gyrus beneath the falx. In some cases, subfalcine herniation can result in compression of the anterior cerebral artery with infarction in the distribution of the callosomarginal branch of the anterior cerebral artery (see **Fig. 7**E).[142] Uncal herniation results in displacement of uncus into the suprasellar cistern or can descend below the tentorium. Descending uncal herniation can result in compression of the posterior cerebral artery against the tentorium and may cause posterior cerebral artery territory infarctions.[143] The compression of the basilar artery from effacement of basal cisterns can result in brain stem ischemia and infarctions.[144] Other potential causes of ischemia and infarctions that result from secondary alterations include vasospasm.[144]

Cerebral herniations can be recognized on CT and MR imaging by a dilatation of the contralateral ventricular system (ventricular entrapment), effacement of the basal cisterns, and midline shift of the brain parenchyma (see **Fig. 3**C).[144–149] MR imaging may be superior in identifying brain herniation in the posterior fossa because of its lack of beam hardening artifacts from the skull base.[10]

SUMMARY

Imaging plays an important role in the management of patients with TBI. CT is the first-line imaging technique allowing rapid detection of primary structural brain lesions that require surgical intervention. CT also detects various deleterious secondary insults allowing early medical and surgical management. Serial imaging is critical to identifying secondary injuries. MR imaging is indicated in patients with acute TBI when CT fails to explain neurologic findings. However, MR imaging is superior in patients with subacute and chronic TBI and also predicts neurocognitive outcome.

REFERENCES

1. Ghajar J. Traumatic brain injury. Lancet 2000;356: 923–9.
2. Cole TB. Global road safety crisis remedy sought: 1.2 million killed, 50 million injured annually. JAMA 2004;291:2531–2.
3. Finfer SR, Cohen J. Severe traumatic brain injury. Resuscitation 2001;48:77–90.
4. Maas AI, Stocchetti N, Bullock R. Moderate and severe traumatic brain injury in adults. Lancet Neurol 2008;7(8):728–41.
5. Kubal WS. Updated imaging of traumatic brain injury. Radiol Clin North Am 2012;50(1):5–41.
6. Thornhill S, Teasdale GM, Murray GD, et al. Disability in young people and adults one year after head injury: prospective cohort study. BMJ 2000; 320:1631–5.
7. Sosin DM, Sniezek JE, Waxweiler RJ. Trends in death associated with traumatic brain injury, 1979 through 1992. Success and failure. JAMA 1995; 273:1778–80.
8. Sosin DM, Sniezek JE, Thurman DJ. Incidence of mild and moderate brain injury in the United States, 1991. Brain Inj 1996;10:47–54.
9. Centers for Disease Control and Prevention (CDC). Traumatic brain injury—Colorado, Missouri, Oklahoma, and Utah, 1990–1993. MMWR Morb Mortal Wkly Rep 1997;46:8–11.
10. Kim JJ, Gean AD. Imaging for the diagnosis and management of traumatic brain injury. Neurotherapeutics 2011;8(1):39–53.
11. Teasdale G, Jennett B. Assessment of coma and impaired consciousness. A practical scale. Lancet 1974;2:81–4.
12. Marshall LF, Gautille T, Klauber MR, et al. The outcome of severe closed head injury. J Neurosurg 1991;75(1S):S28–36.
13. Rimel RW, Giordani B, Barth JT, et al. Moderate head injury: completing the clinical spectrum of brain trauma. Neurosurgery 1982;11(3):344–51.
14. Marshall LF, Marshall SB, Klauber MR, et al. A new classification of head injury based on computerized tomography. J Neurosurg 1991;75(suppl): s14–20.
15. Maas AI, Hukkelhoven CW, Marshall LF, et al. Prediction of outcome in traumatic brain injury with computed tomographic characteristics: a comparison between the computed tomographic classification and combinations of computed tomographic predictors. Neurosurgery 2005;57:1173–82.
16. Bešenski N. Traumatic injuries: imaging of head injuries. Eur Radiol 2002;12(6):1237–52.
17. Faden AI. Pharmacological treatment of central nervous system trauma. Pharmacol Toxicol 1996; 78(1):12–7.
18. Gentry LR. Primary neuronal injuries. Neuroimaging Clin North Am 1991;1:411–32.
19. Kroemer G, Galluzzi L, Brenner C. Mitochondrial membrane permeabilization in cell death. Physiol Rev 2007;87:99–163.
20. National Center for Injury Prevention and Control. Report to Congress on mild traumatic brain injury in the United States: steps to prevent a serious public health problem. Atlanta (GA): Centers for Disease Control and Prevention; 2003.
21. Alves W, Macciocchi SN, Barth JT. Postconcussive symptoms after uncomplicated mild head injury. J Head Trauma Rehabil 1993;8:48–59.
22. Vagnozzi R, Signoretti S, Tavazzi B, et al. Temporal window of metabolic brain vulnerability to concussion: a pilot 1H-magnetic resonance spectroscopic study in concussed athletes–part III. Neurosurgery 2008;62(6):1286–95.
23. Mac Donald CL, Johnson AM, Cooper D, et al. Detection of blast-related traumatic brain injury in U.S. military personnel. N Engl J Med 2011; 364(22):2091–100.
24. Zhou Y, Lui YW, Zuo XN, et al. Characterization of thalamo-cortical association using amplitude and connectivity of functional MRI in mild traumatic brain injury. J Magn Reson Imaging 2014;39(6):1558–68.
25. Sours C, Rosenberg J, Kane R, et al. Associations between interhemispheric functional connectivity and the Automated Neuropsychological Assessment Metrics (ANAM) in civilian mild TBI. Brain Imaging Behav 2014. [Epub ahead of print].
26. George EO, Roys S, Sours C, et al. Longitudinal and prognostic evaluation of mild traumatic brain injury: a 1H-magnetic resonance spectroscopy study. J Neurotrauma 2014;31(11):1018–28.
27. Stokum JA, Sours C, Zhuo J, et al. A longitudinal evaluation of diffusion kurtosis imaging in patients with mild traumatic brain injury. Brain Inj 2015;29:1–11.
28. Grossman EJ, Jensen JH, Babb JS, et al. Cognitive impairment in mild traumatic brain injury: a longitudinal diffusional kurtosis and perfusion imaging study. AJNR Am J Neuroradiol 2013;34(5):951–7.
29. Zhou Y, Milham MP, Lui YW, et al. Default-mode network disruption in mild traumatic brain injury. Radiology 2012;265(3):882–92.
30. Mez J, Stern RA, McKee AC. Chronic traumatic encephalopathy: where are we and where are we going? Curr Neurol Neurosci Rep 2013;13(12):407.

31. Appendix 1: Pathoanatomic terms for definition of TBI lesions and associated findings. Available at: http://commondataelements.ninds.nih.gov/#page=Default.

32. Bazarian JJ, Wong T, Harris M, et al. Epidemiology and predictors of post-concussive syndrome after minor head injury in an emergency population. Brain Inj 1999;13:173–89.

33. McMahon P, Hricik A, Yue JK, et al. Symptomatology and functional outcome in mild traumatic brain injury: results from the prospective TRACK-TBI study. J Neurotrauma 2014;31:26–33.

34. Chaumet G, Quera-Salva MA, Macleod A, et al. Is there a link between alertness and fatigue in patients with traumatic brain injury? Neurology 2008;71:1609–13.

35. Hillary FG, Genova HM, Medaglia JD, et al. The nature of processing speed deficits in traumatic brain injury: is less brain more? Brain Imaging Behav 2010;4:141–54.

36. Immonen RJ, Kharatishvili I, Grohn H, et al. Quantitative MRI predicts long-term structural and functional outcome after experimental traumatic brain injury. Neuroimage 2009;45:1–9.

37. Johansson B, Berglund P, Ronnback L. Mental fatigue and impaired information processing after mild and moderate traumatic brain injury. Brain Inj 2009;23:1027–40.

38. Makley MJ, English JB, Drubach DA, et al. Prevalence of sleep disturbance in closed head injury patients in a rehabilitation unit. Neurorehabil Neural Repair 2008;22:341–7.

39. Mori S, Crain BJ, Chacko VP, et al. Three dimensional tracking of axonal projections in the brain by magnetic resonance imaging. Ann Neurol 1999;45:265–9.

40. Kumar R, Husain M, Gupta RK, et al. Serial changes in the white matter diffusion tensor imaging metrics in moderate traumatic brain injury and correlation with neuro-cognitive function. J Neurotrauma 2009; 26:481–95.

41. Mayer AR, Ling J, Mannell MV, et al. A prospective diffusion tensor imaging study in mild traumatic brain injury. Neurology 2010;74:643–50.

42. Warner MA, Marquez de la Plata C, Spence J, et al. Assessing spatial relationships between axonal integrity, regional brain volumes, and neuropsychological outcomes after traumatic axonal injury. J Neurotrauma 2010;27:2121–30.

43. Arfanakis K, Haughton VM, Carew JD, et al. Diffusion tensor MR imaging in diffuse axonal injury. AJNR Am J Neuroradiol 2002;23:794–802.

44. Messe A, Caplain S, Paradot G, et al. Diffusion tensor imaging and white matter lesions at the subacute stage in mild traumatic brain injury with persistent neurobehavioral impairment. Hum Brain Mapp 2011;32:999–1011.

45. Yuh EL, Mukherjee P, Lingsma HF, et al. Magnetic resonance imaging improves 3-month outcome prediction in mild traumatic brain injury. Ann Neurol 2013;73:224–35.

46. Chu Z, Wilde EA, Hunter JV, et al. Voxel-based analysis of diffusion tensor imaging in mild traumatic brain injury in adolescents. AJNR Am J Neuroradiol 2010;31:340–6.

47. Wilde EA, McCauley SR, Hunter JV, et al. Diffusion tensor imaging of acute mild traumatic brain injury in adolescents. Neurology 2008;70:948–55.

48. Jensen JH, Helpern JA. MRI quantification of non-Gaussian water diffusion by kurtosis analysis. NMR Biomed 2010;23:698–710.

49. Jensen JH, Helpern JA, Ramani A, et al. Diffusional kurtosis imaging: the quantification of non-Gaussian water diffusion by means of magnetic resonance imaging. Magn Reson Med 2005;53:1432–40.

50. Grossman EJ, Ge Y, Jensen JH, et al. Thalamus and cognitive impairment in mild traumatic brain injury: a diffusional kurtosis imaging study. J Neurotrauma 2012;29:2318–27.

51. Christodoulou C, DeLuca J, Ricker JH, et al. Functional magnetic resonance imaging of working memory impairment after traumatic brain injury. J Neurol Neurosurg Psychiatry 2001;71:161–8.

52. McAllister TW, Flashman LA, McDonald BC, et al. Mechanisms of working memory dysfunction after mild and moderate TBI: evidence from functional MRI and neurogenetics. J Neurotrauma 2006;23: 1450–67.

53. McAllister TW, Saykin AJ, Flashman LA, et al. Brain activation during working memory 1 month after mild traumatic brain injury: a functional MRI study. Neurology 1999;53:1300–8.

54. Sanchez-Carrion R, Gomez PV, Junque C, et al. Frontal hypoactivation on functional magnetic resonance imaging in working memory after severe diffuse traumatic brain injury. J Neurotrauma 2008;25:479–94.

55. Soeda A, Nakashima T, Okumura A, et al. Cognitive impairment after traumatic brain injury: a functional magnetic resonance imaging study using the Stroop task. Neuroradiology 2005;47:501–6.

56. Maruishi M, Miyatani M, Nakao T, et al. Compensatory cortical activation during performance of an attention task by patients with diffuse axonal injury: a functional magnetic resonance imaging study. J Neurol Neurosurg Psychiatry 2007;78: 168–73.

57. Fischer BL, Parsons M, Durgerian S, et al. Neural activation during response inhibition differentiates blast from mechanical causes of mild to moderate traumatic brain injury. J Neurotrauma 2014;31: 169–79.

58. Smits M, Dippel DW, Houston GC, et al. Postconcussion syndrome after minor head injury: brain

activation of working memory and attention. Hum Brain Mapp 2009;30:2789–803.

59. Chen CJ, Wu CH, Liao YP, et al. Working memory in patients with mild traumatic brain injury: functional MR imaging analysis. Radiology 2012;264: 844–51.

60. Slobounov SM, Gay M, Zhang K, et al. Alteration of brain functional network at rest and in response to YMCA physical stress test in concussed athletes: RsFMRI study. Neuroimage 2011;55:1716–27.

61. Witt ST, Lovejoy DW, Pearlson GD, et al. Decreased prefrontal cortex activity in mild traumatic brain injury during performance of an auditory oddball task. Brain Imaging Behav 2010;4:232–47.

62. Bryer EJ, Medaglia JD, Rostami S, et al. Neural recruitment after mild traumatic brain injury is task dependent: a meta-analysis. J Int Neuropsychol Soc 2013;19:751–62.

63. Biswal B, Yetkin FZ, Haughton VM, et al. Functional connectivity in the motor cortex of resting human brain using echo-planar MRI. Magn Reson Med 1995;34:537–41.

64. Sporns O. The human connectome: a complex network. Ann N Y Acad Sci 2011;1224:109–25.

65. van den Heuvel MP, Hulshoff Pol HE. Exploring the brain network: a review on resting-state fMRI functional connectivity. Eur Neuropsychopharmacol 2010;20:519–34.

66. Calhoun VD, Liu J, Adali T. A review of group ICA for fMRI data and ICA for joint inference of imaging, genetic, and ERP data. Neuroimage 2009;45: S163–72.

67. Raichle ME. Two views of brain function. Trends Cogn Sci 2010;14:180–90.

68. Marquez de la Plata CD, Garces J, Shokri Kojori E, et al. Deficits in functional connectivity of hippocampal and frontal lobe circuits after traumatic axonal injury. Arch Neurol 2011;68:74–84.

69. Kasahara M, Menon DK, Salmond CH, et al. Altered functional connectivity in the motor network after traumatic brain injury. Neurology 2010;75: 168–76.

70. Shumskaya E, Andriessen TM, Norris DG, et al. Abnormal whole-brain functional networks in homogeneous acute mild traumatic brain injury. Neurology 2012;79:176–82.

71. Tang L, Ge Y, Sodickson DK, et al. Thalamic resting-state functional networks: disruption in patients with mild traumatic brain injury. Radiology 2011;260:831–40.

72. Mayer AR, Mannell MV, Ling J, et al. Functional connectivity in mild traumatic brain injury. Hum Brain Mapp 2011;32:1825–35.

73. Hillary FG, Slocomb J, Hills EC, et al. Changes in resting connectivity during recovery from severe traumatic brain injury. Int J Psychophysiol 2011; 82:115–23.

74. Sours C, Zhuo J, Janowich J, et al. Default mode network interference in mild traumatic brain injury - A pilot resting state study. Brain Res 2013;1537: 201–15.

75. Sharp DJ, Beckmann CF, Greenwood R, et al. Default mode network functional and structural connectivity after traumatic brain injury. Brain 2011;134:2233–47.

76. Kim J, Whyte J, Patel S, et al. Resting cerebral blood flow alterations in chronic traumatic brain injury: an arterial spin labeling perfusion FMRI study. J Neurotrauma 2010;27:1399–411.

77. Ashwal S, Holshouser BA, Shu SK, et al. Predictive value of proton magnetic resonance spectroscopy in pediatric closed head injury. Pediatr Neurol 2000;23:114–25.

78. Garnett MR, Blamire AM, Corkill RG, et al. Early proton magnetic resonance spectroscopy in normal-appearing brain correlates with outcome in patients following traumatic brain injury. Brain 2000;123(Pt 10):2046–54.

79. Govind V, Gold S, Kaliannan K, et al. Whole-brain proton MR spectroscopic imaging of mild-to-moderate traumatic brain injury and correlation with neuropsychological deficits. J Neurotrauma 2010;27:483–96.

80. Babikian T, Marion SD, Copeland S, et al. Metabolic levels in the corpus callosum and their structural and behavioral correlates after moderate to severe pediatric TBI. J Neurotrauma 2010;27: 473–81.

81. Friedman SD, Brooks WM, Jung RE, et al. Proton MR spectroscopic findings correspond to neuropsychological function in traumatic brain injury. AJNR Am J Neuroradiol 1998;19:1879–85.

82. Friedman SD, Brooks WM, Jung RE, et al. Quantitative proton MRS predicts outcome after traumatic brain injury. Neurology 1999;52:1384–91.

83. Gasparovic C, Yeo R, Mannell M, et al. Neurometabolite concentrations in gray and white matter in mild traumatic brain injury: an 1H-magnetic resonance spectroscopy study. J Neurotrauma 2009; 26:1635–43.

84. Kelly AB, Zimmerman RD, Snow RB, et al. Head trauma: comparison of MR and CT—experience in 100 patients. AJNR Am J Neuroradiol 1988;9: 699–708.

85. Ahmadi J, Destian S. Head trauma. Top Magn Reson Imaging 1989;2(1):17–24.

86. Glauser J. Head injury: which patients need imaging? Which test is best? Cleve Clin J Med 2004;71: 353–7.

87. Gentry LR, Thompson B, Godersky JC. Traumatic brain stem injury: MR imaging. Radiology 1989; 171:177–87.

88. Gentry LR, Godersky JC, Thompson B. MR imaging of head trauma: review of the distribution and

radiopathologic features of traumatic lesions. AJR Am J Roentgenol 1988;150(3):663–72.

89. Gentry LR, Thompson B, Godersky JC. Trauma to the corpus callosum: MR features. AJNR Am J Neuroradiol 1988;9:1129–38.

90. Study Group on Head Injury of the Italian Society for Neurosurgery. Guidelines for minor head injured patients' management in adult age. J Neurosurg Sci 1996;40:11–5.

91. Vos PE, Battistin L, Birbamer G, et al. EFNS guideline on mild traumatic brain injury: report of an EFNS task force. Eur J Neurol 2002;9:207–19.

92. UK National Institute for Health and Clinical Excellence. Head injury. Triage, assessment, investigation and early management of head injury in infants, children and adults. Partial update of NICE clinical guideline 4 (June, 2003). 2007. Available at: http://www.nice.org.uk/nicemedia/pdf/CG56NI CEGuideline.pdf. Accessed June 12, 2008.

93. Fainardi E, Chieregato A, Antonelli V, et al. Time course of CT evolution in traumatic subarachnoid haemorrhage: a study of 141 patients. Acta Neurochir (Wien) 2004;146:257–63.

94. Ogawa T, Sekino H, Uzura M, et al. Comparative study of magnetic resonance and CT scan imaging in cases of severe head injury. Acta Neurochir Suppl (Wien) 1992;55:8–10.

95. Doezema D, King JN, Tandberg D, et al. Magnetic resonance imaging in minor head injury. Ann Emerg Med 1991;20:1281–5.

96. Maas A, Dearden M, Teasdale GM, et al. EBIC guidelines for management of severe head injury in adults. European Brain Injury Consortium. Acta Neurochir (Wien) 1997;139:286–94.

97. Servadei F, Murray GD, Penny K, et al. The value of the "worst" computed tomographic scan in clinical studies of moderate and severe head injury. European Brain Injury Consortium. Neurosurgery 2000;46:70–7.

98. Chang EF, Meeker M, Holland MC. Acute traumatic intraparenchymal hemorrhage: risk factors for progression in the early post-injury period. Neurosurgery 2006;58:647–56.

99. Narayan RK, Maas AI, Servadei F, et al. Progression of traumatic intracerebral hemorrhage: a prospective observational study. J Neurotrauma 2008;25:629–39.

100. Sifri ZC, Livingston DH, Lavery RF, et al. Value of repeat cranial computed axial tomography scanning in patients with minimal head injury. Am J Surg 2004;187:338–42.

101. Figg RE, Burry TS, Vander Kolk WE. Clinical efficacy of serial computed tomographic scanning in severe closed head injury patients. J Trauma 2003;55:1061–4.

102. Servadei F, Nasi MT, Giuliani G, et al. CT prognostic factors in acute subdural haematomas: the value of the 'worst' CT scan. Br J Neurosurg 2000;14:110–6.

103. Kent DL, Haynor DR, Longstreth WT Jr, et al. The clinical efficacy of magnetic resonance imaging in neuroimaging. Ann Intern Med 1994;120:856–71.

104. Provenzale JM. Imaging of traumatic brain injury: a review of the recent medical literature. AJR Am J Roentgenol 2010;194(1):16–9.

105. Lee H, Wintermark M, Gean AD, et al. Focal lesions in acute mild traumatic brain injury and neurocognitive outcome: CT versus 3T MRI. J Neurotrauma 2008;25:1049–56.

106. Smits M, Hunink MG, van Rijssel DA, et al. Outcome after complicated minor head injury. AJNR Am J Neuroradiol 2008;29:506–13.

107. Macpherson BC, Macpherson P, Jennett B. CT incidence of intracranial contusion and hematoma in relation to the presence, site and type of skull fracture. Clin Radiol 1990;42:321–6.

108. Leestma JE, Grčević N. Impact injuries to the brain and head. In: Leestma JE, Kirckpatrick JB, editors. Forensic neuropathology. New York: Raven Press; 1988. p. 409–16.

109. West OC, Mirvis SE, Shanmuganathan K. Transsphenoid basilar skull fracture: CT patterns. Radiology 1993;188(2):329–38.

110. Biffl WL, Moore EE, Offner PJ, et al. Blunt carotid and vertebral arterial injuries. World J Surg 2001; 25(8):1036–43.

111. Borczuk P. Mild head trauma. Emerg Med Clin North Am 1997;15:563–79.

112. Zimmerman RA, Bilaniuk LT. Computed tomographic staging of traumatic epidural bleeding. Radiology 1982;144(4):809–12.

113. Bullock MR, Chesnut R, Ghajar J, et al. Surgical management of acute epidural hematomas. Neurosurgery 2006;58(3):S2–7.

114. Gean AD, Fischbein NJ, Purcell DD, et al. Benign anterior temporal epidural hematoma: indolent lesion with a characteristic CT imaging appearance after blunt head trauma. Radiology 2010;257(1):212–8.

115. Al-Nakshabandi NA. The swirl sign. Radiology 2001;218(2):433.

116. Greenberg J, Cohen WA, Cooper PR. The "hyperacute" extraaxial intracranial hematoma: computed tomographic findings and clinical significance. Neurosurgery 1985;17(1):48–56.

117. Sullivan TP, Jarvik JG, Cohen WA. Follow-up of conservatively managed epidural hematomas: implications for timing of repeat CT. AJNR Am J Neuroradiol 1999;20:107–13.

118. Lowenhielm P. On the mechanism of cortical bridging vein rupture. Proceedings of the 1st IRCOBI B1 Conference. Amsterdam, The Netherlands, June 26–27, 1973. p. 423–9.

119. Schneider RC, Reifel E, Crisler HO. Serious and fatal neurosurgical football injuries. JAMA 1961;177:362.

120. Reed D, Robertson WD, Graeb DA, et al. Acute subdural hematomas: atypical CT findings. AJNR Am J Neuroradiol 1986;7:417–21.

121. Lee KS, Bae WK, Bae HG, et al. The computed tomographic attenuation and the age of subdural hematomas. J Korean Med Sci 1997;12:353–9.

122. Zumkeller M, Behrmann R, Heissler HE, et al. Computed tomographic criteria and survival rate for patients with acute subdural hematoma. Neurosurgery 1996;39:708–12.

123. Murray GD, Teasdale GM, Braakman R, et al. The European Brain Injury Consortium survey of head injuries. Acta Neurochir (Wien) 1999;141(3): 223–36.

124. Noguchi K, Ogawa T, Inugama A, et al. Acute subarachnoid hemorrhage: MR imaging with fluid attenuated inversion recovery pulse sequences. Radiology 1995;196:773–7.

125. Drew LB, Drew WE. The contrecoup-coup phenomenon. Neurocrit Care 2004;1(3):385–90.

126. Orrison WW, Gentry LR, Stimac GK, et al. Blinded comparison of cranial CT and MR in closed head injury evaluation. AJNR Am J Neuroradiol 1994; 15:351–6.

127. Beaumont A, Gennarelli T. CT prediction of contusion evolution after closed head injury: the role of pericontusional edema. Acta Neurochir Suppl 2006;96:30–2.

128. Yamaki T, Hirakawa K, Uequchi T, et al. Chronological evaluation of acute traumatic intracerebral haematoma. Acta Neurochir (Wien) 1990;103(3–4): 112–5.

129. Galloway NR, Tong KA, Ashwal S, et al. Diffusion-weighted imaging improves outcome prediction in pediatric traumatic brain injury. J Neurotrauma 2008;25:1153–62.

130. Schaefer PW, Huisman TA, Sorensen AG, et al. Diffusion-weighted MR imaging in closed head injury: high correlation with initial Glasgow coma scale score and score on modified Rankin scale at discharge. Radiology 2004;233:58–66.

131. Schroder ML, Muizelaar JP, Bullock MR, et al. Focal ischemia due to traumatic contusions documented by stable xenon-CT and ultrastructural studies. J Neurosurg 1995;82:966–71.

132. Parizel PM, Ozsarlak O, Van Goethem JW, et al. Imaging findings in diffuse axonal injury after closed head trauma. Eur Radiol 1998;8(6):960–5.

133. Smith DH, Meaney DF, Shull WH. Diffuse axonal injury in head trauma. J Head Trauma Rehabil 2003;18(4):307–16.

134. Adams JH, Graham DI, Gennarelli TA. Head injury in man and experimental animals: neuropathology. Acta Neurochir Suppl (Wien) 1983;32:15–30.

135. Adams H, Mitchell DE, Graham DI, et al. Diffuse brain damage of immediate impact type. Its relationship to 'primary brain-stem damage' in head injury. Brain 1977;100(3):489–502.

136. Haacke EM, Mittal S, Wu Z, et al. Susceptibility-weighted imaging. Part 1. Technical aspects and clinical applications. AJNR Am J Neuroradiol 2009;30:19–30.

137. Scheid R, Ott DV, Roth H, et al. Comparative magnetic resonance imaging at 1.5 and 3 Tesla for the evaluation of traumatic microbleeds. J Neurotrauma 2007;24:1811–6.

138. Akiyama Y, Miyata K, Harada K, et al. Susceptibility-weighted magnetic resonance imaging for the detection of cerebral microhemorrhage in patients with traumatic brain injury. Neurol Med Chir (Tokyo) 2009;49:97–9.

139. Bodanapally UK, Shanmuganathan K, Saksobhavivat N, et al. MR imaging and differentiation of cerebral fat embolism syndrome from diffuse axonal injury: application of diffusion tensor imaging. Neuroradiology 2013;55(6):771–8.

140. Firsching R, Woischneck D, Diedrich M, et al. Early magnetic resonance imaging of brain stem lesions after severe head injury. J Neurosurg 1998;89: 707–12.

141. Hashimoto T, Nakamura N, Richard KE, et al. Primary brain stem lesions caused by closed head injury. Neurosurg Rev 1993;16:291–8.

142. Shibita Y, Matsumura A, Meguro K, et al. Differentiation of mechanism and prognosis of traumatic brain stem lesions detected by magnetic resonance imaging in the acute stage. Clin Neurol Neurosurg 2000;102:124–8.

143. Rothfus WE, Goldberg AL, Tabas JH, et al. Callosomarginal infarction secondary to transfalcial herniation. AJNR Am J Neuroradiol 1987;8:1073–6.

144. Wernick S, Wells RG. Sequelae of temporal lobe herniation: MR imaging. J Comput Assist Tomogr 1989;13:323–5.

145. Mirvis SE, Wolf AL, Numaguchi Y, et al. Posttraumatic cerebral infarction diagnosed by CT: prevalence, origin, and outcome. AJR Am J Roentgenol 1990;154:1293–8.

146. Lee B, Newberg A. Neuroimaging in traumatic brain imaging. NeuroRx 2005;2(2):372–83.

147. Johnson PL, Eckard DA, Chason DP, et al. Imaging of acquired cerebral herniations. Neuroimaging Clin North Am 2002;12:217–28.

148. Hahn FJ, Gurney J. CT signs of central descending transtentorial herniation. AJNR Am J Neuroradiol 1985;6:844–5.

149. Feldmann E, Gandy SE, Becker R, et al. MRI demonstrates descending transtentorial herniation. Neurology 1988;38:697–701.

Easily Missed Fractures of the Upper Extremity

Scott Tyson, MD, Stephen F. Hatem, MD*

KEYWORDS

- Fracture • Upper extremity • Missed diagnosis • Diagnostic error

KEY POINTS

- Radiographs remain the mainstay for fracture assessment; their assessment remains challenging.
- Error rates can decrease by review of missed fractures.
- Three categories of challenging injuries are reviewed: common but challenging; out of mind, out of sight; and satisfaction of search.

INTRODUCTION

Interpretation of radiographs may not have the glamour of newer, high-tech imaging techniques, but remains the staple in the evaluation for acute orthopedic injury. It is difficult: experimental studies spanning a half century have consistently documented a roughly 30% error rate in radiographic interpretation.[1] "Misses" may result in a delay in diagnosis, increased patient pain and suffering, and delay in appropriate therapy.[2] Detriment may not be limited to the patient; in addition to emotional angst, disbelief, and self-doubt, radiologists may be faced with a claim of malpractice. In a recent review of closed malpractice claims in the United States, radiology was the sixth most frequent specialty despite making up less than 5% of United States physicians.[3] Nearly 3 out of 4 claims against diagnostic radiologists cite errors in interpretation resulting in missed diagnoses.[1] A 2013 study found that claims against radiologists related to an error in diagnosis outpaced the next most common cause by nearly 10-fold.[3]

Interpretation errors in radiology can broadly be classified into 2 categories: cognitive and perceptual. Cognitive errors might be owing to a lack of knowledge or mistaken judgment, for example, and are the minority. Perceptual errors, in which an abnormality is simply not seen, account for up to 80% of radiologic errors.[4] Perceptual errors in the identification of fractures are related to many factors, including not just the subtlety of the finding,[2,5] but the amount of clinical information available,[1] technical factors such as the quality of the images and the views obtained,[1] and poorly understood factors seemingly inherent to "human nature."[5]

Given that diagnostic errors in skeletal radiology, along with mammography, are the leading causes of claims against radiologists,[1,3] it is unsurprising that missed fractures are a particular problem in emergency and trauma care. A recent Canadian study showed that fractures accounted for 70% of missed injuries in a level 1 trauma center.[6] Another study has shown emergency physicians' radiographic interpretations for fracture had an 8% false-negative rate.[7] Missed fractures also were the most common discrepancy upon staff review of radiology resident interpretations for the emergency department, accounting for 62.5% in a recent study.[8] This is in keeping with other studies, which have shown that 70% of missed fractures are identifiable in retrospect.[2] In addition, radiologists may change their own interpretations up to 20% of the time.[9] These observations suggest that there may be ways to improve performance, and a recent study has shown just that: Itri and colleagues[10] were able to decrease

Department of Radiology, Imaging Institute, Cleveland Clinic, 9500 Euclid Avenue, Desk A-21, Cleveland, OH 44195, USA
* Corresponding author.
E-mail address: Hatems@ccf.org

Radiol Clin N Am 53 (2015) 717–736
http://dx.doi.org/10.1016/j.rcl.2015.02.013

resident misinterpretation of musculoskeletal emergency films at the Hospital of the University of Pennsylvania after giving a series of upper and lower extremity focused missed case conferences. In 1 year, resident misinterpretations of shoulder and elbow injuries decreased by 80%.[10]

We prefer to think of this as cognitive training to minimize perceptual error: it is easier to see what you know to look for, and easy to miss what you do not. Knowledge of what is missed is paramount, because it allows the generalization of what one learns from his own errors to others. Thankfully, there is a wealth of quality information available on missed fractures in the emergency department, whether by emergency physicians, radiology residents, or staff radiologists. With respect to the subject at hand, upper extremity fractures consistently have accounted for just under one-half (43%–48%) of all missed fractures independent of the group of readers investigated.[2,7,8] A closer look at these studies provides a road map both for what to look for when interpreting films and for this review, with the goal of minimizing errors.

The Wei and colleagues[2] study included more than 3000 extremity fractures. One hundred fifteen missed fractures were identified for an overall missed fracture rate of 3.7%, in keeping with other reports.[4] Subtlety (37%) and imperceptibility (33%) were by far the most common reasons. Less common reasons were obscuring devices and artifacts, multiplicity, osteoporosis, lack of clinical information, and poor technique. It is noteworthy that 5% of the misses were later diagnosed using specialized views, underscoring the importance of knowing how to supplement or tailor the radiographic study to the question at hand. The rate of missed extremity fractures was similar between the upper and lower extremity. Nearly one-third (30.4%) of all missed extremity fractures were in the hand and wrist, and these sites accounted for nearly 2 out of 3 (65%) of missed upper extremity fractures. Per anatomic site, however, fractures were most likely to be missed in the following order: elbow (6.0%) more often than hand (5.4%) more often than wrist (4.1%) more often than shoulder (1.9%).

Of upper extremity fractures missed even on retrospective review, the distal radius was the most common site. Including missed proximal radius fractures at the elbow, the radius alone accounted for one-third of missed diagnoses. Other retrospectively missed upper extremity fracture sites included the clavicle, humeral head, distal humerus, olecranon, scaphoid, hamate, trapezium, ulnar styloid, and phalanges.

Similar results were reported by Kung and colleagues.[8] Fractures were missed by radiology residents in the upper extremity in 1.6% of patients, slightly more than in the lower extremity. The radius as a whole accounted for one-half (50%) of these, split between the head and distally. Sixty-four percent were in the hand and wrist, with other sites of misses including the clavicle, humerus, triquetrum, metacarpals, and phalanges. Misinterpretation of hand and wrist films for fracture was also the leading cause of misdiagnosis in a study of emergency physician interpretations.[7]

In addition to this foreknowledge of the injuries likely to be missed on radiographs, optimizing clinical information, radiographic technique, and views are all important to improving diagnostic performance. In each, the radiology technologist can play a valuable role. With adequate clinical history and high-quality images, attention can be directed to the basics of fracture evaluation at the appropriate sites: cortical disruption, buckling, or crimping; lucent fracture lines; sclerotic fracture lines (overlap, impaction, or intramedullary callus); and double densities owing to overlap by displaced fragments. Careful attention to soft tissue findings such as swelling, laceration, or effusion can direct attention to the injured area.

Our review of easily missed upper extremity fractures in adults emphasizes the following 3 categories of pitfalls, with particular attention to their epidemiology, imaging findings, and optimal radiographic evaluation:

- "Common but challenging": we know to look for it but the findings may be subtle
- "Out of mind, out of sight": the uncommon injuries that are beyond the normal search pattern and hence, "out of mind"
- "Satisfaction of search": the less common or more diagnostically challenging injuries that occur in association with more obvious ones.

COMMON BUT CHALLENGING
Isolated Fracture of the Greater Tuberosity of the Humerus

Almost one-half of all humeral fractures involve the proximal humerus, with isolated greater tuberosity fractures comprising about 20% of all proximal humeral fractures (**Fig. 1**).[11,12] Unlike other proximal humerus fractures, which generally affect older populations with medical comorbidities, isolated greater tuberosity fractures tend to affect younger, healthier patients. In a reported series of 610 proximal humeral fractures, Kim and colleagues[13] compared demographics of patients with isolated greater tuberosity fractures with all other proximal humerus fractures, and showed that mean age

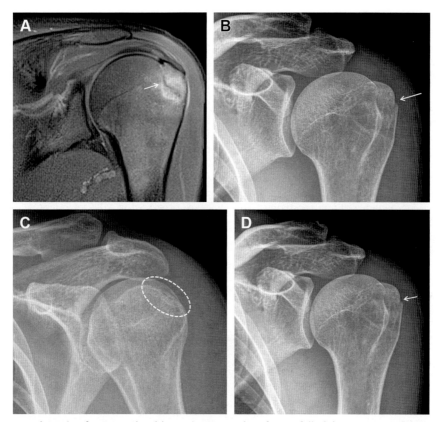

Fig. 1. **Greater tuberosity fracture**. Shoulder pain 2 months after a fall. (*A*) Fat-suppressed proton density weighted oblique coronal MR imaging and (*B*) true anteroposterior (AP) view with external rotation. Initial (*C*) AP internal rotation and (*D*) true AP external rotation radiographs. MR imaging (*A*) obtained to evaluate for rotator cuff tear shows nondisplaced linear fracture (*arrow*) of the greater tuberosity with surrounding bone marrow edema. (*B*) True AP shoulder radiograph with external rotation of the humerus confirmed the fracture (*arrow*) with typical resorption about the fracture in the subacute phase of healing. (*C, D*) Initially interpreted as normal, in retrospect subtle greater tuberosity fracture with cortical disruption (*arrow*) is more apparent on the external rotation view with the greater tuberosity seen in profile. In internal rotation, there is a very subtle double density (*dashed oval*).

(42.8 years greater tuberosity fractures vs 54.2 years all others) differed significantly.

Traditionally, greater tuberosity fractures have been described as either impaction or shear/avulsion injuries.[11,14] Impaction may result from direct trauma to the tuberosity or from impaction against the acromion or superior glenoid with the arm in hyperabduction. Shear/avulsion injury typically occurs in association with anterior glenohumeral dislocation. As the humeral head is displaced forward, the rotator cuff counteracts this force, resulting in avulsion of the greater tuberosity.

Despite being a well-recognized clinical entity, isolated greater tuberosity fractures are missed commonly. Ogawa and colleagues[15] reported a series in which 58 of 99 shoulders (59%) with confirmed isolated fracture of the greater tuberosity that had been overlooked initially. The majority of these were isolated to the supraspinatus facet.[15] The failure to recognize the fracture initially can lead the clinician to an alternative and incorrect diagnosis, and ultimately lead to a poor clinical outcome. Nondisplaced greater tuberosity fractures are not uncommonly diagnosed on MR imaging obtained for suspected posttraumatic rotator cuff tear, owing to pain at the greater tuberosity and with abduction.[16] When a greater tuberosity fracture is identified, treatment is guided by the amount of displacement of the fracture fragment. Although guidelines vary, most authors advocate for surgical treatment for fractures displaced by greater than 5 mm in the general population, and by greater than 3 mm in younger patients and athletes.[14,17]

Evaluation of acute shoulder injury typically culminates with radiographic examination. Because the greater tuberosity overlaps the humeral head on the internal rotation anteroposterior (AP) view, an external rotation AP projection is important to evaluate the greater tuberosity tangentially, separate from the humeral head.[18] Because pain in the acute setting may preclude external rotation occasionally, Ogawa and colleagues[15] advocate for a true lateral view for evaluation of the greater tuberosity.

Nondisplaced Radial Head or Neck Fracture

The majority of elbow fractures in the adult patient are radial head and neck fractures, comprising approximately 33% to 50% of elbow fractures, about one-half of which are nondisplaced (**Fig. 2**).[19] As a result, they are easily missed, which can lead to increased patient morbidity. The typical mechanism is a fall on an outstretched hand resulting in axial loading and valgus stress with radiocapitellar impaction.[20]

Because AP and flexed lateral radiographs alone have a high rate of missed elbow fracture in acute trauma, obtaining additional views has been emphasized, including internal and external obliques as well as the radial head–capitellum view.[21–23] Although there are a few published studies that question the usefulness of additional views of the elbow,[24] most authors support either routine or selected use of supplemental views in the setting of acute injury. In a small series by Grundy and colleagues,[22] the radial head–capitellum view yielded the diagnosis of radial head fracture when the traditional AP and lateral views did not in 21% of patients. These results validated an earlier study by Greenspan and colleagues,[23] which demonstrated additional diagnostic information regarding fracture presence or extent in 20% of patients. Because the treatment of radial head fractures depends on not only confirmation of the fracture, but also on accurate characterization of the fracture, in our practice we routinely obtain oblique and radial head–capitellum views in the setting of trauma when a joint effusion is identified on a routine AP and lateral series.

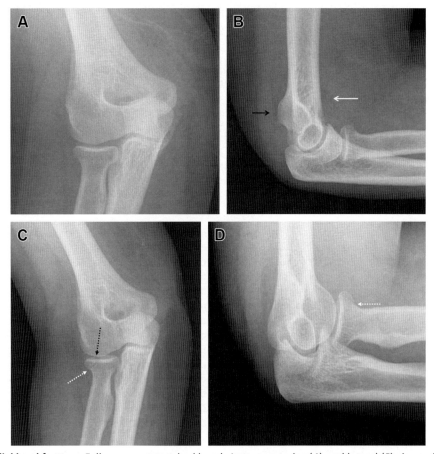

Fig. 2. Radial head fracture. Fall on an outstretched hand. Anteroposterior (*A*) and lateral (*B*) views of the elbow are normal except for the subtle visualization of the uplifted posterior fat pad (*black arrow*), and "sail sign" of an uplifted anterior fat pad (*white arrow*). Subsequent external oblique (*C*) and radial head–capitellar (*D*) views show the intraarticular fracture line (*dashed black arrow*) of the radial head and crimped radial neck (*dashed white arrow*).

Elbow joint effusion in the setting of trauma, as demonstrated on the lateral view by visualization of the posterior fat pad and/or an elevated anterior fat pad, traditionally is considered pathognomic for acute bony injury.[25,26] Recent studies with MR imaging have confirmed fat pad displacement to be a sensitive sign of bony injury (95%) and occult fracture.[27] Thus, after an elbow injury, recognition of a displaced fat pad should prompt further inquiry, including additional careful review of routinely obtained radiographs, obtaining additional views, or obtaining short interval follow-up radiographs. Although MR imaging is typically not used in the acute evaluation of isolated radial head fracture, it is the diagnostic test of choice to characterize comprehensively all coexistent injuries in the traumatic setting.[27]

Distal Radius Fracture

Fractures of the distal radius are the most common fracture of the skeleton and account for an estimated 1 of every 6 acute fractures in the emergency setting (**Fig. 3**).[28] The most common mechanism is a fall on an outstretched hand, particularly in younger patients.[29] In the setting of acute trauma, a routine wrist radiographic series includes posteroanterior (PA), lateral, and pronated oblique views. Although the majority of distal radius fractures are not challenging in terms of identification, nondisplaced fractures, particularly of the radial styloid, are occasionally the exception.

The radial styloid fracture is an oblique fracture, usually extending to the articular surface at the radiocarpal joint; colloquially, it is known as the chauffeur fracture. It is the result of axial loading or direct blow. Although these fractures are often displaced owing to pull from strong radiocarpal ligaments,[30] occasionally they can be nondisplaced and subtle or imperceptible.

Although there are several proposed classification systems regarding distal radial fractures, none are accepted universally. Indeed, it has been shown that interobserver variance between radiologists and orthopedists in fracture classification is poor.[31] In this light, we prefer a detailed description of the fracture with reporting of salient features: fracture location and extent, accurate characterization of the amount of displacement of the articular component, degree of comminution, and identification of coexisting injuries. In particular, the degree of articular displacement has important treatment implications. Prior studies have shown that greater than 2 mm of intraarticular fracture displacement is associated with a high incidence of posttraumatic osteoarthritis.[32]

Scaphoid Fractures

The scaphoid fracture is the most common carpal fracture (**Fig. 4**).[33] It is also one of the most commonly missed fractures.[34] As the primary osseous limiter to wrist extension, a fall on an outstretched hand with resultant hyperextension translates excessive force across the scaphoid, leading to injury.[34] With up to 20% of scaphoid fractures occult radiographically, the diagnosis is often delayed, leading to an increased incidence of avascular necrosis (AVN), malunion, and nonunion.[35]

Scaphoid fractures are generally described by their anatomic location; 60% to 70% involve the scaphoid waist, 15% the proximal pole, 10% the distal pole, and 8% the distal articular surface.[36] The primary blood supply to the scaphoid is via dorsal branches arising from the radial artery entering at the scaphoid waist.[31] Thus, blood supply to the proximal pole is vulnerable. The incidence of AVN after scaphoid fracture is 30% after fractures through the middle third of scaphoid, increasing to nearly 100% after fracture through the proximal fifth.[31,33] Displacement of fracture fragments also increases the risk of AVN. For similar reasons, tenuous blood supply of the proximal scaphoid contributes to lengthier healing times following acute fracture and increases the propensity for delayed healing or nonunion. Although beyond the scope of this discussion, MR imaging in particular has been considered an important tool for early detection of both scaphoid fractures and AVN, with the goal of minimizing the risk of, and sequelae from, AVN.[31]

As with the distal radius, radiographic evaluation begins with PA, lateral, and oblique views of the wrist, with the addition of a "scaphoid view" when clinical signs (anatomic snuffbox tenderness) and history alert the clinician to possible scaphoid fracture. The scaphoid view is a PA radiograph of the wrist centered over the scaphoid with the wrist in ulnar deviation. This view reduces the palmar flexion and foreshortening of the scaphoid seen on neutral views, improving visualization, especially of the waist, and likely increasing sensitivity of fracture identification. The presence of displacement and/or edema of the scaphoid fat stripe along its radial aspect has been advocated by some as a useful sign of occult scaphoid fracture,[37] although this has been brought into question, because others have shown it to be a poor predictor of underlying pathology.[38]

In the setting of wrist injury and anatomic snuff box tenderness, it cannot be overemphasized that negative radiographs do not preclude scaphoid fracture. Most commonly, radiographic

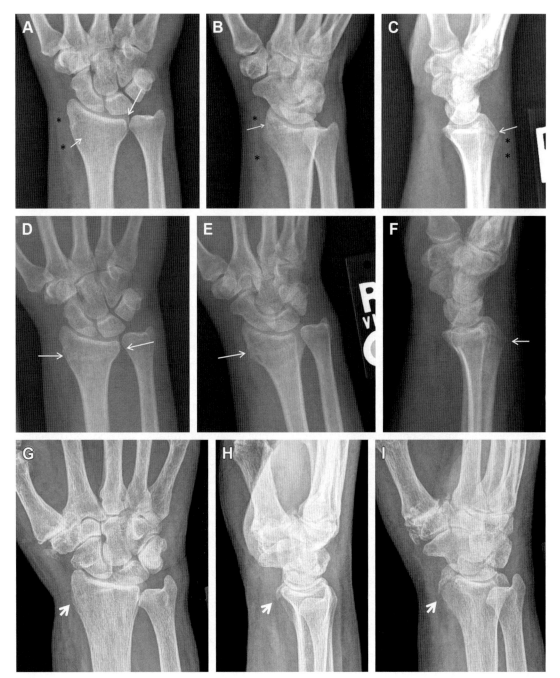

Fig. 3. **Distal radius fracture**. (*A–F*) 57F with radial styloid tenderness after falling on an outstretched hand. (*A–C*) Posteroanterior (PA), oblique, and lateral wrist radiographs at the time of presentation show very subtle soft tissue swelling (*) and hairline fracture (*white arrows*). (*D–F*) PA, oblique, and lateral wrist radiographs 2 weeks later. The fracture (*arrows*) is now readily apparent as a mixed lucent and sclerotic line owing to intramedullary callus deposition. (*G–I*) Different patient. Radial styloid fracture (*thick white arrows*) is barely perceptible on PA (*G*) and lateral (*H*) views, but is better seen on oblique (*I*).

follow-up is obtained for at least 2, and up to 6 weeks, after injury. Some authors have advocated for early MR imaging[39] or CT[40] to speed conclusive diagnosis.

Volar Plate Fractures

The volar plate is a fibrous structure at the volar aspect of the joint capsule at each

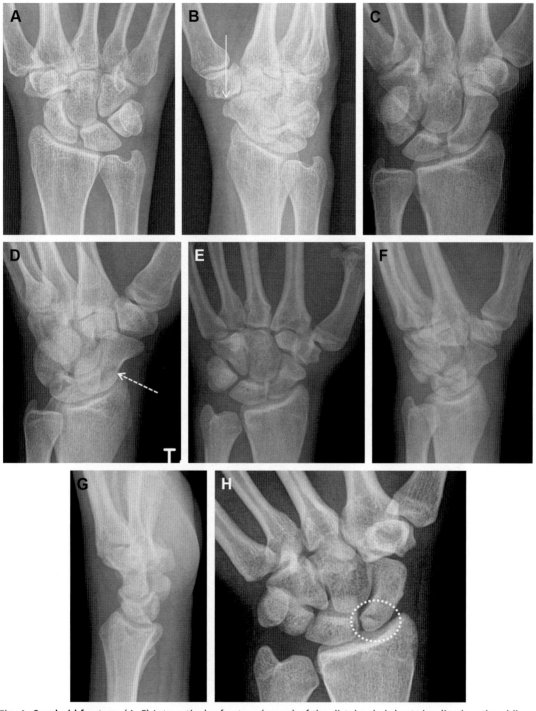

Fig. 4. Scaphoid fracture. (*A, B*) Intraarticular fracture (*arrow*) of the distal pole is best visualized on the oblique view (*B*). (*C, D*) Scaphoid waist fracture (*dashed arrow*) in a different patient is visualized on the oblique view (*D*) only. (*E–H*) In a third patient, proximal pole fracture (*dotted circle*) is not seen on the routine series (*E–G*), but only the dedicated scaphoid view in ulnar deviation (*H*).

metacarpophalangeal and interphalangeal joint space (**Fig. 5**). It serves to prevent hyperextension.[41] The distal aspect of the volar plate is characterized by a dense fibrocartilaginous component centrally that attaches to the volar base of the phalanx. The lateral aspects of this distal attachment fuse with the fibers of the accessory collateral ligaments.[41] During acute

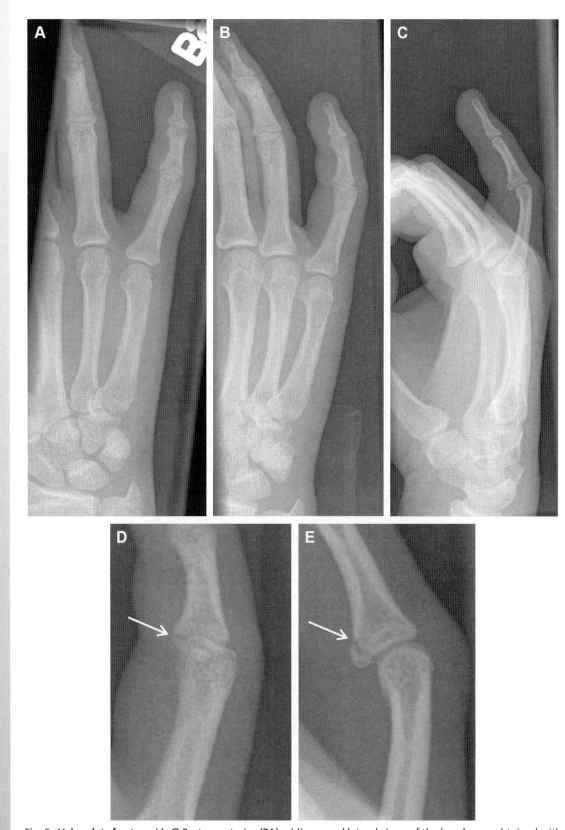

Fig. 5. **Volar plate fracture**. (*A–C*) Posteroanterior (PA), oblique, and lateral views of the hand were obtained with attention to the little finger. Soft tissue swelling directs attention to the proximal interphalangeal joint. The volar plate fracture is difficult to visualize on the PA view owing to its position and characteristic mild flexion resulting in overlapping structures. Magnified oblique (*D*) and lateral (*E*) views show the characteristic appearance of a volar plate fracture fragment (*white arrow*) as a bony sliver of the radial aspect of the articular surface of the base of the middle phalanx on the oblique view (*D*) and as a small volar triangle on the lateral view (*E*). Commonly, the fracture is only seen on either the oblique or lateral; both need careful inspection.

hyperextension, a distal volar plate injury can result in avulsion of the adjacent osseous attachment. Because there is almost always an ulnar component to the force, radial-sided avulsions predominate. In a series of 58 proximal interphalangeal joint volar plate fractures by Nance and colleagues,[41] the majority of the patients (76%) were under the age of 30. Of the volar plate fractures in this series, 51% were sports-related injuries.

Although the presence of a volar plate injury is typically readily apparent clinically, radiographs are performed to evaluate for an associated avulsion fracture. Complications related to volar plate fracture include posttraumatic osteoarthritis, flexion contraction/deformity, and joint instability. AP, lateral, and pronated oblique views should be performed when a volar plate injury is suspected. In the series by Nance and colleagues, approximately two-thirds of the fractures were best seen on the lateral view, and one-third best seen on the oblique view, which best shows the volar radial attachment site to the base of the middle phalanx.

OUT OF MIND, OUT OF SIGHT
Scapula Fractures

Scapula fractures are uncommon entities, representing only up to 1% of all fractures, and typically occur in association with other injuries in the setting of high energy trauma (**Fig. 6**).[42] As such, they have the potential to be missed:

1 Owing to satisfaction of search when other more obvious injuries are identified
2 When only peripherally imaged directly in the acute trauma patient on other studies, such as a chest x-ray
3 When the scapula or shoulder is the primary area of concern but are not associated with a high-energy traumatic injury.

Preferred radiologic evaluation begins with true AP and lateral scapular views to evaluate the glenoid rim and neck, scapular body, acromion, and coracoid, although not uncommonly only shoulder films are requested. As with greater tuberosity fractures, scapular fractures are increasingly identified as unsuspected injuries on shoulder MR imaging.

The scapula is a complex bone, consisting of an articular component, the glenoid, and an unusually shaped body component to which muscles of the shoulder girdle attach. The combination of the complex geometry, obscuring adjacent structures, and the rarity of fracture contribute to the difficulty in detection of a scapular fracture. To add to this challenge, there are noteworthy anatomic variations that are confused easily with a scapula fracture, particularly in the young adult population most likely to suffer athletic or vehicular trauma. Basic awareness of the ossification pattern of the scapula is important to keep from mistaking epiphyseal lines for fractures, especially at the acromion and coracoid. What is more, the ossification centers may be asymmetric, rendering comparison films less useful, do not appear and fuse until

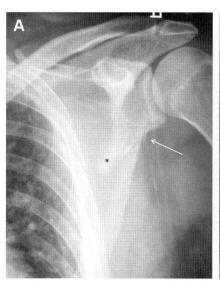
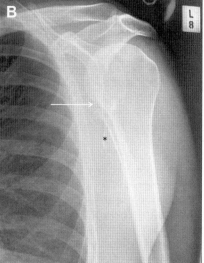

Fig. 6. **Scapula fracture.** Anteroposterior (AP; *A*) and lateral (*B*) views of the scapula. (*A*) The predominant finding on the AP is the V-shaped increased radiodensity owing to overlying fragments (*). Small cortical fragment (*arrow*) is present at the inferior scapular neck. Cortical disruption (*arrow*) and displaced fragment (*) are difficult to visualize through overlying humerus.

late adolescence and young adulthood, and may remain unfused throughout adulthood. There are 2 to 3 acromial ossification centers that become apparent radiographically in the mid teenage years, and coalesce and fuse to the scapula spine by the age of 20 to 25 years.[43] Failure of fusion results in an unfused accessory ossification center at the acromion, the os acromiale, which is seen in approximately 8% of the population.[44] Likewise, the glenoid fossa ossifies from the coracoid base, deep portion of the coracoid process, scapular body, and the lower scapular pole; from the teen years into young adulthood, the glenoid border may normally be irregular.[43] Although less commonly a radiologic quandary, the scapular inferior angle ossification center has a similarly late appearance and incorporation.

Coracoid Fractures

The coracoid process serves as a point of attachment for several myotendinous and ligamentous structures and provides additional anterosuperior stability to the glenohumeral joint (Fig. 7).[45] Coracoid fractures comprise 3% to 13% of all scapula fractures[46] and are frequently missed initially.[47] The mechanisms of fracture include a direct external force, contact from a dislocating humeral head, and avulsion by the short head of the biceps or coracobrachialis tendons. Coracoid base fractures are the most common type and are the result of a direct blow or anterior glenohumeral dislocation. Fracture lines may extend into the upper glenoid, and can be confused with an accessory ossification center, as discussed. They are nondisplaced typically and treated nonsurgically. Fractures of the coracoid at the tip are avulsion fractures, and are also typically treated nonsurgically, even in the setting of significant displacement.[45]

In addition to the scapula and shoulder radiographic views described, additional views such as the axillary view and Stryker view, in which the arm is abducted and the x-ray beam is centered on the coracoid process with 10° cephalad angulation, can better isolate the coracoid from adjacent osseous structures.[48] Weight bearing views in the setting of coexistent acromioclavicular separation may be helpful: the observation of a normal coracoclavicular distance in the setting of a high riding clavicle may be a clue to a coexistent coracoid fracture.[43] In the setting of continued shoulder pain following glenohumeral dislocation and reduction, follow-up radiographs to evaluate for missed coracoid fracture have been advocated,[49] although in our practice MR imaging is increasingly used for its ability to give a comprehensive review of both osseous and soft tissue integrity.

Acromion Fractures

The acromion has 3 roles[45]: (1) articulate with the clavicle, (2) serve as a myotendinous and ligamentous attachment site, and (3) provide posterosuperior stability to the glenohumeral joint (Fig. 8). Fractures of the acromion represent about 8% of all scapular fractures.[50] These fractures most commonly occur in young to middle-aged adults as a result of high-energy trauma, and are often associated with other shoulder injuries.[51] The acromion is most commonly injured via direct trauma; however, avulsion fractures and stress fractures have been reported.[43,51] In addition to the standard radiographic views discussed previously, the Rockwood view (AP with caudal x-ray beam angulation) can be a useful supplement, in particular for evaluation of the inferior aspect of the acromion and the subacromial space.[48]

As mentioned, the unfused acromial ossification center can simulate an acromial fracture. Radiographic findings that favor an os acromiale over a fracture include rounded borders, positioning at, or superior to, the level of the posterior acromion on the AP view, and bilaterality.[43]

Kuhn and colleagues[52] have proposed a classification system for acromial fractures, that although not used universally, is illustrative in terms of potential treatment implications. Nondisplaced (type I) and displaced fractures with preservation of the subacromial space (type II) are generally treated conservatively. Type III fractures narrow the subacromial space and are typically treated surgically.

Carpometacarpal Fracture Dislocation

The carpometacarpal (CMC) articulations are a series of interlocking joints consisting of curved and irregular articular surfaces. Dislocations at the CMC joints are generally a result of high-energy trauma, and commonly are associated with neurovascular injury (Fig. 9).[53] The injury pattern is generally that of dislocation with fracture involving the metacarpal bases, carpal bones, or both. Because of the undulating articular surfaces and overlap of structures on lateral radiographs, the CMCs are notoriously difficult to evaluate radiographically.[43] In general, CMC fracture–dislocations with minimally displaced fractures that are able to maintain reduction can be treated with splinting or closed reduction and internal fixation. However, closed reduction may prove difficult if delayed, demonstrating the importance of early diagnosis.[43]

Particular attention should be directed ulnarly. Simultaneous fourth and fifth CMC dislocations are often subtle and initially missed on standard

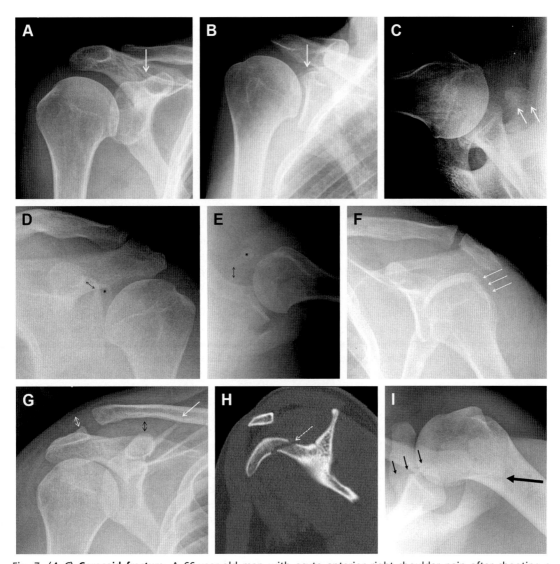

Fig. 7. (A–C) **Coracoid fracture**. A 66-year-old man with acute anterior right shoulder pain after shooting a shotgun. Coracoid base fracture (*white arrow*) is faintly visualized owing to oblique projection on the anteroposterior (AP) internal rotation view (A), overlapping structures on the true AP external rotation projection (B), but is nicely demonstrated on the axillary projection (C). (D–F) **Coracoid fracture and Hill–Sachs lesion**. Chronic shoulder pain with history of prior anterior dislocations. Coracoid process fracture fragment (*) is distracted anterolaterally (*double arrow*) and can be seen on the true AP external rotation (D) and axillary (E) views. It is obscured on the AP internal rotation (F) view, which profiles a Hill–Sachs lesion (*arrows*) of the humeral head in the typical posterolateral location. (G, H) **Coracoid fracture with acromioclavicular joint separation**. AP radiograph (G) shows acromioclavicular joint separation with downward displacement (*white double arrowhead*). A normal coracoclavicular distance (*black double arrowhead*) should prompt careful evaluation of the coracoid. An unusual spike of cortical bone (*white arrow*) parallel to the scapular spine represents medial extension of the coracoid fracture (*dashed white arrow*) readily seen on sagittal CT reconstruction (H). (I) **Coracoid and acromion ossification centers**. Acromion (*large black arrow*) and coracoid (*small black arrows*) ossification centers can both persist into young adulthood and can mimic fractures. A contralateral view can be helpful.

radiographs[54]; however, they are unstable injuries with potentially severe consequences to their misdiagnosis.[55] These dislocations are the most common of CMC dislocations and may occur after less severe trauma; a common mechanism is a punch against a hard surface.[55] We refer to these as "boxer fracture variants," to emphasize the importance of looking for these whenever a search for the ubiquitous fourth and/or fifth metacarpal "boxer's fractures" is negative.

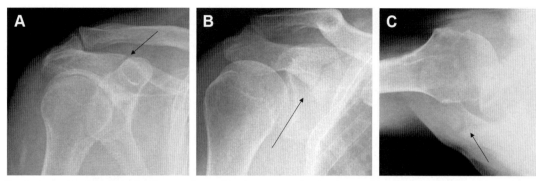

Fig. 8. Acromion fracture. The fracture (*arrow*) is almost completely obscured by the coracoid process on the anteroposterior (AP) internal rotation view (*A*), but can be visualized on the true AP (*B*) and axillary (*C*) projections.

A systematic approach as described by Fisher and colleagues[54] may increase identification of CMC fracture dislocations. On the AP view, careful assessment for interruption of the normally smoothly undulating and parallel articular surfaces (disrupted "parallel M" sign), joint space asymmetry, articular cortex disruption, and articular surface overlap are keys to identifying an abnormality.[54] The lateral view of the wrist demonstrates prominent dislocations at the CMC; however, owing to overlapping structures, more subtle subluxations can be missed easily. Particular attention should be directed to metacarpal angulation on the lateral projection: increased palmar angulation of the involved metacarpals is seen with the common dorsal dislocation.[56] On the PA view, subtle metacarpal angulation radially can be assessed by evaluating metacarpal convergence, as described by Hodgson and Shrewing.[55] In the normal patient, the long axes of the metacarpals ("the metacarpal cascade") converge to a point just proximal to the distal radius articular surface. With CMC dislocations, the cascade lines either do not converge to a single point, or the point of convergence is displaced.[55]

Because of the importance of early and clinically appropriate treatment, either clinical suspicion alone or identification of a CMC fracture dislocation on initial radiographs should prompt consideration of CT evaluation to characterize more fully the injury and look for associated injuries.[31] Associated fractures of the fourth metacarpal base, fifth metacarpal base, and/or hamate are often obscured on radiographs by overlapping structures and are better demonstrated on CT, analogous to tarsometatarsal Lisfranc injuries of the foot.

Hamate Fractures

Fractures of the hamate represent approximately 2% of all carpal fractures (**Fig. 10**)[57] and are generally categorized as either affecting the body or the hook. Fractures involving the hamate body are less common than hook fractures, with variable mechanisms of injury, including fourth and fifth CMC dislocation, as discussed. Nondisplaced fractures can typically be treated conservatively, whereas displaced and nonreducible fractures require operative intervention.[43] The hamate hook can be injured either via direct force or avulsion through the transverse carpal ligament.[58] These injuries can occur as a result of a fall on an outstretched hand but most commonly occur in the grasping athlete: baseball players, golfers, tennis players, and so on. Hook of hamate fractures often present as a subacute injury with persistent pain, but can occur acutely. In minimally displaced hook fractures, conservative therapy with immobilization is used typically, although the rate of delayed healing and nonunion is high (50%).[59,60] For displaced fractures or fractures associated with ulnar neuropathy, resection of the fracture fragment is often used rather than open reduction and internal fixation.[57]

Described findings on the PA view include failure to visualize the hook, indistinctness of its cortical margins, and sclerosis or double density.[61,62] Oblique views should be scrutinized carefully dorsally and distally for fractures of the body. Nonetheless, standard radiographs of the wrist or hand are often negative for fracture, because the hook and the body of the hamate overlap.[57]

Numerous supplemental views have been advocated for evaluation of the hamate. The carpal tunnel view nicely depicts the hook of the hamate axially without overlap from osseous structures, and is likely the most widely added. Other authors favor modified lateral projections to see the entirety of the hook longitudinally without overlapping structures: these include the 30° tilted lateral view with palmar abduction of the thumb[61] and a neutral lateral view with radial deviation of the wrist and thumb abduction.[63]

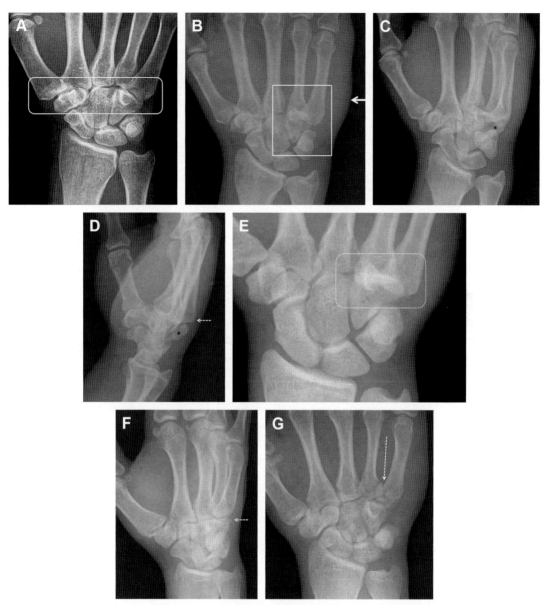

Fig. 9. Fracture dislocation of the fourth and fifth carpometacarpal joints. (*A*) Normal carpometacarpal joints (*box*) show smoothly undulating, parallel, and congruent articular surfaces. Posteroanterior (PA; *B*), oblique (*C*), and lateral (*D*) views of the wrist. Soft tissue swelling adjacent to the proximal fifth metacarpal (*white arrow*) directs attention to the fourth and fifth carpometacarpal joints (*white box*). The articular surfaces are overlapping owing to the coronally oriented, dorsally impacted shear fracture of the hamate (*) with double density on the PA and oblique views. A tiny fracture fragment is confirmed at the base of the fourth metacarpal (*dashed arrow, D*). Note characteristic volar angulation of the fourth and fifth metacarpals. (*E–G*) **Spectrum of Boxer's variant injuries.** (*E*) Dorsal dislocation of the fourth and fifth carpometacarpal joints without fracture (*box*), with hamate flake fracture (*short dashed arrow, F*), and intraarticular fourth metacarpal base fracture (*long dashed arrow, G*).

Triquetrum Fractures

Triquetrum fractures are the second most common carpal fracture following the scaphoid (approximately 15%; **Fig. 11**).[64,65] Dorsal triquetrum fractures are most commonly owing to avulsion from the attachments of dorsal radiocarpal

ligaments. Transverse or sagittal fractures of the triquetral body are far less common, but have been described in association with a variety of different mechanisms, including crush injuries and perilunate fracture dislocations.[57]

The routine wrist series is usually sufficient for fracture identification. Dorsal triquetrum fractures

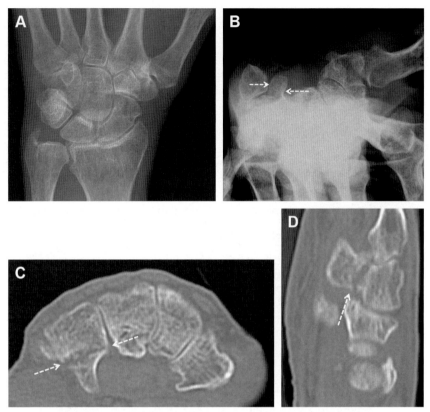

Fig. 10. Hamate fracture. Golfer with acute pain after striking the ball. Routine wrist series normal. Posteroanterior view shown (*A*). Carpal tunnel view faintly visualizes the transverse fracture of the hook (*dashed arrow*), as seen on follow-up CT (axial *C*, sagittal *D*).

typically are visualized clearly on the lateral view as a small osseous fragment dorsally with overlying soft tissue swelling. Fractures of the triquetrum body may be more challenging to identify because there is significant osseous overlap on the PA and lateral views. A 45° oblique radiograph can help to isolate the triquetrum from the adjacent pisiform, potentially improving fracture identification. Dorsal triquetrum fractures seldom require operative intervention; occasionally, symptomatic fractures

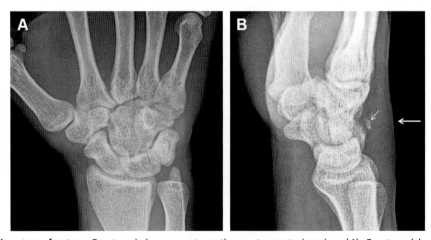

Fig. 11. Triquetrum fracture. Fracture is inapparent on the posteroanterior view (*A*). Fracture (*short arrow*) is only seen on the lateral view (*B*), with associated dorsal soft tissue swelling (*long arrow*).

may necessitate excision of the bone chip for symptomatic relief.[66]

SATISFACTION OF SEARCH
Fractures Associated with Glenohumeral Instability

Although the shoulder complex provides a remarkable range of motion for the upper extremity, this flexibility comes with a cost: the glenohumeral joint is the most frequently dislocated joint in the body (**Figs. 12** and **13**).[67] Concomitant injuries associated with glenohumeral dislocation include neurologic and vascular injury, injuries to the rotator cuff and glenoid labrum, and osseous injuries related to impaction, shear, and avulsive forces.[43,68] Although the goal of prereduction and postreduction radiographs is to diagnose a dislocation and confirm reduction, an important secondary objective is to evaluate for these associated injuries.[69] The humeral head, greater tuberosity, glenoid rim, acromion, and coracoid should be assessed carefully. The presence of these injuries has been associated with increased risk of recurrent dislocation.[69] Greater tuberosity, coracoid, and acromial fractures have been discussed elsewhere in this article; humeral head fractures and glenoid rim fractures are discussed subsequently.

Evaluation of acute suspected shoulder dislocation typically includes radiographic evaluation of the shoulder, and typically includes an AP view in internal rotation, true AP (Grashey view) in external rotation, a lateral (scapular Y) view, and often an axillary or modified axillary view.[48] Prereduction radiographs in the context of clinically obvious anterior shoulder dislocation may not always be necessary; some authors contend that they may be detrimental owing to increased time to reduction, additional radiation, and increased health care costs.[70,71] Shuster and colleagues[70] found that when an experienced emergency physician is confident of anterior shoulder dislocation, prereduction radiographs do not alter management.

In anterior dislocations, impaction of the posterolateral aspect of the humeral head on the anteroinferior glenoid and can result in an osteochondral humeral head fracture known as a Hill–Sachs lesion. In contradistinction, in posterior dislocations the anteromedial humeral head impacts on the posterior glenoid and may develop a reverse Hill–Sachs lesion. Both of these fractures can be seen on AP views, and are often apparent on axillary projections. A Hill–Sachs lesion is best depicted on the AP view with internal rotation of the humerus as an area with lateral notching or flattening of the normal, circular appearance of

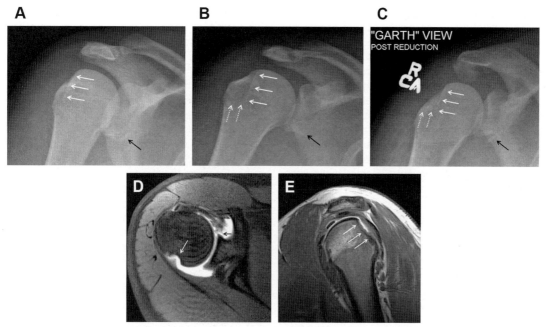

Fig. 12. Anterior dislocation sequelae of Hill–Sachs and Bankart lesions. The medial (*white arrows*) margin of the posterolateral impaction fracture (*white arrows, A-C*) of the humeral head is profiled on the internal rotation view (*A*). In external rotation (*B*) the inferior margin (*dotted white arrows*) of the V-shaped impaction is seen through overlying structures. Axial projections such as the Garth view (*C*) may also show the Hill–Sachs lesion (*dotted and solid white arrows*), but are particularly useful in identifying the osseous Bankart lesion (*black arrow*). Findings confirmed on subsequent MR arthrogram (*D*, axial fat-suppressed T1 and *E*, oblique sagittal T1 images).

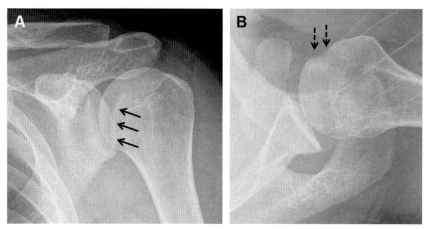

Fig. 13. Posterior dislocation sequelae of reverse Hill–Sachs lesion. History of prior posterior shoulder disloca-tions owing to seizures. (*A*) The anteroposterior view in external rotation shows a linear line of sclerosis (*arrows*) in the humeral head, the "trough sign," which roughly parallels the humeral head articular surface. The impac-tion fracture (*dashed arrows*) is profiled on the axillary projection (*B*).

the humeral head in this position. The trough sign of a reverse Hill–Sachs lesion describes a sclerotic line parallel and lateral to the articular surface of the humerus on the AP view with humeral external rotation.[69] Both of these fractures can worsen if the joint remains dislocated, as persistent muscle spasm can further exacerbate the impaction of the humeral head onto the glenoid.[43]

Owing to the same impaction mechanisms, asso-ciated fractures of the glenoid also occur. The osseous Bankart lesion describes such a lesion of the anterior inferior glenoid in the context of anterior shoulder dislocation.[72] The reverse osseous Bank-art lesion is the posterior glenoid fracture in the setting of posterior dislocation. Glenoid rim fracture fragments may be small, and, owing to overlapping structures, difficult to see radiographically.

Postreduction radiographs are important not just to verify reduction but to look for these fractures: some fractures in the setting of shoulder dislocation are seen only on the postreduction series.[73,74] Hen-dey and colleagues looked at 175 anterior shoulder dislocations and found 17 fractures (14 Hill–Sachs deformities, 2 Bankart fractures, and 1 greater tu-berosity fracture) that were seen only on the postre-duction views. In another study, Kahn and colleagues looked at 57 patients with anterior dislo-cations, and found that the although the majority of fractures associated with dislocation could be iden-tified on prereduction views, more than one-third of fractures (37.5%) were seen only after postreduction imaging.

Essex–Lopresti Fracture–Dislocation

The Essex–Lopresti injury involves fracture of the radial head with dislocation of the distal radioulnar joint (DRUJ; **Fig. 14**). As discussed, nondisplaced

radial head fractures can be extremely subtle. Radial head fractures associated with the Essex–Lopresti fracture dislocation usually are not; they are typically comminuted (although not always) and impacted. This leads to radial shortening, resulting in inteross-eous membrane disruption and injury to the DRUJ, with subsequent DRUJ instability.[75] They are included in this discussion because, although the fractured radial head may be apparent, the impor-tant, associated DRUJ injury can be easily missed.

The totality of this injury is often missed initially in the setting of acute trauma because much of the focus is directed to the fractured radial head, and the symptoms in the wrist are often minimal in the acute stage.[76] In addition, the radiographic fea-tures of distal radioulnar dislocation can be subtle. Although it has been reported that a greater than 5 mm discrepancy between the radioulnar distance on the injured versus noninjured wrist on lateral views is considered diagnostic for dislocation,[77] in our experience this has been difficult to repro-duce. Because the majority of Essex–Lopresti in-juries require surgical treatment, and surgical outcomes are improved with early intervention,[76] once the suggestion of possible distal radioulnar injury in the setting of a comminuted radial head fracture is raised, further investigation, including a focused physical examination, and dedicated CT should be considered. Owing to the subtlety of DRUJ subluxation, we prefer to image both wrists together and, if tolerated, in maximally supinated and pronated as well as neutral positions.

Carpal Instability and the Zone of Vulnerability

Perilunate dislocations and perilunate fracture dis-locations are typically a result of a fall on an

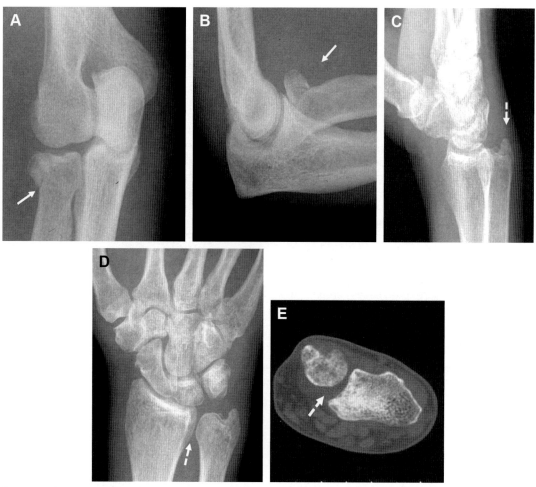

Fig. 14. Essex–Lopresti. (*A, B*) Anteroposterior (*A*) and lateral (*B*) radiographs at presentation after a fall on an outstretched hand show mildly impacted intraarticular fracture of the radial head (*solid white arrow*). (*C–E*) On follow-up visit 1 month later, the patient complained of wrist pain and dorsal subluxation of the distal radioulnar joint (*dashed white arrow*) was suspected radiographically (*D, E*) and confirmed on CT (*E*).

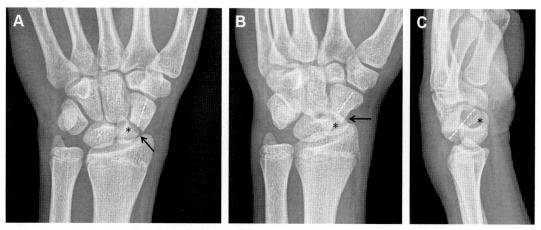

Fig. 15. Trans-scaphoid perilunate fracture dislocation. (*A–C*) Posteroanterior (PA), oblique, and lateral views of the wrist. Scaphoid waist fracture is obvious on the PA and oblique (*black arrows*) views and is the site of disruption of the first and second carpal arcs of Gilula. The proximal pole scaphoid fragment (*) remains in normal apposition with the lunate and the distal pole (*dashed line*) is dislocated dorsally around the lunate with the remainder of the carpus. Note the pie slice–shaped configuration of the lunate–proximal pole scaphoid unit owing to mild palmar flexion.

outstretched hand, with resultant hyperextension and axial loading. Unfortunately, they are missed radiographically in up to 25% of patients (**Fig. 15**).[29] When left untreated, these injuries lead to unacceptable morbidity, including chronic pain and disability.[78]

Perilunate dislocations and perilunate fracture–dislocations have been described by Mayfield and colleagues,[79] who described the mechanism of injury as a sequential process across the perilunate carpus in which both ligamentous and osseous injuries occur. This "zone of vulnerability" includes the radial styloid, trapezium, scaphoid, proximal capitate, proximal hamate, lunate border of the triquetrum, and ulnar styloid.[80,81] These injuries occur in stages, beginning at the radial aspect of the wrist, and propagate in sequence ulnarly. As the injury progresses around the carpus, the potential for multiple fracture–dislocations increases. The transcaphoid fracture–dislocation is the most common of the carpal fracture–dislocation and typically involves the scaphoid waist, with the distal fracture fragment displacing with the rest of the dislocated carpus.[29] This characteristic pattern of injury progression directs a search pattern for wrist fractures in the setting of carpal instability.

SUMMARY

The radiographic assessment for upper extremity fractures remains a challenge. Missed diagnoses potentially have significant consequences for patients, clinicians, and radiologists. By reviewing 3 different categories of missed fractures—the common but challenging, the out of mind out of sight, and the satisfaction of search—we hope to have provided a framework for the reader to use not only when reviewing a study that initially seems to be normal, but for associated injuries when there is an obvious abnormality. Knowledge of what is commonly missed can only aid our diagnostic performance by prompting additional attention to these areas. The use of radiologic signs and the importance of additional views has been emphasized as an additional strategy to minimize mistakes.

REFERENCES

1. Berlin L, Berlin JW. Malpractice and radiologists in Cook County, IL: trends in 20 years of litigation. AJR Am J Roentgenol 1995;165(4):781–8.
2. Wei CJ, Tsai WC, Tiu CM, et al. Systematic analysis of missed extremity fractures in emergency radiology. Acta Radiol 2006;47(7):710–7.
3. Whang JS, Baker SR, Patel R, et al. The causes of medical malpractice suits against radiologists in the United States. Radiology 2013;266(2):548–54.
4. Berlin L. Defending the "missed" radiographic diagnosis. AJR Am J Roentgenol 2001;176(2):317–22.
5. Berlin L, Hendrix RW. Perceptual errors and negligence. AJR Am J Roentgenol 1998;170(4):863–7.
6. Leeper WR, Leeper TJ, Vogt KN, et al. The role of trauma team leaders in missed injuries: does specialty matter? J Trauma Acute Care Surg 2013; 75(3):387–90.
7. Er E, Kara PH, Oyar O, et al. Overlooked extremity fractures in the emergency department. Ulus Travma Acil Cerrahi Derg 2013;19(1):25–8.
8. Kung JW, Melenevsky Y, Hochman MG, et al. On-call musculoskeletal radiographs: discrepancy rates between radiology residents and musculoskeletal radiologists. AJR Am J Roentgenol 2013;200(4): 856–9.
9. Berlin L. Malpractice issues in radiology. Perceptual errors. AJR Am J Roentgenol 1996;167(3):587–90.
10. Itri JN, Kang HC, Krishnan S, et al. Using focused missed-case conferences to reduce discrepancies in musculoskeletal studies interpreted by residents on call. AJR Am J Roentgenol 2011; 197(4):W696–705.
11. Gruson KI, Ruchelsman DE, Tejwani NC. Isolated tuberosity fractures of the proximal humeral: current concepts. Injury 2008;39(3):284–98.
12. Kristiansen B, Barfod G, Bredesen J, et al. Epidemiology of proximal humerus fractures. Acta Orthop Scand 1987;58:75–7.
13. Kim SH, Szabo RM, Marder RA. Epidemiology of humerus fractures in the United States: nationwide emergency department sample, 2008. Arthritis Care Res (Hoboken) 2012;64(3):407–14.
14. George MS. Fractures of the greater tuberosity of the humerus. J Am Acad Orthop Surg 2007;15(10): 607–13.
15. Ogawa K, Yoshida A, Ikegami H. Isolated fractures of the greater tuberosity of the humerus: solutions to recognizing a frequently overlooked fracture. J Trauma 2003;54(4):713–7.
16. Reinus WR, Hatem SF. Fractures of the greater tuberosity presenting as rotator cuff abnormality: magnetic resonance demonstration. J Trauma 1998; 44(4):670–5.
17. Platzer P, Kutscha-Lissberg F, Lehr S, et al. The influence of displacement on shoulder function in patients with minimally displaced fractures of the greater tuberosity. Injury 2005;36(10):1185–9.
18. De Smet AA. Anterior oblique projection in radiography of the traumatized shoulder. AJR Am J Roentgenol 1980;134(3):515–8.
19. Radin EL, Riseborough EJ. Fractures of the radial head. A review of eighty-eight cases and analysis of the indications for excision of the radial head

and non-operative treatment. J Bone Joint Surg Am 1966;48(6):1055–64.

20. Sonin A. Fractures of the elbow and forearm. Semin Musculoskelet Radiol 2000;4(2):171–91.

21. McGinley JC, Roach N, Hopgood BC, et al. Nondisplaced elbow fractures: a commonly occurring and difficult diagnosis. Am J Emerg Med 2006;24(5):560–6.

22. Grundy A, Murphy G, Barker A, et al. The value of the Radial Head-Capitellum view in radial head trauma. Br J Radiol 1985;58(694):965–7.

23. Greenspan A, Norman A, Rosen H. Radial head-capitellum view in elbow trauma: clinical application and radiographic-anatomic correlation. AJR Am J Roentgenol 1984;143(2):355–9.

24. Manns RA, Lee JR. Critical evaluation of the radial head-capitellum view in acute elbow with an effusion. Clin Radiol 1990;42(6):433–6.

25. Norell HG. Roentgenologic visualization of the extracapsular fat; its importance in the diagnosis of traumatic injuries to the elbow. Acta Radiol 1954; 42(3):205–10.

26. Bohrer SP. The fat pad sign following elbow trauma. Its usefulness and reliability in suspecting "invisible" fractures. Clin Radiol 1970;21(1):90–4.

27. O'Dwyer H, O'Sullivan P, Fitzgerald D, et al. The fat pad sign following elbow trauma in adults: its usefulness and reliability in suspecting occult fracture. J Comput Assist Tomogr 2004;28(4):562–5.

28. Owen RA, Melton LJ, Johnson KA, et al. Incidence of Colles' fracture in a North American community. Am J Public Health 1982;72(6):605–7.

29. Herzberg G, Comtet JJ, Linscheid RL, et al. Perilunate dislocations and fracture-dislocations: a multi-center study. J Hand Surg Am 1993;18(5):768–79.

30. Mayfield JK. Wrist ligament anatomy and biomechanics. In: Gilula LA, editor. The traumatized hand and wrist: radiographic and anatomic correlation. Philadelphia: W B Saunders Co; 1992. p. 335.

31. Goldfarb CA, Yin Y, Gilula LA, et al. Wrist fractures: what the clinician wants to know. Radiology 2001; 219(1):11–28.

32. Knirk JL, Jupiter JB. Intra-articular fractures of the distal end of the radius in young adults. J Bone Joint Surg Am 1986;68(5):647–59.

33. Dobyns JH, Linsheid RL. Fractures and dislocations of the wrist. In: Rockwood CA Jr, Green DP, editors. Fractures in adults. 2nd edition. J.B.Lippincott Company; 1984. p. 411–509.

34. Perron AD, Brady WJ, Keats TE, et al. Orthopedic pitfalls in the ED: scaphoid fracture. Am J Emerg Med 2001;19(4):310–6.

35. Ahn JM, El-Khoury GY. Occult fractures of extremities. Radiol Clin North Am 2007;45(3):561–79, ix.

36. Cooney WP, Linsheid RL, Dobyns JH. Fractures and dislocations of the wrist. In: Rockwood CA, Green DP, editors. Fractures in adults. Philadelphia: Lippincott; 1996. p. 745–867.

37. Terry DW, Ramin JE. The navicular fat stripe: a useful roentgen feature for evaluating wrist trauma. Am J Roentgenol Radium Ther Nucl Med 1975;124(1): 25–8.

38. Annamalai G, Raby N. Scaphoid and pronator fat stripes are unreliable soft tissue signs in the detection of radiographically occult fractures. Clin Radiol 2003;58:798–800.

39. Hunter JC, Escobedo EM, Wilson AJ, et al. MR imaging of clinically suspected scaphoid fractures. AJR Am J Roentgenol 1997;168:1287–93.

40. Welling RD, Jacobson JA, Jamadar DA, et al. MDCT and radiography of wrist fractures: radiographic sensitivity and fracture patterns. AJR Am J Roentgenol 2008;190:10–6.

41. Nance EP, Kaye JJ, Milek MA. Volar plate fractures. Radiology 1979;133:61–4.

42. Voleti PB, Namdari S, Mehta S. Fractures of the scapula. Adv Orthop 2012;2012:903850.

43. Tornetta P III, Court-Brown C, Heckman JD, et al, editors. Rockwood and Green's fractures in adults: two volumes plus integrated content website (Rockwood, Green, and Wilkins' Fractures), 7th edition. Philadelphia: Lippincott Williams & Wilkins; 2009.

44. Kaplan PA, Dussault R, Helms CA, et al. Musculoskeletal MRI. Philadelphia: Saunders; 2001.

45. Goss TP. The scapula: coracoid, acromial, and avulsion fractures. Am J Orthop (Belle Mead NJ) 1996; 25(2):106–15.

46. McGinnis M, Denton JR. Fractures of the scapula: a retrospective study of 40 fractured scapulae. J Trauma 1989;29(11):1488–93.

47. Güleç A, Kütahya H, Göncü RG, et al. Isolated fracture of the coracoid process. Case Rep Orthop 2014;2014:482130.

48. Goud A, Segal D, Hedayati P, et al. Radiographic evaluation of the shoulder. Eur J Radiol 2008;68(1):2–15.

49. Garcia-Elias M, Salo J. Non-union of a fractured coracoid process after dislocation of the shoulder. A case report. J Bone Joint Surg Br 1985;67(5): 722–3.

50. Kurdy NM, Shah SV. Fracture of the acromion associated with acromioclavicular dislocation. Injury 1995;26(9):636–7.

51. Ogawa K, Naniwa T. Fractures of the acromion and the lateral scapular spine. J Shoulder Elbow Surg 1997;6(6):544–8.

52. Kuhn JE, Blasier RB, Carpenter JE. Fractures of the acromion process: a proposed classification system. J Orthop Trauma 1994;8(1):6–13.

53. Gurland M. Carpometacarpal joint injuries of the fingers. Hand Clin 1992;8(4):733–44.

54. Fisher MR, Rogers LF, Hendrix RW, et al. Carpometacarpal dislocations. Crit Rev Diagn Imaging 1984; 22(2):95–126.

55. Hodgson PD, Shewring DJ. The 'metacarpal cascade lines'; use in the diagnosis of dislocations

of the carpometacarpal joints. J Hand Surg Eur Vol 2007;32(3):277–81.

56. Parkinson RW, Paton RW. Carpometacarpal dislocation: an aid to diagnosis. Injury 1992;23(3):187–8.

57. Suh N, Ek ET, Wolfe SW. Carpal fractures. J Hand Surg Am 2014;39(4):785–91 [quiz: 791].

58. Cohen MS. Fractures of the carpal bones. Hand Clin 1997;13(4):587–99.

59. Failla JM. Hook of hamate vascularity: vulnerability to osteonecrosis and nonunion. J Hand Surg Am 1993;18(6):1075–9.

60. Carroll RE, Lakin JF. Fracture of the hook of the hamate: acute treatment. J Trauma 1993;34(6): 803–5.

61. Akahane M, Ono H, Sada M, et al. Fracture of hamate hook–diagnosis by the hamate hook lateral view. Hand Surg 2000;5(2):131–7.

62. Norman A, Nelson J, Green S. Fractures of the hook of hamate: radiographic signs. Radiology 1985; 154(1):49–53.

63. Papilion JD, DuPuy TE, Aulicino PL, et al. Radiographic evaluation of the hook of the hamate: a new technique. J Hand Surg Am 1988;13(3):437–9.

64. Levy M, Fischel RE, Stern GM, et al. Chip fractures of the os triquetrum: the mechanism of injury. J Bone Joint Surg Br 1979;61B:355–7.

65. Garcia-Elias M. Dorsal fractures of the triquetrum-avulsion or compression fractures? J Hand Surg Am 1987;12(2):266–8.

66. Bryan RS, Dobyns JH. Fractures of the carpal bones other than lunate and navicular. Clin Orthop Relat Res 1980;(149):107–11.

67. Kroner K, Lind T, Jensen J. The epidemiology of shoulder dislocations. Arch Orthop Trauma Surg 1989;108(5):288–90.

68. Robinson CM, Shur N, Sharpe T, et al. Injuries associated with traumatic anterior glenohumeral dislocations. J Bone Joint Surg Am 2012;94(1):18–26.

69. Ridpath CA, Wilson AJ. Shoulder and humerus trauma. Semin Musculoskelet Radiol 2000;4(2): 151–70.

70. Shuster M, Abu-Laban RB, Boyd J. Prereduction radiographs in clinically evident anterior shoulder dislocation. Am J Emerg Med 1999;17(7):653–8.

71. Shuster M, Abu-Laban RB, Boyd J, et al. Prospective evaluation of a guideline for the selective elimination of pre-reduction radiographs in clinically obvious anterior shoulder dislocation. CJEM 2002; 4(4):257–62.

72. Bankart AS. Recurrent or habitual dislocation of the shoulder-joint. Br Med J 1923;2(3285):1132–3.

73. Hendey GW, Kinlaw K. Clinically significant abnormalities in postreduction radiographs after anterior shoulder dislocation. Ann Emerg Med 1996;28(4): 399–402.

74. Kahn JH, Mehta SD. The role of post-reduction radiographs after shoulder dislocation. J Emerg Med 2007;33(2):169–73.

75. Sheehan SE, Dyer GS, Sodickson AD, et al. Traumatic elbow injuries: what the orthopedic surgeon wants to know. Radiographics 2013;33(3):869–88.

76. Jungbluth P, Frangen TM, Arens S, et al. The undiagnosed Essex-Lopresti injury. J Bone Joint Surg Br 2006;88(12):1629–33.

77. Nakamura R, Horii E, Imaeda T, et al. Distal radioulnar joint subluxation and dislocation diagnosed by standard roentgenography. Skeletal Radiol 1995; 24(2):91–4.

78. Perron AD, Brady WJ, Keats TE, et al. Orthopedic pitfalls in the ED: lunate and perilunate injuries. Am J Emerg Med 2001;19(2):157–62.

79. Mayfield JK, Johnson RP, Kilcoyne RK. Carpal dislocations: pathomechanics and progressive perilunar instability. J Hand Surg Am 1980;5(3):226–41.

80. Johnson RP. The acutely injured wrist and its residuals. Clin Orthop Relat Res 1980;(149):33–44.

81. Scalcione LR, Gimber LH, Ho AM, et al. Spectrum of carpal dislocations and fracture-dislocations: imaging and management. AJR Am J Roentgenol 2014; 203(3):541–50.

Easily Missed Fractures in the Lower Extremity

Joseph S. Yu, MD

KEYWORDS

- Trauma • Hip • Femur • Knee • Ankle • Fractures • Injury • Ligaments

KEY POINTS

- A systematic approach is useful when evaluating radiographs of patients with acute trauma to their lower extremity.
- Recalling high-risk areas in the hip, knee, and ankle allows the radiologist to quickly evaluate key locations in each projection for findings that are frequently subtle and may be evident in only 1 view.
- The technique is simple and sufficiently comprehensive to maximize fracture detection.
- However, the key to success is meticulous attention to detail and remembering to not overlook regions that frequently hide fractures.

HIP

The hip joint is a stable spheroidal joint composed of the femoral head and the cup-shaped acetabulum. The capsule that encloses the joint attaches to the rim of the acetabulum and the femoral neck. Within the joint, the fibrocartilaginous labrum deepens the socket by adding to the surface area by 10% to 15% and is integral to both function and stability.[1] Three capsular condensations, the iliofemoral, pubofemoral, and ischiofemoral ligaments, also contribute to joint stability.

The hip joint is frequently injured in trauma. Dislocations are relatively common in high-energy trauma and tend to occur in younger people.[2] These dislocations are associated with a high incidence of cartilaginous and osteochondral lesions. Femoral neck fractures are important injuries in the elderly population but may be difficult to detect owing to arthritis, obesity, osteoporosis, or external rotation of the leg.

Radiographic Evaluation

A recurring scenario in the emergency department is hip pain after falling or motor vehicle collision. Evaluation of the hip joint starts with adequate radiographs that include an anteroposterior (AP) pelvic radiograph with accompanying AP and frog leg views of the hip.

Assessment includes close scrutiny for symmetry of the femoral heads and joint spaces, integrity of the acetabular arc and radiographic pelvic "teardrop," and continuity of 4 critical osseous landmarks. The osseous landmarks are the iliopectineal line, ilioischial line, anterior acetabular rim line, and posterior acetabular rim line. These reference lines allow inspection of the quadrilateral plate, the anterior and posterior columns, and the acetabular walls. Shenton line, which is drawn along the superior margin of the obturator ring and laterally along the medial cortex of the femoral neck, is helpful in identifying dislocations.

Even with careful inspection, the incidence of radiographically occult hip fractures ranges from 4% to 9% in patients presenting with pain after trauma.[3,4] In these situations, MRI is the most appropriate follow-up imaging study owing to its exquisite sensitivity to edema in the bone marrow (**Fig. 1**). The reported sensitivity and specificity of MRI for occult fractures is 100%.[5,6]

Acetabular fractures

Fractures of the acetabulum are often complex, and the Judet-Letournel classification is useful when reporting findings.[7,8] By carefully evaluating

Dr J.S. Yu has no financial disclosure.
Department of Radiology, The Ohio State University Wexner Medical Center, 395 West 12th Avenue, Suite 481, Columbus, OH 43210, USA
E-mail address: Joseph.yu@osumc.edu

Radiol Clin N Am 53 (2015) 737–755
http://dx.doi.org/10.1016/j.rcl.2015.02.003

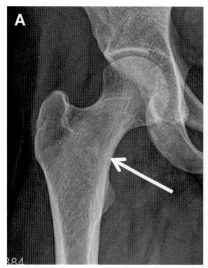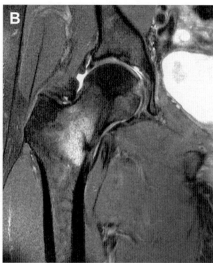

Fig. 1. Occult femur stress fracture in distance runner. (*A*) Radiograph of the hip shows no obvious fracture but there is a faint linear area of sclerosis at the base of the neck medially (*arrow*). (*B*) Coronal short tau inversion recovery (STIR) magnetic resonance image shows a unicortical linear low-signal-intensity abnormality on the compressive side of the femoral neck surrounded by intensely bright marrow edema.

the osseous landmarks and pelvic symmetry, most acetabular fractures may be easily identified and appropriately classified.

The most common type of fracture of the acetabulum is a posterior acetabular wall fracture, which comprises nearly one-fourth of fractures in this joint, and it is usually produced by a posterior hip dislocation. Unlike the shoulder, nearly 85% of dislocations of the hip are directed posteriorly, occurring with hip flexion so that the head of the femur is driven toward the back of the acetabulum.[2]

Visualizing the fracture may be quite subtle owing to overlapping osseous structures. Disruption of the posterior rim line is characteristic of a posterior wall fracture (**Fig. 2**).[9] The fracture may involve the posterior acetabular rim and/or a portion of the retroacetabular surface. Oblique (Judet) views are optimal for diagnosis, but when there are large or numerous fragments, computed tomography (CT) is preferred for comprehensive evaluation for instability.[10]

Pubic fractures

Pubic bone fractures typically are associated with other fractures in the pelvis. Fractures in the rami may be subtle, particularly in patients with osteoporosis who have sustained trauma (**Fig. 3**). Meticulous attention to cortical disruption and changes in bone density is required.

Long-distance runners are susceptible to stress fractures of the pubic arch usually in the inferior ramus near the symphysis pubis.[11] Because these fractures are nondisplaced, they are easy to overlook.

Pediatric considerations

Avulsion injuries that involve the ossification centers in skeletally immature patients constitute an important group of injuries that affect the muscular, tendinous, and ligamentous attachments about the hip joint (**Fig. 4**).[12] These injuries frequently occur as a manifestation of strong muscular contractions during athletic events. In the hip, important areas to consider include the ischium (hamstring), pubis (adductors), and anterior inferior iliac spine (rectus femoris) (**Fig. 5**).

Femoral head fractures

Femoral head fractures most commonly are associated with hip dislocations. The incidence of femoral head fractures is about 7% in patients with posterior dislocation and ranges from 10% to 68% in patients with anterior dislocation.[13,14]

Note that fractures may be the result of either a shearing injury or a direct impaction. Both types of fractures may be extremely subtle. CT is advocated not only to confirm the diagnosis and identify other fractures but also to assess the presence of intra-articular fragments (**Fig. 6**).

Proximal femoral fracture

Fractures of the femoral neck are generally a condition of elderly people.[15] Subcapital fractures are most common, but these may be difficult to detect when the femur is externally rotated or there is significant osteophyte formation from arthritis. Obesity and osteopenia may further compromise an already challenging hip radiograph, so meticulous inspection is required.

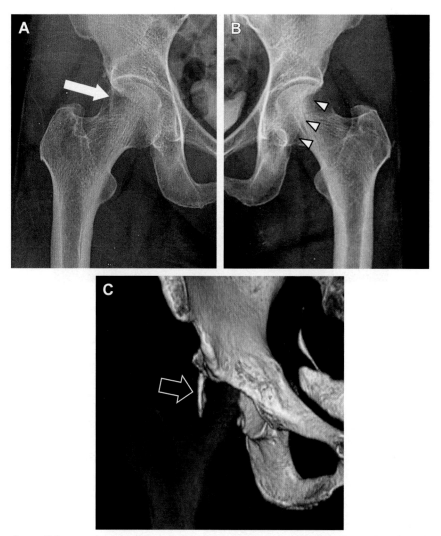

Fig. 2. Posterior wall fracture in a patient with hip dislocation. (*A*) Radiograph of right hip shows a linear fragment of bone posterior to the femoral head (*arrow*) and absence of the posterior rim line. (*B*) Left hip comparison shows the posterior rim line (*arrowheads*). (*C*) Computed tomographic three-dimensional reconstruction image shows the defect in the posterior wall and the displaced and rotated fragment of bone (*arrow*).

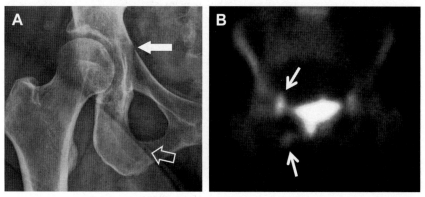

Fig. 3. Lateral compression anterior column/pubic fracture after bike accident. (*A*) Frontal radiograph shows subtle disruption of the right iliopectineal line (*arrow*), which was not detected initially. There is also a subtle fracture of the right inferior pubic ramus (*open arrow*). (*B*) Bone scintigraphy 10 days later confirms the anterior column fracture and the right inferior pubic ramus fracture (*arrows*). Note that the left anterior column was also abnormal.

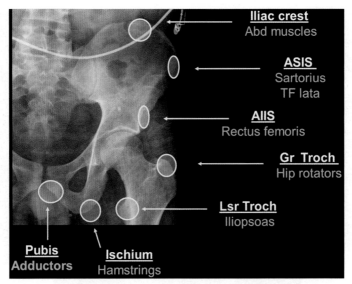

Fig. 4. Risk areas for pediatric avulsion fractures. Asymmetry of the apophyseal plates should be viewed as suspicious in the setting of trauma and overuse. Abd, abdominal; AIIS, anterior inferior iliac spine; ASIS, anterior superior iliac spine; Gr Troch, greater trochanter; Lsr Troch, lesser trochanter; TF, tensor fascia.

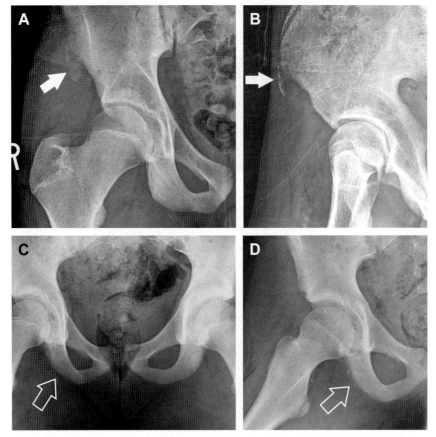

Fig. 5. Pediatric avulsion fractures. Frontal (*A*) and oblique (*B*) radiographs show distracted fragments of bone that have pulled off the anterior superior iliac spine (*arrows*). Frontal (*C*) and frogleg lateral right (*D*) hip radiographs in a different patient show irregularity of the right ischial cortex consistent with a right hamstring tendon avulsion injury (*open arrows* in *C* and *D*).

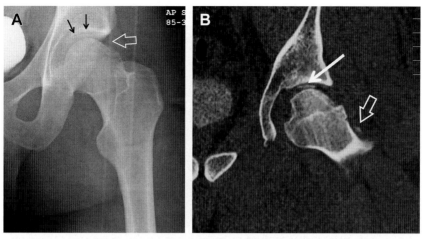

Fig. 6. Femoral head fracture from a hip dislocation. (*A*) Radiograph shows contour defect in the superolateral aspect of the femoral head (*open arrow*). Note the entrapped fragment of bone in the superior joint space (*black arrows*). (*B*) Coronal CT multiplanar reformatted (MPR) image confirms the osteochondral fragment of bone (*white arrow*) as well as a second fragment (*open arrow*) in the joint superior to the zona orbicularis.

Trochanteric fractures may be difficult to visualize when they are minimally displaced. Because bone overlap may provide a significant distraction, having an additional view often alleviates errors by offering a different perspective to the tubercles (**Fig. 7**).

Femoral neck stress fractures
Stress fractures of the femoral neck are common in athletes who participate in endurance activities, and these usually develop on the compressive side of the neck. A linear, sclerotic band oriented perpendicular to the medial cortex at the base of the neck is diagnostic of this type of fatigue fracture (**Fig. 8**). When present, no other imaging is necessary.

Stress fractures occurring on the tensile side of the neck, however, may progress to a complete fracture (**Fig. 9**).[16] These fractures may be caused by overuse or may occur because of an underlying osseous abnormality. These fractures involve the outer cortex of the midportion of the neck, and a subtle linear lucency may be the only abnormality. Tensile stress fractures usually require surgical fixation.

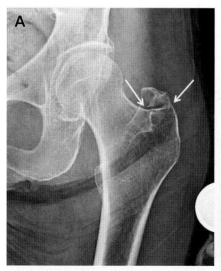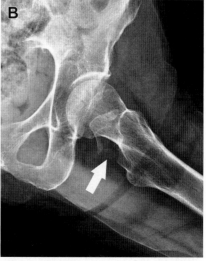

Fig. 7. Greater trochanteric fracture after a fall. (*A*) Frontal radiograph does not reveal an obvious fracture as initially reported. But closer inspection shows disruption of the cortex in the superior margin of the greater trochanter (*arrows*). (*B*) Frog leg lateral view shows that the fracture distracted, particularly posteriorly (*arrow*). This view was neglected on initial inspection because the area of interest, the femoral neck, was not optimally depicted.

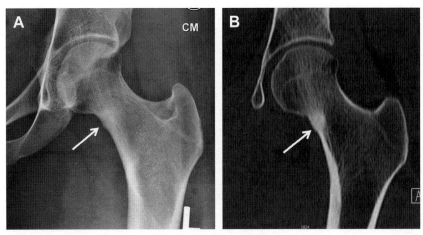

Fig. 8. Compressive side femoral neck stress fracture in a distance runner. Radiograph (*A*) and coronal CT multiplanar reformatted (MPR) (*B*) image show a transverse lucency through the medial cortex of the femoral neck (*arrows*) with surrounding sclerosis. The fracture is oriented perpendicular to the cortex.

Bisphosphonate insufficiency fracture

Another important insufficiency fracture that affects the femur is related to long-term bisphosphonate use. Some investigators have referred to this condition as an atypical shaft fracture. The abnormality characteristically involves the lateral cortex of the middle 50% of the shaft sparing the subtrochanteric region proximally and the supracondylar region distally (**Fig. 10**).[17] This fracture is seen in patients who have been on bisphosphonate therapy for over 3 years.[18] Prodromal symptoms occur in 60% to 75% of patients as either groin or thigh pain that often is erroneously attributed to arthritis of the hip or back.

The characteristic radiographic appearance of this insufficiency fracture is a volcano-like elevation of the periosteum associated with a transverse lucency through the lateral cortex. It is noteworthy that more than 50% of patients present with a complete fracture of the shaft. Because the condition is bilateral in 50% to 60% of cases, evaluation of the contralateral leg is required once the diagnosis is confirmed in one extremity.

KNEE

Most ligament injuries of the knee are caused by low-energy trauma, such as from those that occur in sports, whereas many fractures are caused by high-energy trauma. Avulsion and impaction fractures may imply the presence of an underlying ligament abnormality.[19–21] As many of these fractures are subtle, accurate detection of these fractures depends on knowledge of the anatomic high-risk

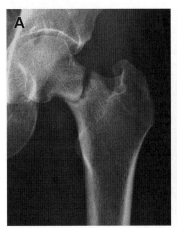
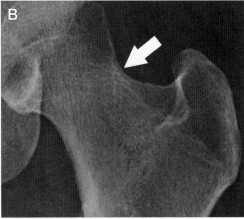

Fig. 9. Tensile side femoral neck stress fracture in a patient with eating disorder. (*A*) Frontal radiograph shows a complete fracture of the femoral neck with varus angulation. (*B*) A radiograph done 2 weeks earlier shows focal osteopenia in the lateral cortex where the fracture eventually occurred (*arrow*).

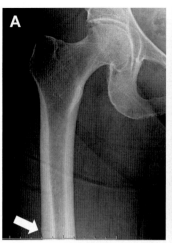
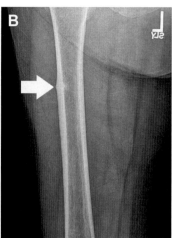
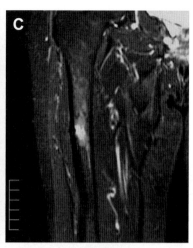

Fig. 10. Bisphosphonate-related insufficiency fracture in an elderly patient. (A) Radiograph of hip shows classic edge-of-film finding that was missed. There was a transverse cortical lucency in the lateral cortex (arrow). (B) Follow-up femur radiograph shows focal endosteal reaction and a volcano-like periosteal elevation (arrow) characteristic of this insufficiency fracture. (C) Coronal short tau inversion recovery (STIR) magnetic resonance image shows associated bone marrow edema at the level of the fracture.

areas as well as careful inspection of the radiographs. A mechanistic approach is often useful.[21]

Mechanisms of Injury

In general, unidirectional mechanisms result in unidirectional instability and complex mechanisms result in multidirectional instability. Hyperextension, posterior (dashboard) tibial translation, anterior tibial translation, valgus stress, and varus stress are considered simple or one-vector force mechanisms.

Complex injury mechanisms have multiple vector forces. External rotation and valgus stress with knee flexion, flexion with internal rotation and varus stress, hyperextension with valgus stress, and hyperextension with varus stress and internal rotation are complex types.

The pivot shift injury pattern is the most common mechanism of injury in the knee accounting for 46% of anterior cruciate ligament (ACL) tears.[19] This injury occurs with rapid deceleration and a simultaneous change in direction so that the lateral femoral condyle strikes against the posterolateral margin of the lateral tibial plateau when the ACL fails.[22,23]

Flexion-internal rotation-varus accounts for about 1% of injury mechanisms that affect the knee.[19] The Segond fracture occurs with this mechanism of injury. Hyperextension injuries are responsible for about 8% of ACL tears.[19]

Tibial eminence anterior cruciate ligament avulsion fractures

Avulsion of the ACL usually occurs at the tibial eminence (Fig. 11). Although this injury is more common in adolescents, it is not considered uncommon in adults. There are 4 types of ACL avulsion fractures in the Meyers and McKeever classification system.[24]

In type I, there is incomplete osseous avulsion that shows no or minimal displacement of the tibial eminence fragment. In type II, the fragment is anteriorly elevated but the fracture is still not complete. In type III, there is complete separation of the fragment, and in type IV, the fragment is displaced and rotated.

Impacted condylopatellar sulcus (deep lateral notch)

The condylopatellar sulcus is a natural depression in the condylar region of the femur that separates the patellar articular surface from the tibial surface. A pivot shift mechanism may produce impaction of the lateral notch causing the sulcus to deepen (Fig. 12). In the lateral radiograph, when the depth exceeds 1.5 mm, it is associated with a torn ACL in 70% of the patients and when the depth exceeds 2.0 mm, 100% of patients reportedly have a torn ACL.[25,26]

Posterolateral tibial chip fracture

A posterolateral compression fracture involving a small portion of the cortex may be the only evidence of a pivot shift injury mechanism (Fig. 13).[27] This fracture is a rare finding on conventional knee radiographs but when suspected, the small fracture fragment may be visible on an internally rotated oblique radiograph.

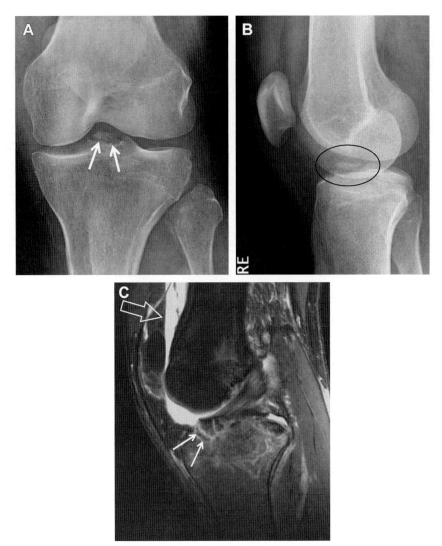

Fig. 11. ACL avulsion fracture from a motorcycle accident. (*A*) Frontal radiograph shows a fracture through the base of the medial tibial spine (*arrows*). It is important not to mistake the bone fragment as an intra-articular body. (*B*) The lateral radiograph shows a typical elongated bone fragment above the tibia (*oval*). (*C*) Sagittal T2-weighted magnetic resonance image shows that the ACL attaches to the avulsed fragment (*arrows*). Note the surrounding marrow edema and the lipohemarthrosis (*open arrow*).

Segond fracture

The Segond fracture is a vertically oriented avulsion fracture occurring at the lateral tibial plateau several millimeters below the articular surface of the plateau (**Fig. 14**). This fracture is best depicted on AP radiographs, and it involves that region of the tibia where the middle third of the lateral capsular ligament, anterior oblique band of the fibular collateral ligament, and the posterior fibers of the iliotibial tract converge.[28]

Avulsion of the cortical bone occurs when a varus force is introduced on the knee when the foot is firmly planted as the femur internally

rotates, a common maneuver in running athletes. This injury produces bone contusions in the medial femoral condyle and the posteromedial tibial plateau, and it is associated with tears of the ACL in 75% to 100% of patients and lateral meniscal tears in 33% of patients and can lead to anterolateral rotational instability.[29]

Medial Segond fracture

An avulsion fracture that arises from the cortex of the medial tibial plateau has been referred to as a medial or reverse Segond fracture. The rotational mechanism that causes the avulsion of the deep

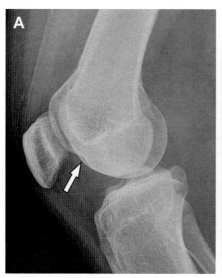
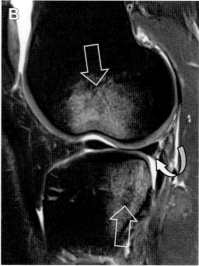

Fig. 12. Deep lateral notch sign after a twisting injury. (A) Lateral radiograph shows a deepened lateral condy-lopatellar sulcus (*arrow*). (B) Sagittal T2-weighted magnetic resonance image shows bone contusions in the lateral femoral condyle and the posterolateral tibia (*open arrows*). Anterior tibial translation from an ACL tear exposes the posterior horn of the lateral meniscus (*curved arrow*).

capsular component of the medial collateral liga-ment is the opposite of that which creates the classic Segond fracture.[30] This fracture is associ-ated with tears of the posterior cruciate ligament (PCL) and the root of the medial meniscus.[31,32]

The medial Segond fracture is best depicted in the AP view of the knee appearing as a small linear fracture fragment involving the corner of the tibia (**Fig. 15**).

Avulsion fracture of the fibular styloid process (arcuate sign)

A transversely oriented fracture of the fibular styloid occurs when there is direct impact to the anteromedial tibia when the knee is extended referred to as an arcuate sign (**Fig. 16**),[33] which is an important indicator of posterolateral knee instability. A concomitant tear of either the ACL or the PCL has been reported with this fracture.

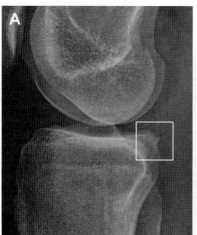
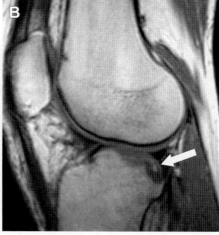

Fig. 13. Posterolateral tibial chip fracture. (A) Lateral radiograph shows a small compression chip fracture in the posterolateral tibia (*square*). This occurs in pivot shift injury mechanisms when the tibia strikes the lateral femoral condyle. (B) Sagittal T1-weighted magnetic resonance image in another patient shows a posterolateral fracture fragment (*arrow*) and an anterior drawer sign from a torn ACL.

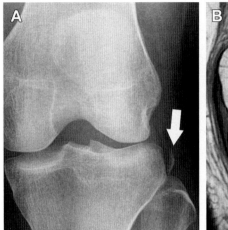
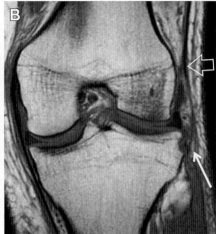

Fig. 14. Segond fracture in a football player. (*A*) Frontal radiograph shows an avulsion of the lateral tibial cortex below the joint line (*arrow*). (*B*) Coronal T1-weighted magnetic resonance image shows that the fragment is attached to the iliotibial band (*open arrow*) and the anterior oblique band of the lateral collateral ligament (not shown).

If the arcuate sign is unrecognized or left untreated, reconstruction of an ACL ligament tear is likely to fail.[34] The structures that attach to the fibular styloid include the popliteofibular, fabellofibular, and arcuate ligaments.[35]

Posterior tibial eminence posterior cruciate ligament avulsion fractures

Up to 6% of PCL tears are associated with an osseous avulsion fracture.[24] Like the ACL, avulsions fractures of the PCL arise at the distal tibial attachment.[36] The most common mechanism of injury is a dashboard injury, although occasionally other mechanisms may be responsible. Nearly all injuries that produce a tibial avulsion fracture are caused by motor vehicle accidents.[37]

The characteristic radiographic appearance is a variable-sized triangular fragment of bone that is displaced superiorly into the joint seen on lateral knee radiographs (**Fig. 17**).

Avulsion fracture of the fibular head

The lateral aspect of the knee contains the iliotibial tract, biceps femoris muscle and tendon, lateral capsular ligament, and lateral collateral ligament (LCL). The LCL is the primary stabilizer against excessive varus force.[38] When there is sufficient varus force, an isolated ligament rupture or avulsion fracture of the fibular head at the insertion of the conjoined occurs.[38]

Radiographically, the fracture orients vertically in the lateral aspect of the fibular head (**Fig. 18**).

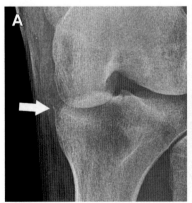
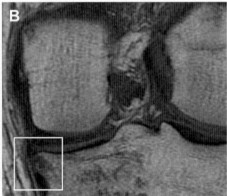

Fig. 15. Reverse Segond fracture in a soccer player. (*A*) Frontal radiograph shows a small flake of bone in the medial tibia at the joint line (*arrow*). (*B*) Coronal T1-weighted magnetic resonance image shows that the fragment arises at the attachment of the deep capsular component of the medial collateral ligament (*square*).

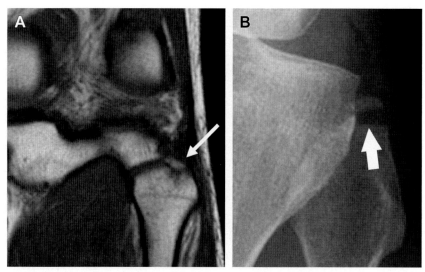

Fig. 16. Fibular styloid fracture sustained during a fall. (*A*) Coronal T1-weighted magnetic resonance image shows an avulsion fracture of the styloid process of the fibula (*arrow*). The arcuate ligament attaches to the bone fragment, whereas the conjoined tendon passes lateral to it. (*B*) Frontal radiograph close-up shows the transverse orientation of the fracture (*arrow*).

The fracture fragment is usually larger than that associated with a fibular styloid fracture. The fragment often migrates superiorly, producing a ribbonlike deformity of the LCL on MRI.

ANKLE

Low-energy trauma accounts for three-fourths of injuries to the ankle, and often such trauma is from athletic activity.[39] Ankle pain is one of the most common problems encountered by emergency physicians, and radiography remains the mainstay diagnostic tool for diagnosing fractures.

About 85% of ankle sprains are the result of an inversion mechanism, although eversion, internal and external rotation, excessive dorsiflexion, as well as adduction and abduction stresses on the foot are also forces that can produce fractures.[40,41] Diagnosis often depends on the knowledge of high-risk areas, so it is useful to have a search strategy that is based on anatomic landmarks (**Fig. 19**).[42]

Fractures of the Posterior Tibial Malleolus

The ankle joint is considered a ring, thus the medial and lateral malleoli ought to be scrutinized together.[43] Fractures involving the attachments of the deltoid ligament and the LCL complex

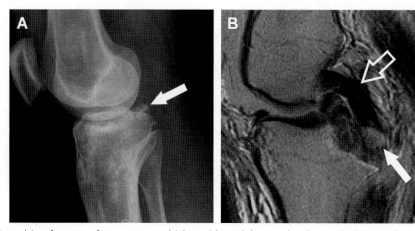

Fig. 17. PCL avulsion fracture after a motor vehicle accident. (*A*) Lateral radiograph shows a displaced triangular fragment of bone in the posterior joint space (*arrow*). (*B*) Sagittal proton density magnetic resonance image shows that the fragment of bone (*arrow*) is attached to the posterior cruciate ligament (*open arrow*).

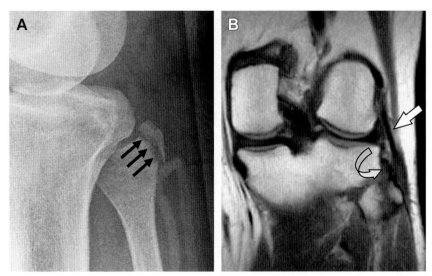

Fig. 18. Fibular head avulsion fracture from hyperextension injury. (*A*) Lateral radiograph close-up shows a vertically oriented fracture (*arrows*) through the lateral aspect of the fibular head. (*B*) Coronal T1-weighted magnetic resonance image shows that the fragment is attached to both the lateral collateral ligament (*arrow*) and the arcuate ligament (*curved arrow*).

generally are not difficult to detect, particularly when there is overlying soft tissue swelling.

However, fractures involving the posterior tibial malleolus caused by tension from the posterior tibiofibular ligament may be difficult to visualize.[44] These fractures can vary in size (**Fig. 20**); they are important because they are associated with a distal tibial spiral fracture or can be present as part of a trimalleolar fracture complex.[45]

Fractures of the Anterior Tibial Tubercle

The Tillaux fracture, an avulsion fracture of the anterior tibial tubercle, occurs when tension from the anterior tibiofibular ligament overwhelms the bone. This fracture occurs from external rotation and abduction of the foot.[46] The appearance is characteristic on an oblique radiograph appearing as a vertically oriented fracture line that extends

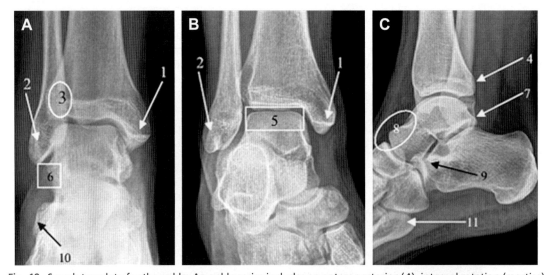

Fig. 19. Search template for the ankle. An ankle series includes an anteroposterior (*A*), internal rotation (mortise) view (*B*), and a lateral view (*C*). There are 11 areas where fractures occur, including the medial (1) and lateral (2) malleoli, anterior tibial tubercle (3) and posterior tibial malleolus (4), talar dome (5), lateral talar process (6), tubercles of the posterior talus process (7), dorsal to the talonavicular joint (8), anterior calcaneus process (9), calcaneal insertion of the extensor digitorum brevis (10), and the base of the fifth metatarsal bone (11). (*From* Yu JS, Cody ME. A template approach for detecting fractures in low energy ankle trauma. Emerg Radiol 2009;16:309–18.)

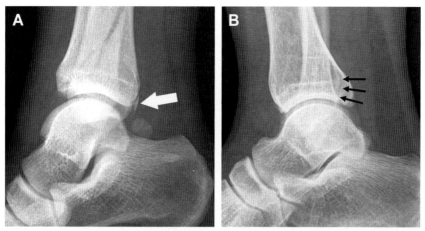

Fig. 20. Posterior tibial malleolus fractures. (*A*) Lateral radiograph shows a small flake of bone arising from the posterior tibial malleolus (*arrow*). This flake occurred from a twisting injury. (*B*) Lateral radiograph in a different patient after a plantar flexion injury shows a fracture (*arrows*) with a larger fragment of bone.

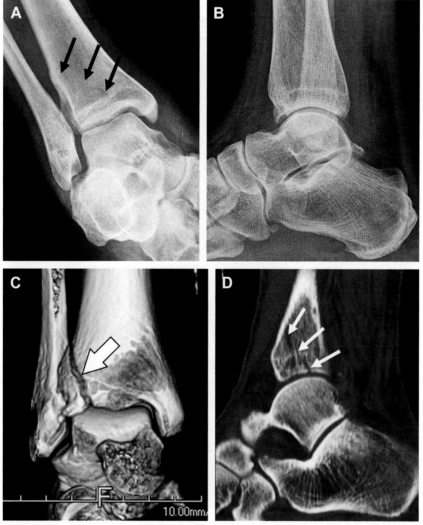

Fig. 21. Anterior tibial tubercle fracture from falling off a curb. (*A*) Frontal radiograph show a subtle oblique fracture line (*arrows*) and soft tissue swelling. (*B*) Lateral view appears normal. (*C*) Coronal three-dimensional CT image more clearly depicts the fracture line and size of the bone fragment (*arrow*). (*D*) Sagittal CT multiplanar reformatted (MRP) image shows the fracture orientation in this projection (*arrows*).

from the tibial articular surface proximally communicating to a horizontal component that extends laterally violating the lateral cortex of the tibia (**Fig. 21**).

Fractures of the Lateral Process of the Talus

A fracture of the lateral process of the talus is either caused by ankle eversion with dorsiflexion so that the superolateral surface of the calcaneus strikes against the inferior margin of the lateral talus process or occasionally by ankle inversion[47]; it is known as a snowboarder's fracture.[48] The fracture is apparent only on frontal views of the ankle, and a tip-off is that the epicenter of the soft tissue swelling is distal to the lateral malleolus (**Fig. 22**).

Fractures of the Posterior Process of the Talus

The posterior talus process has 2 tubercles, the medial and lateral tubercles. Avulsion fracture of the medial tubercle of the posterior process of the talus occurs after forceful dorsiflexion-pronation of the ankle.[49] Chip fractures occur when the ankle is severely plantar flexed so that the posterior tubercle become wedged between the posterior tibial lip and the calcaneus compressing the lateral tubercle.[50] These fractures may be extremely subtle and require differentiation from the os trigonum.

Fractures of the posterior tubercles are best detected in the lateral view, but because these fractures are often difficult to visualize using standard

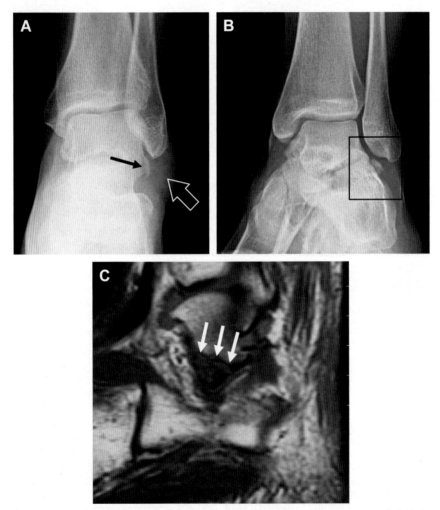

Fig. 22. Lateral talus process fractures. (*A*) Frontal radiograph shows an avulsion fracture of the lateral talus process (*arrow*) from an inversion injury. Note that the soft tissue swelling is distal to the lateral malleolus (*open arrow*). (*B*) Radiograph from another patient shows a larger triangular fragment of bone (*square*) from an eversion injury typical of a snowboarder's fracture. (*C*) Sagittal T1-weighted magnetic resonance image from the second patient showing the transverse fracture orientation (*arrows*).

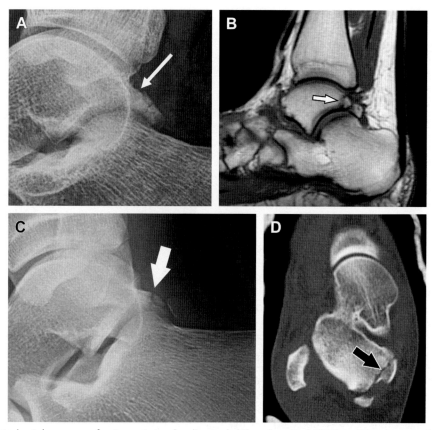

Fig. 23. Posterior talus process fractures. Lateral radiograph (*A*) and sagittal (*B*) T1-weighted magnetic resonance image shows a simple fracture of the posterolateral process (*arrows*). Only in retrospect was the fracture noted on the radiograph. Lateral radiograph (*C*) and axial CT (*D*) image shows a comminuted fracture of the posteromedial process (*arrows*).

radiographic views, shallow and steep external rotation oblique views have been suggested as adjunctive projections when there is a high index of suspicion and CT is not available (**Fig. 23**).[51]

Anterior Calcaneus Process Fracture

The anterior calcaneal process serves as the attachment site of the Y-shaped bifurcate

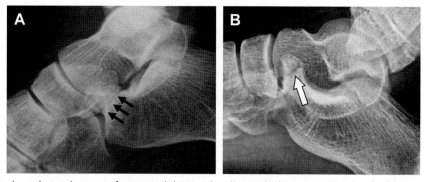

Fig. 24. Anterior calcaneal process fractures. (*A*) Lateral radiograph shows a nutcracker fracture of the anterior calcaneal process (*arrows*). The overlap with the navicular can obscure the fracture. (*B*) Lateral radiograph in another patient shows the fracture from an inversion injury (*arrow*). This mechanism results in smaller bone fragments.

ligament, which consists of 2 components, the calcaneonavicular and calcaneocuboid limbs. The bifurcate ligament is an important stabilizer in plantar and dorsal flexion of the ankle.[52]

Fractures of the anterior calcaneal process may be caused either by tension or by compression.[53] These fractures are often missed on initial radiographic inspection. These fractures occur by tension on the bifurcate ligament during forceful inversion and plantar flexion of the foot, or by compression of the anterior process between the cuboid and the talus during eversion and dorsiflexion. Impaction fractures, or nutcracker lesions, tend to be larger than avulsion fractures.

The lateral projection of the ankle offers the best opportunity for identifying the fracture, and close scrutiny for a break in the cortex is the key to making the correct diagnosis (**Fig. 24**).[42] If the lateral view is equivocal, an oblique projection of the foot may be diagnostic.

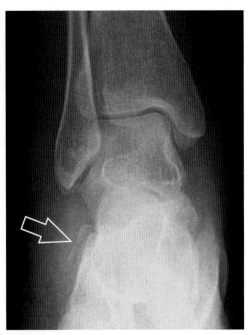

Fig. 25. Extensor digitorum brevis avulsion fracture from skating injury. Frontal radiograph shows 2 fragments of bone (*arrow*) arising from the anterolateral calcaneus at the origin of the extensor digitorum brevis muscle. The soft tissue swelling distal to the lateral malleolus is an important observation.

Extensor Digitorum Brevis Avulsion Fracture

Another important calcaneal avulsion fracture occurs at the origin of the extensor digitorum brevis muscle during forced inversion of the ankle.[54] This fracture is best depicted on the AP projection as a variable-sized fragment or fragments of bone that arise from the dorsolateral aspect of the calcaneus (**Fig. 25**). An important observation is that soft tissue swelling occurs distal to the lateral malleolus.

Lisfranc Joint Complex

The tarsometatarsal (TMT) joints, collectively referred to as Lisfranc joint, are partially stabilized by the intermetatarsal ligaments from the second to the fifth rays. The first and second TMT joints are different in that there is no intermetatarsal ligament between the bases of the first and second metatarsals.[55] Discrete dorsal, interosseous, and plantar ligaments attach the medial cuneiform to the base of the second metatarsal. The Lisfranc ligament is the strongest of these ligaments stabilizing the base of the second metatarsal to the medial cuneiform.

Fractures involving the Lisfranc ligament occur as a result of plantar flexion with either pronation or supination.[56] Although Lisfranc fracture dislocations account for 0.2% of all fractures, the diagnosis is initially missed in approximately 20% of the cases.[57] Initial radiographs may appear normal, but weight-bearing views may show subluxation or dislocation.

The classic finding is an osseous fragment between the second metatarsal base and medial cuneiform associated with widening of the intermetatarsal space from lateral subluxation of the second metatarsal base (partial homolateral type), although this constellation of findings is not common (**Fig. 26**). Subluxation can also occur at the navicular-medial cuneiform articulation, resulting in a divergent type of Lisfranc injury (**Fig. 27**A).

The lateral Lisfranc complex is composed of the bases of the fourth and fifth metatarsal bones, which articulate with the distal surface of the cuboid. The dorsal and plantar cuboideometatarsal, along with the intermetatarsal ligaments, peroneus brevis tendon, and lateral cord of the plantar fascia, contribute to the overall stability of the lateral midfoot region. Direct trauma and forced plantar flexion of the forefoot can disrupt these ligaments.

A small cortical avulsion from the cuboid can be seen on the oblique view of the foot (**Fig. 27**B).[58] Soft tissue swelling proximal to the base of the fifth metatarsal base may be associated with subluxation of the TMT joint.

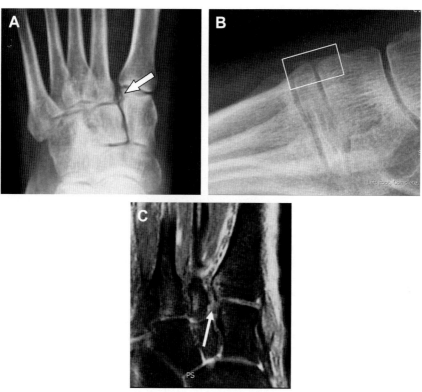

Fig. 26. Lisfranc fracture after falling off a horse. (*A*) Frontal radiograph shows a small bone fragment adjacent to the medial cuneiform bone (*arrow*) and lateral subluxation of the base of the second metatarsal. (*B*) Close-up of weight-bearing lateral view shows subtle dorsal subluxation of the second metatarsal with respect to the middle cuneiform (*rectangle*). (*C*) Axial STIR magnetic resonance image shows disruption of the Lisfranc ligament (*arrow*) as well as marrow edema in the first through third metatarsals and medial and middle cuneiforms.

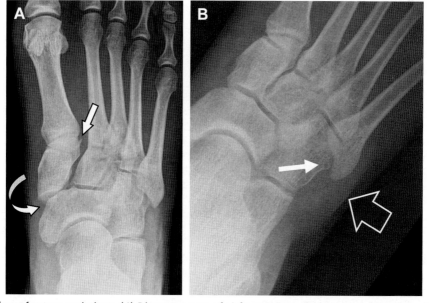

Fig. 27. Lisfranc fracture variations. (*A*) Divergent type of Lisfranc injury with medial subluxation of the medial cuneiform (*curved arrow*) resulting in widening of the space between the first and second metatarsal. Note the fracture adjacent to the medial cuneiform (*arrow*). (*B*) Lateral Lisfranc injury with a cuboid avulsion from the cuboideometatarsal ligament (*arrow*). Note that the soft tissue swelling occurs proximal to the base of the fifth metatarsal (*open arrow*).

SUMMARY

A systematic approach is useful when evaluating radiographs of patients with acute trauma to their lower extremity. Recalling high-risk areas in the hip, knee, and ankle allows the radiologist to quickly evaluate key locations in each projection for findings that are frequently subtle and may be evident on only 1 view. The technique is simple and sufficiently comprehensive to maximize fracture detection. However, the key to success is meticulous attention to detail and remembering not to overlook regions that frequently hide fractures.

REFERENCES

1. Tan V, Seldes RM, Katz MA, et al. Contribution of acetabular labrum to articulating surface area and femoral head coverage in adult hip joint: an anatomic study in cadavera. Am J Orthop 2001;30: 809–12.
2. Epstein HC. Traumatic dislocations of the hip. Clin Orthop 1973;92:116–42.
3. Dominguez S, Liu P, Roberts C, et al. Prevalence of traumatic hip and pelvic fractures in patients with suspected hip fracture and negative initial standard radiographs—a study of emergency department patients. Acad Emerg Med 2005;12: 366–70.
4. Parker MJ. Missed hip fractures. Arch Emerg Med 1992;9:23–7.
5. Perron AD, Miller MD, Brady WJ. Orthopedic pitfalls in the ED: radiographically occult hip fracture. Am J Emerg Med 2002;20:234–7.
6. Haramati N, Staron RB, Barax C, et al. Magnetic resonance imaging of occult fractures of the proximal femur. Skeletal Radiol 1994;23:19–22.
7. Judet R, Judet J, Letournel E. Fractures of the acetabulum. Classification and surgical approaches for open reduction. J Bone Joint Surg Am 1964;46: 1615–46.
8. Letournel E. Acetabular fractures: classification and management. Clin Orthop 1980;151:81–106.
9. Scott WW, Fishman EK, Magid D. Acetabular fractures: optimal imaging. Radiology 1987;165:537–9.
10. Moeb BR, Ajibade DA, Israel H. Computed tomography as a predictor of hip stability status in posterior wall fractures of the acetabulum. J Orthop Trauma 2009;23:7–15.
11. Pavlov H, Nelson TL, Warren RF, et al. Stress fractures of the pubic ramus. A report of twelve cases. J Bone Joint Surg Am 1982;64:1020–5.
12. Sanders TG, Zlatkin MB. Avulsion injuries of the pelvis. Semin Musculoskelet Radiol 2008;12:42–53.
13. DeLee JC, Evan JA, Thomas J. Anterior dislocation of the hip and associated femoral head fractures. J Bone Joint Surg Am 1980;62:960–4.
14. Epstein HC, Wiss DA, Coze L. Posterior fracture-dislocation of the hip with fractures of the femoral head. Clin Orthop 1985;201:9–17.
15. Yu JS. Hip and femur trauma. Imaging of trauma to the extremities. Semin Musculoskelet Radiol 2000;4: 205–20.
16. Malhotra R, Meena S, Digge VK. Tensile type of stress fracture neck of femur: role of teriparatide in the process of healing in a high risk patient for impaired healing of fracture. Clin Cases Miner Bone Metab 2013;10:210–2.
17. Goh SK, Yang KY, Koh JS, et al. Subtrochanteric insufficiency fractures in patients on alendronate therapy: a caution. J Bone Joint Surg Br 2007;89: 349–53.
18. Lenart BA, Lorich DG, Lane JM. Atypical fractures of the femoral diaphysis in postmenopausal women taking alendronate. N Engl J Med 2008; 358:1304–6.
19. Hayes CW, Brigado MK, Jamadar DA, et al. Mechanism-based pattern approach to classification of complex injuries of the knee depicted at MR imaging. Radiographics 2000;20:S121–34.
20. Gottsegen CJ, Eyer BA, White EA, et al. Avulsion fractures of the knee: imaging findings and clinical significance. Radiographics 2008;28:1755–70.
21. Miller L, Yu JS. Radiographic indicators of acute ligament injuries of the knee: a mechanistic approach. Emerg Radiol 2010;17:435–44.
22. Sanders TG, Medynski MA, Feller JF, et al. Bone contusion patterns of the knee at MR imaging: footprint of the mechanism of injury. Radiographics 2000;20:S135–51.
23. Murphy BJ, Smith RL, Uribe JW, et al. Bone signal abnormalities in the posterolateral tibia and lateral femoral condyle in complete tears of the anterior cruciate ligament: a specific sign? Radiology 1992; 182:221–4.
24. Kendall NS, Hsu SY, Chan KM. Fracture of the tibial spine in adults and children: a review of 31 cases. J Bone Joint Surg Br 1992;74:848–52.
25. Cobby MJ, Schweitzer ME, Resnick D. The deep lateral femoral notch: an indirect sign of a torn anterior cruciate ligament. Radiology 1992;184: 855–8.
26. Yu JS, Bosch E, Pathria MN, et al. The deep lateral femoral sulcus: correlation in 124 patients with anterior cruciate ligament tear. Emerg Radiol 1995;2: 129–34.
27. Stallenberg B, Genevois PA, Sintzoff SA Jr, et al. Fracture of the posterior aspect of the lateral tibial plateau: radiographic sign of anterior cruciate ligament tear. Radiology 1993;187:821–5.
28. Campos JC, Chung CB, Lektrakul N, et al. Pathogenesis of the Segond fracture: anatomic and MR imaging evidence of an iliotibial tract or anterior oblique band avulsion. Radiology 2001;219:381–6.

29. Weber WN, Neumann CH, Barakos JA, et al. Lateral tibial rim (Segond) fractures: MR imaging characteristics. Radiology 1991;180:731–4.

30. Hall FM, Hochman MG. Medial Segond-type fracture: cortical avulsion off the medial tibial plateau associated with tears of the posterior cruciate ligament and medial meniscus. Skeletal Radiol 1997; 26:553–5.

31. Escobedo EM, Mills WJ, Hunter JC. The "reverse Segond" fracture: association with a tear of the posterior cruciate ligament and medial meniscus. AJR Am J Roentgenol 2002;178:979–83.

32. Engelsohn E, Umans H, DiFelice GS. Marginal fractures of the medial tibial plateau: possible association with medial meniscal root tear. Skeletal Radiol 2007;36:73–6.

33. Huang GS, Yu JS, Munshi M, et al. Avulsion fracture of the head of the fibula (the "arcuate" sign): MR imaging findings predictive of injuries to the posterolateral ligaments and posterior cruciate ligament. AJR Am J Roentgenol 2003;180:381–7.

34. Fleming RE, Blatz DJ, McCarroll JR. Posterior problems in the knee: posterior cruciate insufficiency and posterolateral rotator insufficiency. Am J Sports Med 1981;9:107–13.

35. Yu JS, Salonen DC, Hodler J, et al. Posterolateral aspect of the knee: improved MR imaging with a coronal oblique technique. Radiology 1996;198: 199–204.

36. Rodriguez W Jr, Vinson EN, Helms CA, et al. MRI appearance of posterior cruciate ligament tears. AJR Am J Roentgenol 2008;191:W155–9.

37. El-Dieb A, Yu JS, Huang GS, et al. Pathologic conditions of the ligaments and tendons of the knee. Radiol Clin North Am 2002;40:1061–79.

38. Recondo JA, Salvador E, Villanua JA, et al. Lateral stabilizing structures of the knee: functional anatomy and injuries assessed with MR imaging. Radiographics 2000;20:S91–102.

39. Long D, Yu JS, Vitellas K. The ankle joint: imaging strategies in the evaluation of ligamentous injuries. Crit Rev Diagn Imaging 1998;39:393–445.

40. Mack RP. Ankle injuries in athletics. Clin Sports Med 1982;1:71–84.

41. Garrick JG, Regua RK. The epidemiology of foot and ankle injuries in sports. Clin Sports Med 1988;7: 29–36.

42. Yu JS, Cody ME. A template approach for detecting fractures in low energy ankle trauma. Emerg Radiol 2009;16:309–18.

43. Nielsen JO, Dons-Jensen H, Sorensen HT. Lauge-Hansen classification of malleolar fractures. An assessment of the reproducibility in 118 cases. Acta Orthop Scand 1990;61:385–7.

44. Haraguchi N, Haruyama H, Toga H, et al. Pathoanatomy of posterior malleolar fractures of the ankle. J Bone Joint Surg Am 2006;88:1085–92.

45. Tornetta P 3rd, Ostrum RF, Trafton PG. Trimalleolar ankle fracture. J Orthop Trauma 2001;15:588–90.

46. Protas JM, Kornblatt BA. Fractures of the lateral margin of the distal tibia. The Tillaux fracture. Radiology 1981;138:55–7.

47. Hawkins LG. Fractures of the lateral process of the talus. J Bone Joint Surg Am 1965;47:1170–5.

48. Funk JR, Srinivasan SC, Crandall JR. Snowboader's talus fractures experimentally produced by eversion and dorsiflexion. Am J Sports Med 2003;31:921–8.

49. Kim DH, Berkowitz MJ, Pressman DN. Avulsion fractures of the medial tubercle of the posterior process of the talus. Foot Ankle Int 2003;24:172–5.

50. Bureau NJ, Cardinal E, Hobden R, et al. Posterior ankle impingement syndrome: MR imaging findings in seven patients. Radiology 2000;215:497–503.

51. Ebraheim NA, Patil V, Frisch NC, et al. Diagnosis of medial tubercle fractures of the talar posterior process using oblique views. Injury 2007;38:1313–7.

52. Robbins MI, Wilson MG, Sella EJ. MR imaging of calcaneal process fractures. AJR Am J Roentgenol 1999;172:475–9.

53. Petrover D, Schweitzer ME, Laredo JD. Anterior process calcaneal fractures: a systematic evaluation of associated conditions. Skeletal Radiol 2007;36: 627–32.

54. Norfray JF, Rogers LF, Adamo GP, et al. Common calcaneal avulsion fracture. AJR Am J Roentgenol 1980;134:119–23.

55. de Palma L, Santucci A, Sabetta SP, et al. Anatomy of the Lisfranc joint complex. Foot Ankle Int 1997;18: 356–64.

56. Vuori JP, Aro HT. Lisfranc joint injuries: trauma mechanisms and associated injuries. J Trauma 1993;35:40–5.

57. Gupta RT, Wadhwa RP, Learch TJ, et al. Lisfranc injury: imaging findings for this important but often-missed diagnosis. Curr Probl Diagn Radiol 2008;37:115–26.

58. Bahel A, Yu JS. Lateral plantar pain: diagnostic considerations. Emerg Radiol 2010;17:291–8.

Imaging of Pancreatic and Duodenal Trauma

Kira Melamud, MD*, Christina A. LeBedis, MD, Jorge A. Soto, MD

KEYWORDS

- Trauma • Pancreatic injury • Duodenal injury • Computed tomography
- Magnetic resonance cholangiopancreatography • Blunt • Penetrating

KEY POINTS

- Pancreatic and duodenal injuries are rare but life-threatening occurrences, often occurring concomitantly and in association with other solid organ injuries.
- Imaging findings of pancreatic and duodenal trauma on computed tomography and MR imaging are often nonspecific, and high levels of clinical suspicion and understanding of mechanism of injury are imperative.
- Familiarity with the grading schemes of pancreatic and duodenal injury is important because they help in assessing for key imaging findings that directly influence management.

INTRODUCTION

Traumatic pancreatic and duodenal injuries are rare, especially in the setting of blunt abdominal trauma. These injuries are reported to make up only 2% of all blunt abdominal trauma.[1] Although exceedingly uncommon, it is imperative for radiologists to be vigilant for these injuries, because delay in diagnosis portends poor outcome with reported mortalities of up to 30% in patients with blunt pancreatic trauma,[2] and up to 25% in patients with duodenal injuries.[3] The rarity of such injuries, the complex anatomy, and the common association with concomitant multiorgan injury, which may obscure the subtlety of the imaging patterns of duodenal and pancreatic injury, pose a unique challenge. Variable imaging findings of pancreatic and duodenal injury, which may range from normal appearance to complete transection in the case of the pancreas or perforation in the case of duodenum, further complicate the situation. In addition, clinical signs and symptoms are also largely nonspecific and unreliable.[1]

Multidetector computed tomography (CT) plays a pivotal role in early injury surveillance in the setting of blunt abdominal trauma. In contrast, ultrasonography (US) and MR imaging play a smaller role in the initial diagnosis of pancreatic or duodenal injury, with their roles reserved for evaluation of potential posttraumatic complications. This article discusses direct and indirect imaging findings of pancreatic and duodenal injuries. CT protocols used in our institution for abdominal imaging in the setting of trauma are also detailed, as optimization of CT technique is imperative, particularly in evaluation of pancreatic trauma, because a poorly timed contrast bolus may compromise detection of pancreatic injury. Knowledge of typical mechanisms of injury and frequently associated patterns of organ injuries may provide important clues in initial assessment of the trauma CT scan, and these are also described. In addition, potential delayed complications of duodenal and pancreatic injuries are reviewed, as well as grading scales of injuries and treatment strategies.

Funding Sources: None.
Conflicts of Interest: None.
Department of Radiology, Boston University Medical Center, 820 Harrison Avenue, FGH Building 3rd Floor, Boston, MA 02118, USA
* Corresponding author.
E-mail address: kira.melamud@bmc.org

EPIDEMIOLOGY

Morbidity and mortality associated with pancreatic and duodenal trauma are high. As previously stated, the mortality for either pancreatic or duodenal injury may be up to approximately 30%. Early mortality is usually related to severe hemorrhage from associated vascular injury[2] and multiple coexisting injuries. In contrast, multiorgan failure and superimposed infections result in delayed deaths and complications. The probability of complications associated with either of these injuries ranges from about 30% to 60%, and, in many cases, is linked to missed findings and delayed diagnosis on initial imaging.[1] Early diagnosis is imperative, because delay by even 24 hours can increase the risk of death 4-fold.[1,4] Common complications of duodenal and pancreatic injuries include pancreatitis, pseudocysts, fistulas, intra-abdominal abscesses, and bowel anastomosis breakdown, and may lead to sepsis and multiorgan failure.

Coexisting injuries are common, caused by high-impact mechanisms typically associated with duodenal and pancreatic trauma, and are reported to occur in 50% to 98% of cases.[1] The most frequently associated solid organ injuries include the liver (47% of cases), spleen (28% of cases), and kidneys (23%).[1]

NORMAL ANATOMY AND PERTINENT RELATIONSHIPS
Pancreas

The pancreas is an endocrine and exocrine gland that is located in the superior retroperitoneum, and is also divided into anatomic sections: head, neck, body, tail, and the uncinate process. It is typically 15 to 20 cm long, and weighs up to 100 g. It is located anterior to the left kidney and several crucial vascular structures. The pancreatic head is intimately associated with the proximal duodenum, which explains why concomitant injuries to both of these organs are so common. In addition, the head of the pancreas has close anatomic relationships with the inferior vena cava (IVC) and the portal vein, often resulting in more severe injuries when the head of the pancreas is involved, as opposed to the body/tail. Injury to the neck and/or uncinate process may result in associated trauma to the superior mesenteric artery and/or vein, because these vessels run posteriorly here. In contrast, the splenic artery and vein run superoposteriorly to the tail of the pancreas, and may become compromised in trauma to the distal pancreas. In addition, the pancreatic duct usually traverses the entirety of the pancreas and, thus, trauma to any anatomic region of the pancreas may result in duct compromise with free leakage of pancreatic enzymes (**Fig. 1**).[1]

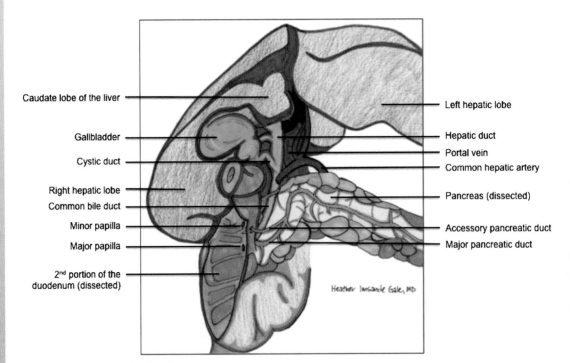

Fig. 1. Pancreatic and duodenal anatomy.

Duodenum

The duodenum is the first portion of the small bowel, extending from the pylorus to the duodeno-jejunal junction at the ligament of Treitz. There are 4 segments to the duodenum, each with complex anatomic relationships. The first segment of the duodenum (D1) encompasses the duodenal bulb, is mostly intraperitoneal, and passes posterosuperiorly toward the neck of the gallbladder. The second or descending segment of the duodenum (D2) is typically 7 to 8 cm long and is retroperitoneal. This segment is the drainage site of the minor and major papillae, which drain the pancreatic and biliary ducts. Because of the complex anatomy of the proximal duodenum, severe injuries of this segment necessitate more complicated surgical approaches than injuries involving the third or fourth portion.[5] The third or transverse portion of the duodenum (D3) extends horizontally and to the left approximately 10 to 12 cm, and is also retro-peritoneal. This segment is located ventral to the lumbar spine, aorta, and IVC, and is thus vulnerable to anteroposterior compression forces. The superior mesenteric vessels run anteriorly to the third portion of the duodenum. The last (fourth) portion of the duodenum (D4) is only approximately 2 to 3 cm long, remains retroperitoneal until the ligament of Treitz, and runs superiorly and to the left.[1] Blunt injuries caused by shearing forces centered at the junctions of the intraperitoneal and retroperitoneal segments of the duodenum have been reported and, thus, a thorough understanding of these anatomic relationships is crucial (see **Fig. 1**).[6]

MECHANISMS OF INJURY
Blunt Trauma

The pancreas and the duodenum are predominantly retroperitoneal in location, which frequently safeguards these organs in the setting of minor trauma. Because of their intimate relationship, the pancreas and duodenum are frequently injured concomitantly. Severe anteroposterior trauma, which compresses these organs against the spine, is the most common mechanism of injury. Familiarity with this typical mechanism of injury is crucial to radiologists, because this may provide the biggest clue to the need for a thorough interrogation of this region on initial imaging.

Classic accidents that have been described include seat-belt injuries, deceleration trauma, and handlebar compression trauma (**Fig. 2**). Presence of flexion/distraction fractures of the L1-L2 vertebrae should alert the radiologist to perform a careful evaluation of the retroperitoneal viscera in this area. Less common mechanisms include

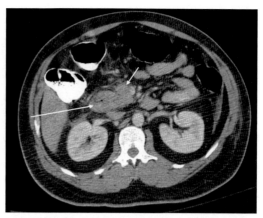

Fig. 2. A 30-year-old man who sustained blunt trauma to the abdomen after a motor vehicle accident. Contrast-enhanced CT (CECT) axial image of the abdomen shows a focal hematoma located at the root of the mesentery, just anterior to the horizontal portion of the duodenum (*short arrow*). There is circumferential wall thickening of the second portion of the duodenum (*long arrow*), concerning for a duodenal contusion. Note the fluid along the right anterior pararenal fascia. The patient was managed conservatively.

direct blows to the upper abdomen, as may happen in sports injuries and falls. The pancreatic body is the most frequently injured portion, accounting for greater than 65% of the injuries.[1]

Penetrating Trauma

The most frequent mechanisms of penetrating injury to the upper retroperitoneum are gunshot injuries and stab wounds. Because of their intimate relationship, a documented injury to either one of these organs should increase suspicion of injury to the other (**Fig. 3**).

IMAGING IN ABDOMINAL TRAUMA

CT is the mainstay initial modality to detect and characterize abdominal injuries in hemodynamically stable patients. In the setting of blunt trauma, such as after a fall or motor vehicle accident, CT is the fastest and most comprehensive technique of evaluating for pancreatic or duodenal injuries, and it helps guide the management algorithm. In a hemodynamically unstable patient or a patient who has a penetrating injury in which severe abdominal injury is suspected clinically, CT can play a role in the immediate post–exploratory laparotomy setting in which subtle injuries, such as those to the pancreas, are not readily recognizable intraoperatively because of the severity of other concomitant injuries. As discussed later, CT also

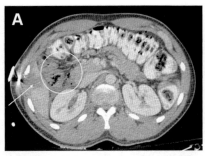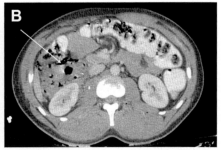

Fig. 3. A 19-year-old man who sustained a gunshot wound to the abdomen. (*A*) Axial CECT image shows a paper clip marking the entry site of the gunshot wound along the right lateral abdomen with the bullet tract extending through hepatic segment VI (*short arrow*) into the region of ascending colon and proximal duodenum. Note the wall thickening and poor enhancement of the ascending colon and second portion of the duodenum (*circle*). There is also hemorrhage in the Morrison pouch. (*B*) Inferiorly, note extraluminal gas in the region of ascending colon and second portion of the duodenum (*arrow*), which indicates penetrating injury. There was no extravasation of rectal contrast. At surgery, injuries to the ascending colon and second portion of the duodenum were found and repaired.

plays an important role in detection of delayed complications of pancreatic and duodenal injuries.

In the immediate posttraumatic period, other diagnostic modalities are much less advantageous and expedient than CT for detection of pancreatic and duodenal injury. For example, diagnostic peritoneal lavage, which is less frequently used now than in the past, is highly unreliable for detection of retroperitoneal injuries. Similarly, although US has been used in the emergency setting for detection of free intraperitoneal fluid with high sensitivity (86%),[7] it remains highly nonspecific in identifying the exact organs injured. Nonetheless, focused abdominal sonogram for trauma designed to assess for free intraperitoneal fluid has a role in the management algorithm of hemodynamically unstable patients after trauma.[8] MR imaging with cholangiopancreatogram (MRCP), plays a limited role in injury surveillance in the setting of acute trauma, but has been adopted as a problem-solving tool for directed questions. It is an important noninvasive imaging modality in evaluating for pancreatic duct or biliary injury.

Computed Tomography Techniques

The use of multidetector CT (MDCT) imaging provides high temporal resolution and the ability to generate high-quality multiplanar and three-dimensional reformations, which improve the ability to diagnose traumatic injuries.[8] Advances in MDCT technology in the early 2000's with the creation of 16 and 64 row MDCT, have been a particular boon in trauma imaging, allowing for improved image quality by minimizing motion related image degradation, due to faster scanning times compared to prior MDCT models. Specific protocols regarding slice thickness, timing of imaging acquisition, volume and types of

intravenous contrast administered, and use of oral contrast vary among institutions. In our level I trauma center, we currently use 64MDCT technology (Lightspeed VCT, GE Medical Systems, Milwaukee, WI). Our routine blunt abdominopelvic trauma protocol uses the following acquisition parameters: reconstruction thickness, 1.25 and 3.75 mm; noise index, 24; pitch, 1:0.984; gantry rotation time, 0.5 seconds. All patients receive a bolus of 100 mL of intravenous contrast (Iopamidol, 370 mg iodine/mL, Isovue; Bracco Diagnostics Inc, Princeton, NJ) at a rate of 4 to 5 mL/s with the use of a power injector through an 18-gauge or 20-gauge cannula in an antecubital vein. We use a dual-syringe power injector to deliver 30 mL of saline solution, also at 5 mL/s, as a chasing bolus to follow the intravenous contrast injection (**Table 1**).[3,9]

Table 1 Abdominal blunt trauma CT protocol	
Landmarks	**Diaphragm to Greater Trochanters**
Intravenous contrast	100 mL, 3 mL/s, with 30-mL saline chasing bolus
Scan delay (s)	70
Slice thickness (mm)	1.25
Reconstruction thickness (mm)	3.75
Noise index	24
Pitch	1:0.984
Delayed acquisition	May be obtained after 5-min delay, if necessary as determined by radiologist

Our routine abdominopelvic CT protocols in the setting of trauma use a standard delay of 70 seconds after injection of intravenous contrast, to acquire images in the portal-venous phase of enhancement. In addition, our trauma examinations are monitored during acquisition by a radiologist in the CT control room, and, in patients with acute injuries identified on the portal-venous–phase images, 5-minute low-radiation-dose delayed images of the abdomen and pelvis are obtained. The delayed images are particularly useful to assess for active abdominopelvic hemorrhage. The acquired axial thin-section images allow for full multiplanar capability. We routinely generate 2.5-mm multiplanar reconstructed images automatically in the coronal and sagittal planes. We do not routinely administer oral contrast for CT of blunt abdominal trauma; instead, we reserve the use of positive oral contrast for some follow-up CT examinations if there is concern for a perforating bowel or duodenal injury.

Special Computed Tomography Protocol Considerations in the Setting of Pancreatic Trauma

A unique CT protocol dilemma posed by imaging of the pancreas is the timing of optimal pancreatic parenchymal enhancement. The pancreatic parenchyma enhances with highest contrast earlier than the other, more frequently injured solid organs, such as the liver and the spleen. The optimal pancreatic parenchymal phase is usually achieved with acquisition of images approximately 35 to 40 seconds after intravenous contrast administration, and may increase sensitivity of often subtle CT pancreatic parenchymal findings in the setting of trauma. However, to date, there is insufficient data to validate routine use of an earlier acquisition in the initial investigation of trauma. However, if the initial trauma imaging raises a question of pancreatic injury, follow-up CT with use of the pancreatic parenchymal phase may be considered.[1,10–12] However, in this setting, MR cholangiopancreatography may be better suited as a follow-up imaging examination, because of the added benefits of not delivering ionizing radiation and providing a more direct evaluation of pancreatic duct integrity.

Another special CT protocol consideration in imaging of possible pancreatic injury pertains to postprocessing after image acquisition. Curved planar reformations and minimum intensity projection have been shown to be useful in depicting the pancreatic ductal structures and may be useful in evaluating the integrity of the pancreatic duct in patients with blunt trauma and CT findings of pancreatic injury (**Fig. 4**).[1,13–15]

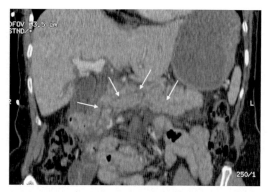

Fig. 4. Curved reformat reconstructed from CECT axial images (same patient as **Fig. 7**) through the axis of the pancreatic duct helps confirm continuity of the duct throughout its course (*arrows*).

PANCREATIC TRAUMA
Clinical and Laboratory Findings

Clinical signs of pancreatic injury are nonspecific, especially in the immediate posttraumatic scenario. The classic triad of leukocytosis, hyperamylasemia, and upper abdominal pain associated with pancreatic injury may take days to develop. In the setting of trauma, subtle findings such as epigastric discomfort out of proportion to physical examination[3] may become overshadowed by other concomitant injuries, or the patient may be altered or intubated/sedated. A seat-belt sign, or contusions and abrasions across the torso and upper abdomen in a restrained passenger related to a seatbelt, is a nonspecific physical sign, but is associated with overall increased intra-abdominal injuries. One study of children involved in motor vehicle collisions found that pancreatic injury was 22 times more common among children with the seat-belt sign,[16] and thus this may provide an early diagnostic clue.

Increase of serum amylase level may be a sign of pancreatic injury, but it may take several hours to days to develop, with some literature suggesting that as many as 40% of patients with pancreatic injury may initially have normal serum amylase.[3] A continuous increase in serum amylase level on serial examinations is a worrisome sign even in established pancreatic injury, and may indicate need for further imaging and intervention.

Computed Tomography Findings in Pancreatic Injury

Signs of pancreatic injury on CT include frank laceration, transection, or comminution of the pancreas; pancreatic hematoma; and active pancreatic or peripancreatic hemorrhage (**Table 2**).

Table 2
Differential considerations of types of pancreatic injury on CT

Types of Pancreatic Injury	Description
Lacerations/fractures/transections	Linear hypoattenuating regions, may be comminuted, possibly with displacement of structures. Lacerations spanning >50% of pancreatic diameter imply ductal injury
Contusion	Diffuse or focal area of nonlinear hypoattenuation
Hematoma	Hyperattenuating region within the pancreatic parenchyma

A jagged, hypoattenuating line that disrupts the pancreatic parenchyma is a typical finding of a pancreatic laceration (**Fig. 5**). Pancreatic contusions are frequently more subtle on imaging, and present as focal hypoattenuation within the parenchyma or focal pancreatic enlargement. Mixed-density pancreatic hematomas may also occur (**Fig. 6**). Localized blood collections interdigitating between the pancreatic parenchyma and the splenic vein is a highly sensitive secondary sign of pancreatic injury (**Box 1**).[1]

In the setting of penetrating injury, pancreatic trauma should be suspected if there is retention of a foreign body (eg, bullet fragments) in close vicinity to the pancreas, even if no obvious laceration or hematoma is seen. If there is no retention of foreign bodies, such as in a through-and-through gunshot wound, extrapolation of likely trajectory through the region of the pancreas, by analyzing adjacent injuries or retained tract of air, is sufficient to suspect pancreatic injury. In our institution, entrance and exit wounds on the skin are marked with radio-opaque objects, such that the CT trajectory of the wound can be estimated.

The most important factor that mandates intervention in the setting of pancreatic trauma is disruption of the pancreatic duct. A laceration of pancreatic parenchyma that extends over more than one-half of the pancreatic diameter is suggestive of pancreatic duct disruption. MRCP and endoscopic retrograde cholangiopancreatography (ERCP) may aid in diagnosis of pancreatic duct injury if the CT findings are not definitive.

Pitfalls of Pancreatic Injury

The most important pitfall in the initial posttraumatic scan is that CT findings of pancreatic injury may be either absent or subtle early after injury. Another pitfall in diagnosis of pancreatic injury is the presence of peripancreatic fluid, which may be related to either aggressive resuscitation efforts or to hemoperitoneum related to injuries of adjacent organs. Because of these confounding factors and the difficulty in detecting pancreatic duct injuries on CT, the severity of pancreatic injury tends to be underestimated on imaging. Nonetheless, the sensitivity and specificity of CT

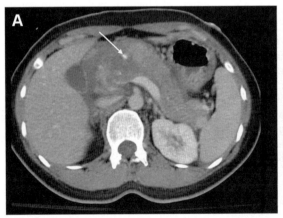 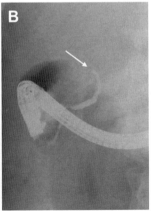

Fig. 5. A 37-year-old woman who sustained a blunt injury to the abdomen from impaction on the steering wheel presented with severe epigastric tenderness. (*A*) Axial CECT image shows an extensive fracture of the pancreatic neck with a large intrapancreatic hematoma with active extravasation (*arrow*). (*B*) Endoscopic retrograde cholangiopancreatography (ERCP) shows abrupt cutoff of the pancreatic duct at the junction of the neck and body of the pancreas (*arrow*), concerning for traumatic duct disruption and stricture. On further injection of contrast at ERCP, there was free leakage of contrast from the pancreatic parenchyma (not shown). The patient subsequently underwent Roux-en-Y pancreaticojejunostomy.

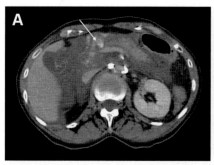
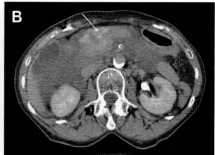

Fig. 6. A 37-year-old woman involved in a motor vehicle accident. (*A*) CECT axial image shows disruption/fracture of the pancreatic head and neck with a large pancreatic hematoma with active extravasation (*arrow*). (*B*) Note the expansion of the hyperdense pancreatic hematoma on a delayed CT image from the same study, confirming active extravasation (*arrow*). The patient was treated with an emergent Whipple procedure.

in detecting these injuries is reported to be approximately 80%.[1,3]

Mimics of Pancreatic Injury

The morphology of the pancreas, with its many clefts, is one of the biggest mimics in diagnosing pancreatic injury. A deep pancreatic cleft, especially in the setting of aggressive intravenous hydration, can easily be mistaken for a pancreatic laceration (**Figs. 7** and **8**). The reverse may also be true, because a laceration, especially one without full pancreatic transection, can be overlooked and deemed to be a pancreatic cleft. A hypodense

or hyperenhancing pancreatic lesion in a patient with trauma may be mistaken for a contusion or hematoma, respectively. Similarly, focal or diffuse pancreatic edema with peripancreatic inflammation of the pancreas related to primary pancreatitis may be mistaken for pancreatic injury. In these cases, familiarity with the severity of mechanism of injury is frequently sufficient to help avoid such pitfalls.[17]

Grading Pancreatic Injury

The American Association for the Surgery of Trauma (AAST) pancreatic injury scoring system is also frequently used by radiologists and trauma surgeons. The major factors that influence the grade of pancreatic injury include the location and severity of injury, and the integrity of the main pancreatic duct.[17] More proximal injuries (located toward the head of the gland) that are definite lacerations or even transections, with involvement of the main pancreatic duct, naturally receive higher scores than injuries that involve the pancreatic tail and are focal contusions without pancreatic duct disruption (**Table 3**).

MR Imaging Findings in Pancreatic Injury

The 2 most important determinants of outcome following pancreatic injury are the time from injury to definitive diagnosis, as discussed earlier, and status of the main pancreatic. If there is no definitive transection that spans the diameter of the pancreas, detection of pancreatic duct injury on MDCT may be challenging. In the past, ERCP was the only method available for determining the integrity of the main pancreatic duct. However, in recent years in hemodynamically stable patients in whom there is concern for pancreatic injury, MRCP has come to the forefront as a noninvasive means to assess pancreatic duct integrity. MRCP sequences use heavily T2-weighted two-dimensional and

---

Box 1
Diagnostic criteria on CT

Imaging findings in pancreatic injuries

Direct findings:

    Laceration (linear region of nonenhancement)

    Diffuse or focal pancreatic enlargement

    Heterogenous enhancement

Indirect findings:

    Peripancreatic fat stranding or fluid

    Fluid between the splenic vein and the pancreas

    Peripancreatic hemorrhage

    Injuries to adjacent organs or vessels

    Trajectory of penetrating injury through the region of the pancreas

Complications:

    Pseudocyst

    Pancreatitis

    Abscess

    Fistula

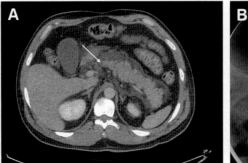
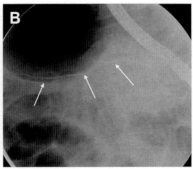

Fig. 7. A 47-year-old man involved in a motor vehicle accident with multiple injuries, including crush injuries of lower extremities resulting in bilateral lower extremity amputations. (A) Initial CECT shows extensive peripancreatic fluid, as well as a linear hypodensity (arrow) through the pancreatic parenchyma in the head/neck junction that was concerning for a laceration. (B) ERCP shows an intact pancreatic duct (arrows). At surgery, no pancreatic laceration was found. The imaging finding likely represent a fluid-filled pancreatic cleft, which is a common imaging pitfall. Given extensive peripancreatic fluid on imaging and increased amylase level, posttraumatic pancreatitis was suspected in this patient.

three-dimensional images, which show biliary anatomy as well as the spatial relationship of fluid-containing structures. The use of secretin may further increase the diagnostic accuracy of MRCP in pancreatic ductal injury by temporarily increasing ductal caliber and allowing improved visualization.[8] In addition to showing the course of the pancreatic duct from the head to the tail, MRCP has the added advantage compared with ERCP in detecting pancreatic parenchymal abnormalities (Fig. 9) and associated adjacent abnormalities, such as concomitant biliary injuries, that may also go undetected on initial trauma CT. MRCP may also play a role in surgical or pre-ERCP planning by elucidating any ductal anomalies.[18] The role of ERCP may be confirmatory in indeterminate cases before definitive surgical intervention or may play a therapeutic role when stenting of the pancreatic duct is a feasible option.[8]

Delayed Complications of Pancreatic Injury

Pancreatic injury is associated with a significant risk of delayed morbidities, ranging from 11% to 62%.[1] Late complications of undetected pancreatic trauma develop in up to one-third of the patients, and may present weeks to years after initial trauma (Fig. 10).[19] Reported complications include posttraumatic pancreatitis, pancreatic abscess, and formation of pseudocysts. Presence of focal peripancreatic fluid collections after trauma implies ductal injury, and necessitates appropriate investigation of the pancreatic duct.[19] Leakage of pancreatic enzymes can predispose to abnormal fistulization between the pancreas and adjacent structures (Fig. 11). Pseudoaneurysm formation of adjacent vascular structures may present as delayed hemorrhage. Posttraumatic strictures of the pancreatic duct, which can predispose to recurrent pancreatitis, have also been reported.[19]

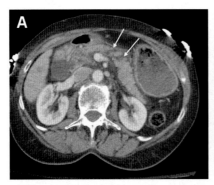
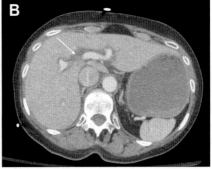

Fig. 8. An 80-year-old woman involved in a motor vehicle accident. (A) Axial CECT immediately after trauma shows 2 adjacent linear hypodensities with the body of the pancreas (arrows), concerning for pancreatic lacerations. Note the small amount of peripancreatic fluid. At surgery, no signs of traumatic injury to the pancreas were found. The findings on CT likely represent an imaging pitfall of pancreatic clefts distended with fluid caused by aggressive resuscitation. (B) Note that the periportal edema (arrow) and fullness of the IVC on the same scan supporting the diagnosis.

Table 3
AAST pancreatic injury grading scale

Grade	Injury	Description
I	Hematoma	Small contusion without duct injury
	Laceration	Small laceration without duct injury
II	Hematoma	Major contusion without duct injury
	Laceration	Major laceration without duct injury
III	Laceration	Distal parenchymal laceration with duct injury
IV	Laceration	Proximal laceration with involvement of the ampulla
V	Laceration	Extensive disruption of the pancreatic head

Adapted from Moore EE, Cogbill TH, Malangoni MA, et al. Organ injury scaling, II: pancreas, duodenum, small bowel, colon, and rectum. J Trauma 1990;30(11):1427.

DUODENAL TRAUMA
Clinical Findings of Duodenal Trauma

Similar to pancreatic injury, clinical signs of traumatic duodenal injury are highly nonspecific, especially in the early posttraumatic setting. Mild upper abdominal tenderness may be the only symptom. In the setting of duodenal perforation, extravasation of duodenal contents into the peritoneal cavity, often via the foramen of Winslow, can present as generalized peritonitis, with worsening abdominal tenderness, but this may take hours to become apparent. Leakage of peritoneal contents contained within the lesser sac may take even longer to be detected clinically. An increase in serum amylase level may also be associated with duodenal perforations, because pancreatic enzymes make up a portion of the duodenal contents.[5]

Computed Tomography Findings in Duodenal Injury

Duodenal injuries may result from penetrating or blunt trauma. The spectrum of duodenal injuries ranges from contusion or intramural hematoma to complete perforation or devascularization

(**Box 2**). Duodenal hematoma or contusion may present on imaging as focal wall thickening (>4 mm) from edema or hyperdense intramural hematoma. If sufficiently large, intramural hemorrhage in the duodenum may present as gastric outlet obstruction, but this is frequently a delayed, rather than immediate, outcome. Secondary signs of duodenal injury, which are less specific, include fluid or hemorrhage in the retroperitoneum and stranding of retroperitoneal fatty tissues, which have been associated with both intramural hematomas and perforations (**Fig. 12**). In the presence of obvious pancreatic injury on CT imaging, duodenal injury should at least be questioned by the radiologists, even if no primary signs are seen.

Duodenal perforations have also been reported in the setting of trauma. Extraluminal gas in the retroperitoneum, discontinuity of the duodenal wall, and extravasation of positive contrast material (if administered) into the retroperitoneum are direct signs of duodenal perforation. More subtle injuries to the duodenum may allow air to escape into the duodenal wall, resulting in focal pneumatosis. Distinction between a duodenal wall hematoma and perforation is critical, because the former

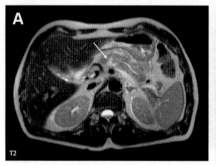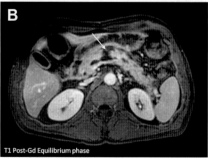

Fig. 9. A 55-year-old man who was found unconscious with increased serum amylase and lipase levels. Initial CT of the abdomen showed a focal area of hypoattenuation in the body of the pancreas, concerning for a laceration (not shown). Subsequent MRCP (*A, B*) confirmed the finding, showing a linear region of increased T2-weighted signal (*arrow* in *A*) with corresponding lack of enhancement on postgadolinium images (*arrow* in *B*). Note the lack of visualization of the pancreatic duct in the region of signal abnormality on the T2 image, which was concerning for traumatic pancreatic duct transection. Trauma history was later confirmed.

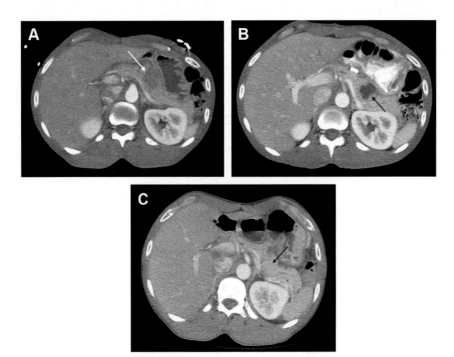

Fig. 10. A 47-year-old man sustained blunt abdominal trauma after a fall down stairs. (*A*) CECT axial image shows a heterogenous hematoma in the body of the pancreas, confirmed at surgery (*arrow*). (*B*) CECT obtained 3 weeks later for worsening abdominal pain reveals an organized fluid collection in the region of previously evacuated hematoma, concerning for a pseudocyst (*arrow*). (*C*) CECT obtained for an unrelated reason 2 years later shows resolution of the pancreatic collection after conservative management (*arrow*).

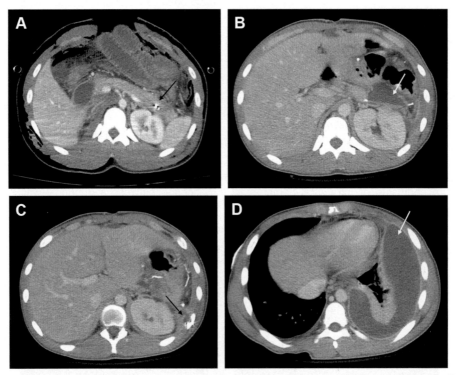

Fig. 11. A 19-year-old man who sustained multiple gunshot wounds to the upper abdomen. (*A*) CECT obtained after exploratory laparotomy shows bullet fragments in the tail of the pancreas (*arrow*) with surrounding hypodensity, indicating a laceration. The patient subsequently underwent distal pancreatectomy and splenectomy. (*B–D*) CECT obtained 3 weeks after injury for persistent fever shows a rim-enhancing fluid collection extending from the pancreatectomy bed (*arrow* in *B*) along a diaphragmatic defect (*arrow* in *C*) and into the left pleural space (*arrow* in *D*) along the trajectory of the bullet tract. Fluid sampling indicated that this was a large pancreatic fluid collection with fluid amylase levels exceeding 3000 U/L. This collection was successfully treated with percutaneous drainage.

Box 2	
Differential considerations of types of duodenal injury	
Contusion	Perforation
• Treated conservatively	• Treated surgically
• Imaging features:	• Imaging features:
○ Focal duodenal wall thickening (>4 mm)	○ Discontinuity of the duodenal wall
○ High-density intramural hematoma	○ Retroperitoneal extraluminal gas
○ Intramural gas (pneumatosis)	○ Retroperitoneal extraluminal oral contrast
○ Periduodenal fluid/stranding	○ Periduodenal fluid/stranding

may be treated conservatively, whereas the latter necessitates surgical intervention. Severe devascularization injuries or avulsions of the ampulla of Vater are even rarer, but have been associated with traumatic duodenal perforations (**Box 3**).[20]

In the setting of penetrating injuries without frank duodenal disruption or perforation on imaging, the presumed trajectory of injury, if it extends through the region of the duodenum, is sufficient to raise concern for duodenal trauma (**Fig. 13**).

Pitfalls and Mimics of Duodenal Trauma on Computed Tomography

There are several common pitfalls that lead to false-positive findings of traumatic bowel injury with regard to the duodenum. For instance, focal underdistention of the duodenum may be mistaken for abnormal wall thickening. In addition, diffuse thickening of the small bowel, including the duodenum, may be related to aggressive intravenous hydration with systemic volume overload causing bowel wall edema (**Fig. 14**). Hypoperfusion complex may present with several small bowel manifestations, including diffuse bowel wall edema or increased bowel wall enhancement,

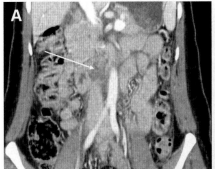
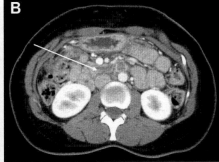
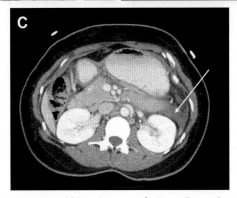

Fig. 12. A 37-year-old woman who sustained blunt trauma after a strike to the epigastrium in a go-cart accident. (*A*) Coronal and (*B*) axial images from the initial CECT shows an irregular hypoattenuation of the third portion of the duodenum (*arrows* in *A* and *B*) and surrounding fat stranding, concerning for a contusion. (*C*) Repeat CT performed 6 hours later shows increasing hyperdense fluid concerning for hemorrhage (42 Hounsfield units) in the retroperitoneum (*arrow*), and similar irregular enhancement of the third portion of the duodenum (not shown). At surgery, a 1-cm perforation was found in the third portion of the duodenum and repaired.

both of which may be mimics of duodenal injury.[7] Associated findings of hypoperfusion complex, including flattening of the IVC and hyperenhancing adrenal glands, can help steer radiologists from making false-positive diagnoses. Importantly, retroperitoneal edema is also a known finding in hypoperfusion complex, and can easily be interpreted as an indirect sign of duodenal or pancreatic injury.[7] In addition, duodenal diverticula, which are common, may be mistaken for extraluminal gas, especially if small, and care should be taken to distinguish the two entities.

Grading Duodenal Injury and Management on Computed Tomography

Duodenal injury grading schemas have been created to help triage patients who require definitive surgical management and distinguish them from those who may be treated conservatively. The most accepted grading system is published by the AAST. The major differentiating factors in the duodenal injury scoring system include the location, severity and extent of duodenal injury, involvement of the ampulla and common bile duct, and vascular injury (**Table 4**).[17]

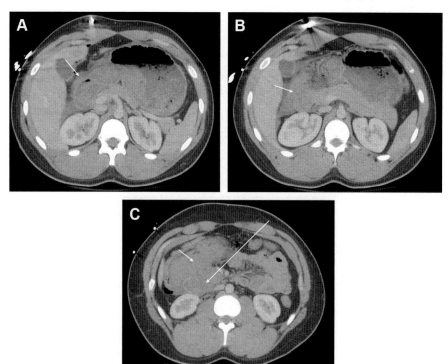

Fig. 13. A 21-year-old man who was hemodynamically stable after a gunshot wound to the upper abdomen. Serial axial CECT images show extensive hyperdense hemorrhage surrounding the pylorus and the proximal duodenum (*short arrows* in A–C). Note the paucity of wall enhancement of the medial aspect of the duodenum at the junction of the second/third portions (*long arrow* in C), which are concerning for injury. Considering the close relationship to the pancreatic head, pancreatic injury was questioned. At surgery, perforations of the pylorus and duodenum were confirmed, as was injury to the pancreas.

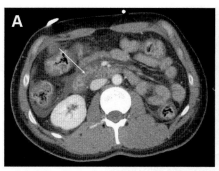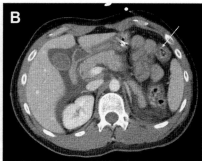

Fig. 14. A 26-year-old man who sustained a blast injury underwent CECT of the abdomen after emergent bilateral above-the-knee amputations. (*A*) Note the heterogeneous attenuation of the duodenum with mucosal hyperenhancement on this CECT axial image, which was concerning for possible duodenal injury (*arrow*). No injury was found at surgery. (*A, B*) Note the extensive simple-appearing periduodenal fluid, which tracks along the right pararenal fascia, Morrison pouch, gallbladder fossa, and right paracolic gutter, and is likely related to aggressive hydration, resulting in pitfall imaging findings of duodenal injury. There was also extensive periportal edema (not shown). Note the wall edema of visualized large bowel, which can be seen in aggressive hydration (*arrow* in *B*).

Overall, higher grades of duodenal injury require more complicated surgical intervention. For example, grade I and II duodenal injuries, presenting as hematomas, may be managed conservatively with close clinical surveillance. Higher grades of injury may necessitate surgical intervention varying from primary anastomosis through a distal duodenal perforation to more complex surgeries such as pancreaticoduodenectomy in patients with massive destructive lesions of the duodenum, pancreas, and common bile duct.[5,20]

When both imaging and clinical findings are nonspecific, such as in the presence of retroperitoneal fluid, but the mechanism of trauma is evokes concern for duodenal injury, close-interval follow-up CT (in our institution we recommend in 6–8 hours) can be useful to assess for possible evolution of injury during expectant management by the surgeon.[8]

Magnetic Resonance Findings of Duodenal Injuries

As in pancreatic injuries, MR imaging plays a limited role in initial diagnosis of duodenal injury, because significant perforating injuries requiring surgery most commonly present as free air on imaging, which is often difficult to identify on MR. Instead, the role of MR imaging is reserved for evaluation of common concomitant injuries, such as to the bile or pancreatic ducts (**Fig. 15**). However, minor injuries, such as an acute duodenal intramural hematoma, may be more evident on MR than on CT, and may present as a hyperintense focus on T1-weighted imaging, with blooming on gradient echo sequences. MRCP may be used in the setting of duodenal trauma to assess for injury of the common bile duct/ampulla, with added advantage provided by hepatobiliary contrast

Table 4
AAST duodenal injury grading scale

Grade	Injury	Description
I	Hematoma, laceration	Involvement of a single portion of the duodenum
II	Hematoma, laceration	Involvement of more than 1 portion, disruption of <50% of the circumference
III	Laceration	Disruption of 50%–75% of the circumference of D2; disruption of 50%–100% of the circumference of D1, D3, and D4
IV	Laceration	Disruption of >75% of the circumference of D2 or involvement of the ampulla or distal common bile duct
V	Laceration, vascular injury	Massive disruption of the duodenopancreatic complex or devascularization of the duodenum

Note: The duodenum is divided into duodenal bulb (D1), descending part (D2), transverse part (D3), and ascending part (D4).

Adapted from Moore EE, Cogbill TH, Malangoni MA, et al. Organ injury scaling, II: pancreas, duodenum, small bowel, colon, and rectum. J Trauma 1990;30(11):1428.

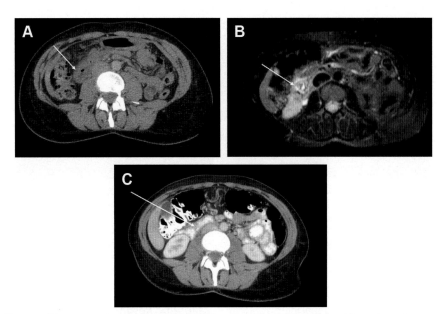

Fig. 15. A 33-year-old woman who sustained blunt abdominal trauma after being blown by a strong gust of wind and striking a metal pole. (*A*) CECT of the abdomen obtained immediately after trauma shows circumferential wall thickening (*arrow*) of the second portion of the duodenum. (*B*) T2-weighted fat-suppressed image from MRCP obtained to evaluate the integrity of the pancreatic duct shows increased T2 signal within the wall of the duodenum (*arrow*), consistent with duodenal contusion with a trace of surrounding free fluid. (*C*) Repeat CECT performed 1 week after trauma shows resolution of circumferential duodenal wall thickening (*arrow*) in this patient who was treated conservatively.

agents such as gadoxetate disodium, which can help localize associated bile leaks.

Delayed Complications of Duodenal Injuries

Several delayed complications have been described in the setting of duodenal injuries. For example, intramural hematomas, which occur in the submucosal or subserosal layers of the duodenal wall, may present with gastric outlet obstructions several days after injury as the contents of the hematoma evolve and expand over time.[5] This delayed complication may be the first diagnosis of an otherwise subtle mural injury. Delayed postoperative complications after repair of duodenal perforations of which a radiologist should be aware include abscess formation and dehiscence of duodenal suture line. The risk of dehiscence is particularly high when the diagnosis of duodenal perforation was delayed; the perforation involves much of the duodenal wall, resulting in undue tension on the suture line; or in the setting of injury to the proximal duodenum, especially with pancreatic injury in which leakage of pancreatic, gastric, and biliary contents precludes healing.[5]

SUMMARY

Pancreatic and duodenal injuries are uncommon but significant sequelae of major abdominal trauma that frequently occur concomitantly in both blunt and penetrating injuries because of their close anatomic relationship. Multidetector CT is the mainstay in imaging of acute abdominal trauma. Awareness of frequently subtle and nonspecific but crucial CT findings of pancreatic and duodenal injury can help guide the management algorithm. In pancreatic injury, evaluation for pancreatic duct integrity is pivotal, and often determines the necessity for intervention. In duodenal injury, identification of perforation, or associated disruption of the biliary or pancreaticoduodenal complex, increases the grade of injury, necessitating surgical intervention. MRCP is a supporting noninvasive imaging modality in the setting of suspected pancreatic and duodenal injury that can help evaluate biliary or pancreatic duct injury, whereas ERCP can play both a diagnostic and therapeutic role.

REFERENCES

1. Linsenmaier U, Wirth S, Reiser M, et al. Diagnosis and classification of pancreatic and duodenal injuries in emergency radiology. Radiographics 2008;28(6):1591–602.
2. Rekhi S, Anderson SW, Rhea JT, et al. Imaging of blunt pancreatic trauma. Emerg Radiol 2010;17(1):13–9.

3. Souba WW, Fink MP, Jurkovich GJ, et al. ACS surgery: principle & practice, 6th edition. Chapter 108: injuries to the pancreas and duodenum. New York: WebMD Professional Publishing; 2007. p. 1326–40.

4. Smego DR, Richardson JD, Flint LM. Determinants of outcome in pancreatic trauma. J Trauma 1985; 25(8):771–6.

5. Degiannis E, Boffard K. Duodenal injuries. Br J Surg 2000;87(11):1473–9.

6. Luther A, Mann C, Hart C, et al. Duodenal rupture secondary to blunt trauma from a football. J Surg Case Rep 2013;2013(1) [pii:rjs041].

7. Brofman N, Atri M, Hanson JM, et al. Evaluation of bowel and mesenteric blunt trauma with multidetector CT. Radiographics 2006;26(4):1119–31.

8. Stuhlfaut JW, Anderson SW, Soto JA. Blunt abdominal trauma: current imaging techniques and CT findings in patients with solid organ, bowel, and mesenteric injury. Semin Ultrasound CT MR 2007; 28(2):115–29.

9. LeBedis CA, Anderson SW, Mercier G, et al. The utility of CT for predicting bile leaks in hepatic trauma. Emerg Radiol 2015;22(2):101–7. Availabe at: http://link.springer.com/article/10.1007%2Fs10140-014-1262-9#.

10. Shanmuganathan K. Multi-detector row CT imaging of blunt abdominal trauma. Semin Ultrasound CT MR 2004;25(2):180–204.

11. McNulty NJ, Francis IR, Platt JF, et al. Multi-detector row helical CT of the pancreas: effect of contrast-enhanced multiphasic imaging on enhancement of the pancreas, peripancreatic vasculature, and pancreatic adenocarcinoma. Radiology 2001; 220(1):97–102.

12. Mullinix AJ, Foley WD. Multidetector computed tomography and blunt thoracoabdominal trauma. J Comput Assist Tomogr 2004;28(Suppl 1):S20–7.

13. Salles A, Nino-Murcia M, Jeffrey RB Jr. CT of pancreas: minimum intensity projections. Abdom Imaging 2008;33(2):207–13.

14. Gong JS, Xu JM. Role of curved planar reformations using multidetector spiral CT in diagnosis of pancreatic and peripancreatic diseases. World J Gastroenterol 2004;10(13):1943–7.

15. Anderson SW, Soto JA. Pancreatic duct evaluation: accuracy of portal venous phase 64 MDCT. Abdom Imaging 2009;34(1):55–63.

16. Sokolove PE, Kuppermann N, Holmes JF. Association between the "seat belt sign" and intra-abdominal injury in children with blunt torso trauma. Acad Emerg Med 2005;12(9):808–13.

17. Moore EE, Cogbill TH, Malangoni MA, et al. Organ injury scaling, II: pancreas, duodenum, small bowel, colon, and rectum. J Trauma 1990;30(11):1427–9.

18. Gupta A, Stuhlfaut JW, Fleming KW, et al. Blunt trauma of the pancreas and biliary tract: a multimodality imaging approach to diagnosis. Radiographics 2004;24(5):1381–95.

19. Patel SV, Spencer JA, el-Hasani S, et al. Imaging of pancreatic trauma. Br J Radiol 1998;71(849): 985–90.

20. Khelif K, De Laet MH. Traumatic duodenal necrosis with avulsion of Vater's papilla in a child. J Pediatr Surg 2006;41(7):e21–3.

Imaging of Urinary System Trauma

Joel A. Gross, MD[a],*, Bruce E. Lehnert, MD[a], Ken F. Linnau, MD[a],
Bryan B. Voelzke, MD, MS[b], Claire K. Sandstrom, MD[a]

KEYWORDS

• Renal trauma • Kidney trauma • Ureter trauma • Bladder trauma • Genitourinary trauma
• Urinary tract trauma • CT cystogram • CT urinoma

KEY POINTS

- Computed tomography (CT) imaging of the kidney, ureter, and bladder permit accurate and prompt diagnosis or exclusion of injuries.
- Review of initial imaging of the kidneys and ureters while the patient is in the CT scanner permits selection of patients who require delayed imaging, and prevents radiation exposure to patients who do not.
- Clinical and imaging criteria permit selective cystography of patients to evaluate for bladder trauma.
- Use of the appropriate imaging techniques in the initial imaging for urologic trauma or during follow-up imaging results in lower radiation dose than evaluation with standard imaging protocols.

INTRODUCTION

The urinary system consists of the kidneys, ureters, bladder, and urethra. In this article, we focus on imaging of blunt urinary system trauma with specific references to penetrating trauma where appropriate. We review imaging of the kidneys, ureters, and bladder and refer the reader to an excellent article on male pelvic trauma for a review of imaging of the male urethra and penis.[1] Imaging plays a limited role in the evaluation of the female urethra after trauma and is not discussed herein.

The organs of the urinary system differ from other solid and hollow organs in the body based on their ability to create urine (kidneys), transmit urine (ureters and urethra), or store urine (bladder). Consequently, fluid located adjacent to these structures may represent hematoma or urine, and specific imaging may be necessary to determine whether urinary extravasation is present.

RENAL TRAUMA
Epidemiology

Urinary tract injuries occur in 8% to 10% of traumatic injuries to the abdomen[2,3] with the kidney affected most often.[4] Most significant renal trauma is accompanied by injuries to other organs.[4] Most isolated renal injuries are considered minor and can be managed conservatively.[4] Penetrating trauma accounts for approximately 10% of renal injuries, and the vast majority of injuries are attributed to blunt trauma.[4,5]

The kidney is the third most commonly injured organ in adults after blunt abdominal trauma, but is the most commonly injured organ in children.[6]

Disclosure Statement: The authors have no relevant financial disclosures related to this paper.
[a] Department of Radiology, Harborview Medical Center, University of Washington School of Medicine, Box 359728, 325 Ninth Avenue, Seattle, WA 98104-2499, USA; [b] Department of Urology, Harborview Medical Center, University of Washington School of Medicine, Box 359868, 325 Ninth Avenue, Seattle, WA 98104-2499, USA
* Corresponding author.
E-mail address: jagross@uw.edu

Radiol Clin N Am 53 (2015) 773–788
http://dx.doi.org/10.1016/j.rcl.2015.02.005
0033-8389/15/$ – see front matter © 2015 Elsevier Inc. All rights reserved.

The pediatric kidney is proposed to be at increased risk of injury due to its greater size relative to the pediatric abdomen and less robust protection from minimal perinephric fat, weaker abdominal muscles, and unossified ribs.[6,7] Abnormal kidneys, such as those with hydronephrosis, cysts, masses, horseshoe configuration, or ectopic location, are also at greater risk of sustaining blunt traumatic injury.[7,8]

Renal Imaging Technique

Contrast-enhanced computed tomography (CT) is the preferred method of imaging renal trauma in hemodynamically stable patients.[9] On CT, the renal cortex and medulla enhance maximally at different times. Although oncologic imaging might best be performed during the nephrographic phase,[10] when the attenuation of the cortex and medulla is similar, most renal trauma imaging is performed in the late corticomedullary phase, when the cortex enhances more robustly than the medulla. This phase corresponds with the portal venous contrast phase, which optimizes enhancement of the organs most commonly injured (the liver and spleen) while providing reasonable enhancement of the other torso structures, including the kidney. Although arterial phase imaging is occasionally helpful in diagnosing or further characterizing traumatic vascular lesions, it is not necessary for the vast majority of patients and can be excluded from routine initial trauma imaging to minimize radiation dose.

For the remainder of this article, we refer to the contrast-enhanced phase obtained to evaluate the renal parenchyma as the parenchymal phase, whether this occurs during the corticomedullary phase or nephrographic phase.

On the parenchymal phase, it is usually impossible to determine whether any fluid around the urinary tract represents hematoma, urine, or other fluid (bowel contents, serous fluid, etc). When fluid is identified around the urinary tract or a renal injury is identified on the parenchymal phase, delayed images are obtained to evaluate for urinary extravasation. On the delayed phase, intravenous (IV) contrast will have been excreted into the collecting system. A full-thickness collecting system injury manifests as fluid with higher attenuation than adjacent or surrounding hematoma due to extravasation of concentrated contrast in the urine. The optimal time to wait between the injection of contrast and delayed phase imaging has not been demonstrated clearly. Although a number of institutions perform delayed phase imaging after 5 minutes, we typically wait 10 minutes (if the patient is stable to do so). Longer delays permit more excreted contrast to traverse the kidneys and ureters, which we believe improves injury detection. Regardless of delay time, technologists can use this time to process the current study (or prepare for the next study) and clinicians can access the patient for monitoring and treatment. If a CT cystogram is indicated, it can be set up during the delay.

Delayed phase imaging should be performed as low dose studies, because identifying high-density contrast outside of the collecting system does not require the high contrast resolution and low noise necessary for the parenchymal phase images. This can be accomplished by increasing the noise index, by decreasing the reference or equivalent milliampere-seconds (mAs), or by other techniques available on the large variety of scanners in use. Axial image slice thickness can also be increased (eg, from 2–3 to 5 mm). In our experience, these techniques can cut radiation dose by more than 50%, and by scanning only the relevant area (eg, only the kidneys and excluding the pelvis), dose can be further reduced to less than 25% of the original scan of the abdomen and pelvis.

Real-time review of the parenchymal phase images by the radiologist permits selection of patients who require delayed imaging (or additional studies), allowing the patient to complete their imaging and return more expeditiously from radiology. This also avoids the unnecessary radiation dose that would otherwise be incurred if all patients routinely underwent delayed imaging.

Alternative Imaging Studies

Although ultrasound is portable, rapid, less expensive, and does not expose the patient to ionizing radiation and contrast agents, it is much less sensitive than CT, detecting only 48% of renal injuries.[9]

Before the availability of CT, IV pyelograms (IVPs) were performed to evaluate for renal injury, but this study is less sensitive than CT and should be used only when CT is not available.[2,11]

One-shot IVPs are very rarely used, especially given the increased accessibility, availability, and speed of CT imaging. This study is obtained to confirm the presence of a contralateral functioning kidney in a patient taken to the operating room without imaging and in whom renal exploration or nephrectomy is considered.[2] In such cases, IV contrast is injected (2 mL/kg), and a radiograph of the kidneys is obtained 10 to 15 minutes later to determine whether an enhancing and excreting contralateral kidney is identified. In lieu of a 1-shot IVP, manual palpation of the contralateral kidney can suffice.

Although MRI was reported to be as effective as CT in correctly staging renal injury,[12] its utility in the acute imaging of renal trauma is limited by the longer imaging time required, limited access to the patient during imaging, and increased cost. CT remains the imaging study of choice for acute renal trauma.[12,13]

Indications for Imaging

Indications for imaging of renal trauma exist (**Table 1**), but many of these criteria were developed before the widespread use of CT in the imaging of trauma patients. For blunt trauma, the 2014 American Urologic Association (AUA) guidelines recommend imaging of adults either with gross hematuria or with both microscopic hematuria and systolic blood pressure less than 90 mm Hg.[2] These guidelines also recommend imaging for children using the same criteria, while acknowledging that children do not exhibit hypotension in the same manner as adults. More specific criteria for imaging children were published previously, proposing imaging for children with higher degrees of hematuria (>50 red blood cells per high power field or gross hematuria) regardless of blood pressure[6,14]; however, this has not been explicitly addressed in the 2014 AUA guidelines. Many of these publications also recommend imaging of patients with clinical findings or mechanisms of injury suspicious for renal injury (such as deceleration injuries, flank ecchymosis, or rib fractures[2]), thus limiting the value of the more specific criteria proposed.

These specific criteria for imaging of renal trauma are not routinely utilized in our practice, because patients with penetrating trauma (who are stable for imaging) and patients with blunt trauma and hematuria or episodes of hypotension are typically imaged based on more general criteria for imaging after torso trauma.

Renal Injuries

In 1989, the American Association for the Surgery of Trauma (AAST) published a grading system for renal injuries[15] that is widely used by surgeons and frequently by radiologists (**Table 2**). After reviewing the injuries described by this system, we review some limitations and proposed improvements.

A renal contusion (**Fig. 1**) may be radiologically occult or may manifest as areas of decreased attenuation on the parenchymal phase and may demonstrate increased attenuation on delayed phase images.[16] It may be difficult to differentiate from medullary tissue, which enhances less avidly than cortical tissue on parenchymal phase images. Contusions are presumed to be present if patients demonstrate new hematuria without radiologic evidence of urinary tract trauma. These injuries are of little clinical significance and are generally treated conservatively.

A subcapsular hematoma (**Fig. 2**) demonstrates smooth convex margins away from the kidney. Compression or flattening of the underlying parenchyma is a specific finding of subcapsular hematoma, but is frequently absent or subtle. Evaluation for an expanding subcapsular hematoma is impossible on a single phase CT, and diagnosis is difficult even with delayed images. In the absence of other findings that upgrade the renal injury (such as visible lacerations), isolated subcapsular hematomas should be reported as grade I injuries.

Blood around the kidney that is more diffuse or streaky and that does not demonstrate findings of a subcapsular hematoma represents a perinephric hematoma. This hematoma is typically more irregular than a subcapsular hematoma, because it dissects through the perinephric fat within Gerota's fascia. Expansion of a perinephric hematoma on CT is identified rarely (unless a change in size is noted between 2 phases of the examination), and most perinephric hematomas are reported as grade II injuries.

Perinephric hematomas are frequently caused by renal lacerations. A renal laceration appears

Table 1 Renal trauma imaging indications		
Trauma	**Population**	**Indications**
Blunt trauma	Adult	One or more of 1. Gross hematuria 2. Microhematuria and SBP <90 mm Hg 3. Clinical suspicion of urinary tract injury
	Pediatric	>50 red blood cells/ HPF
Penetrating trauma	Adult and pediatric	One or both of 1. Any degree of hematuria 2. Clinical suspicion of urinary tract injury

Abbreviations: HPF, high power field; SBP, systolic blood pressure.

Data from Santucci RA, Wessells H, Bartsch G, et al. Evaluation and management of renal injuries: consensus statement of the renal trauma subcommittee. BJU Int 2004;93(7):937–54.

Table 2
Renal injury grading

Grade[a]	Type	Description[b]
I	Contusion	Microscopic or gross hematuria; urologic studies normal
	Hematoma	Subcapsular, nonexpanding without parenchymal laceration
II	Hematoma	Nonexpanding perirenal hematoma confined to renal retroperitoneum
	Laceration	<1.0 cm parenchymal depth of renal cortex without urinary extravasation
III	Laceration	>1.0 cm parenchymal depth of renal cortex without collecting system rupture or urinary extravasation
IV	Laceration	Parenchymal laceration extending through the renal cortex, medulla, and collecting system
	Vascular	Main renal artery or vein injury with contained hemorrhage
V	Laceration	Completely shattered kidney
	Vascular	Avulsion of renal hilum that devascularizes the kidney

[a] Advance 1 grade for multiple injuries to the same organ.
[b] Based on most accurate assessment at autopsy, laparotomy, or radiologic study.
From Moore EE, Shackford SR, Pachter HL, et al. Organ injury scaling: spleen, liver, and kidney. J Trauma 1989;29(12):1665, 1666.

as a linear or jagged defect in the parenchyma, with lower attenuation on parenchymal phase images than the surrounding, normally enhancing parenchyma. Note that the AAST grading system does not measure the length of the laceration, but instead utilizes the depth of the laceration to differentiate grade II lesions (**Fig. 3**) from grade III lesions (**Fig. 4**). Other common sources of low attenuation lesions in the kidney include cysts and scars. Although round/oval cysts are easily differentiated from lacerations, the frequently encountered thin, low attenuation lesions in the kidneys can be more challenging. In general, these are likely to represent collapsed cysts or scars if

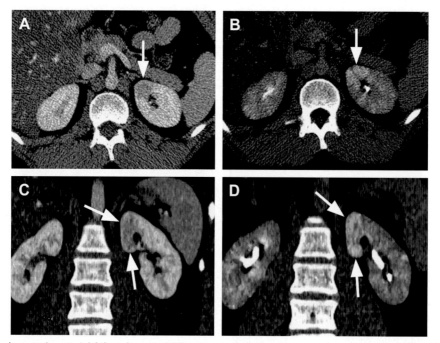

Fig. 1. Renal contusion. Axial (*A*) and coronal (*C*) parenchymal phase images demonstrate an area of decreased enhancement representing a renal contusion (*arrows*). Delayed phase axial (*B*) and coronal (*D*) images demonstrate relative persistent enhancement ("staining") in the contused region (*arrows*).

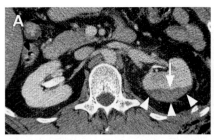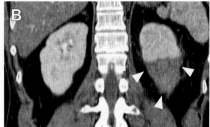

Fig. 2. Subcapsular hematoma. (A) Axial CT image demonstrates posterior subcapsular hematoma (*arrowheads*) with compression and flattening of the underlying renal parenchyma (*arrow*). (B) Coronal CT image demonstrates the well-defined posterior subcapsular hematoma (*arrowheads*).

they demonstrate smooth margins and do not have adjacent perinephric or subcapsular hematoma. However, a (sub)segmental infarct could have a similar appearance and should be considered as a possible diagnosis.

After identification of a laceration or perinephric fluid, delayed images are required to determine whether perinephric fluid represents hematoma, urine, or both. Urinary extravasation cannot be excluded on standard parenchymal phase images. Although low-density fluid is suggestive of extravasated urine, high-density fluid does not exclude urinary extravasation because blood may be intermixed with urine. Delayed images allow the kidneys to concentrate and excrete contrast through the collecting system and ureters. If these structures have been well-distended during the delay period, contrast-opacified urine should leak out through a collecting system defect into surrounding tissues (Fig. 5). The high density contrast is distinguishable from less dense surrounding hematoma. A rare situation that may prove challenging is active vascular or bowel contrast extravasation into this region. Fortunately, bowel contrast is almost never administered in the initial imaging for blunt trauma, and

vascular contrast extravasation should also be visible on the parenchymal phase.

Although the AAST definition of a grade IV injury requires a "parenchymal laceration extending through the renal cortex, medulla, and collecting system," we not infrequently identify urinary extravasation without a laceration through the cortex and medulla. These injuries may be due to occult renal lacerations or may represent isolated collecting system injuries. Either way, we designate them as grade IV injuries with urinary extravasation to ensure that the clinical team recognizes and manages the urinary extravasation appropriately.

A complete traumatic renal artery occlusion (Fig. 6) is a grade IV injury under a strict interpretation of the AAST classification. These injuries are diagnosed rarely within the 4-hour window necessary to be considered for revascularization, and thus these kidneys usually go on to infarction.[17] It seems surprising to us that an injury that can result in complete loss of a kidney is only considered a grade IV injury, rather than grade V. Perhaps it was assigned a lower grade because this injury is not life threatening, because there is no significant hemorrhage, in contrast with the injuries listed as grade V. However, many consider

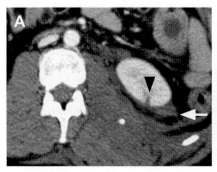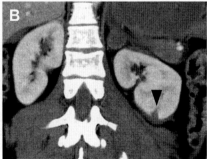

Fig. 3. Grade II renal laceration. Axial (A) and coronal (B) parenchymal phase CT images demonstrate a superficial laceration (*black arrowheads*) less than 1 cm deep, with adjacent subcapsular and perinephric hematoma (*white arrow*).

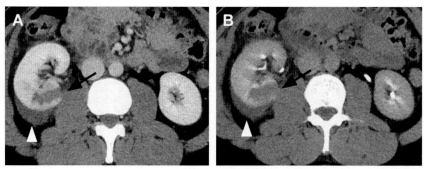

Fig. 4. Grade III renal laceration. (*A*) Axial parenchymal phase CT image demonstrates a laceration more than 1 cm deep (*black arrow*) with adjacent fluid collection (*white arrowhead*). At this time, urinary extravasation cannot be excluded, and the injury cannot be graded appropriately. (*B*) Axial delayed phase CT image demonstrates the laceration (*black arrow*) and adjacent fluid collection (*white arrowhead*). Contrast is present in the collecting systems bilaterally, without evidence of contrast-enhanced urinary extravasation into the laceration or adjacent fluid collection, confirming that the fluid represents a hematoma. With this additional knowledge, the injury can now be designated a grade III laceration.

this to be a grade V injury, focusing on the devascularization of the kidney, even though the renal hilum is not truly avulsed. As a result of this confusion, we prefer to describe the injury without assigning an injury grade. Other, less severe injuries to the main renal artery and vein are also considered grade IV injuries.

The AAST grade V classification does not clearly identify what is meant by a "completely shattered kidney" and there may be variability in how a kidney with extensive lacerations is graded. In the absence of specific guidance, we call the kidney shattered (**Fig. 7**) if there are deep lacerations involving the upper and lower poles and interpolar

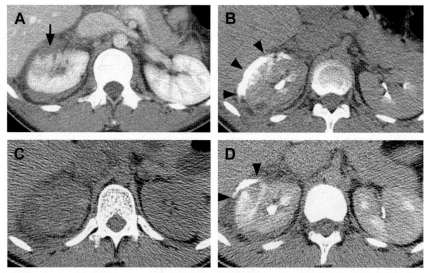

Fig. 5. Grade IV laceration and CT urinoma. (*A*) Axial parenchymal phase CT demonstrates renal laceration and perinephric fluid (*arrow*). (*B*) Axial delayed phase CT image from the same study demonstrates moderate urinary extravasation along the anterior lateral aspect of the right kidney (*arrowheads*). A CT urinoma study was obtained consisting of a low dose axial noncontrast CT (*C*) and 10-minute delayed phase CT (*D*). There is contrast-enhanced urine external to the collecting system (*arrowheads*) on delayed images (*D*), which could be due to partial resolution of the leak seen on the initial CT (*B*) or which could represent a persistent leak. The noncontrast images (*C*) show that there is no contrast in this location, proving that the contrast in (*D*) represents a persistent leak. This diagnosis is made easily despite the noisy images resulting from the low radiation dose utilized in the CT urinoma study.

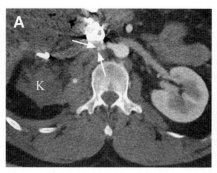
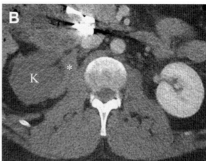

Fig. 6. Acute renal infarct. Arterial (A) and venous (B) phase axial CT images demonstrate acute renal infarction. Right kidney (K) is completely nonenhancing. The right main renal artery is abruptly occluded just distal to its origin (arrows), and there is a right retroperitoneal hematoma (*). High-density material anterior to the kidney, right renal artery, and inferior vena cava is intraperitoneal packing from preceding laparotomy.

areas, resulting in no large portions of intact parenchyma (≥25% of the kidney, but this is an arbitrary number used by the authors).

The final injury specified is an avulsion of the renal hilar vessels, which devascularizes the kidney. This rare injury can result in renal infarction and severe hemorrhage from the avulsed vessels.

Challenges in renal injury classification and proposed updates

Although the AAST grading system includes many of the common injuries, a number of injuries are not included explicitly or may cause confusion. Active arterial extravasation and vascular injuries such as pseudoaneurysms (**Fig. 8**) and arteriovenous fistulas are not included if not accompanying a grade IV or V vascular injury. Similarly, segmental renal artery injuries and segmental infarctions of

the kidney are not described explicitly. Ureteropelvic junction avulsions are also omitted from the renal trauma grading system.

These limitations have been recognized, and a revised classification has been proposed[18] addressing many of these issues. However, this revised classification has yet to be accepted and incorporated by the AAST. The revised classification is essentially the same for grade I through III injuries. The major changes are listed herein.

Grade IV injuries in the revised system include any laceration into the collecting system, whether involving the parenchyma or directly lacerating the collecting system or renal pelvis, including a ureteropelvic junction disruption. It also includes injuries to segmental renal arteries or veins, which are often the cause of segmental renal infarcts. Shattered kidneys are downgraded from grade V to IV.

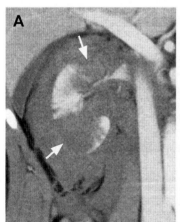
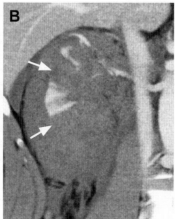
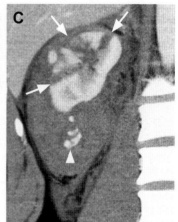

Fig. 7. Shattered kidney. (A–C) Coronal CT images during the parenchymal phase demonstrate multiple deep lacerations (arrows) throughout the kidney, with no large intact portions of renal parenchyma. A large perinephric hematoma fills the perinephric space secondary to active arterial extravasation from multiple locations, most evident inferior to the kidney (C, arrowhead).

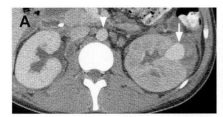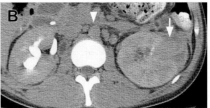

Fig. 8. Renal pseudoaneurysm. (A) Axial parenchymal phase CT image demonstrates left renal pseudoaneurysm as an oval collection of contrast (arrow) projecting between lacerated renal parenchyma and into a subcapsular hematoma. (B) Contrast washes out of this collection on delayed phase images (arrow). Pseudoaneurysm has similar enhancement to the aorta (arrowhead) on both phases (A, B).

Grade V injuries in the revised system are expanded to include main renal artery or vein lacerations, avulsions, and thrombosis.

A final source of confusion with the AAST classification is the instruction to "advance one grade for multiple injuries to the same organ"[15] or to "advance one grade for bilateral injuries up to grade III."[19] This is not followed commonly, perhaps because many are unaware of this instruction or because they find it confusing.

Segmental or subsegmental renal infarctions present as low-density, triangular lesions without adjacent hematoma. If unilateral, particularly if multiple, they may be due to a renal artery injury with distal emboli. Bilateral infarctions or unilateral infarctions accompanied by infarctions in other organs suggest a more central source of emboli, such as an aortic injury or cardiac thrombus (Fig. 9).

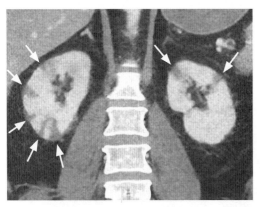

Fig. 9. Subsegmental renal infarctions. Coronal parenchymal phase CT image demonstrates bilateral wedge-shaped (sub)segmental perfusion defects (white arrows) representing infarcts caused by thoracic aortic injury showering emboli to both kidneys. A central source such as the aorta or heart should be considered when bilateral infarcts are noted. When unilateral infarcts are present, the etiology is more likely to be due to injury of the main renal artery, segmental, or subsegmental artery.

Follow-up imaging

Patients with urinary extravasation (without suspicion for renal pelvis or proximal ureteral avulsion) are often initially treated conservatively, as recommended by the 2014 AUA guidelines.[2] To evaluate for the resolution (or decrease) of urinary extravasation, patients should undergo a CT urinoma study. The optimal time for reimaging has not been determined. However, AUA guidelines recommended repeat CT imaging "after 48 hours" and imaging is obtained 2 to 3 days after injury at our institution.

A CT urinoma protocol differs from a trauma CT of the abdomen and pelvis and from a CT IVP. It is not intended to diagnose acute parenchymal injuries and thus does not require the high contrast and spatial resolution that would necessitate higher radiation dose. It is simply intended to evaluate for the resolution of urinary contrast extravasation. A low-dose, nonenhanced CT is obtained through the abdomen to evaluate for any residual contrast from earlier studies. IV contrast is administered, and low-dose delayed images are obtained 10 minutes later to identify urinary extravasation (see Fig. 5). Note that parenchymal phase images are not obtained routinely as a part of this study (although they can be added if there are specific indications). New or increased contrast external to the collecting system on the delayed images confirms the presence or persistence of urinary extravasation.

A CT urinoma study may also be performed for some high-risk patients without evidence of urinary extravasation on their initial trauma CT. Some patients with severe grade III injuries with multiple deep lacerations but no evidence of urinary extravasation initially may develop urinary extravasation over a few days. Theories as to the cause of delayed extravasation include occlusion of the initial collecting system injury by clot or compression by edematous or displaced tissues. Over time, thrombolysis, perhaps due to urokinase in the urine, and decreased swelling unmask the collecting system injury and result in the development of urinary extravasation. Determination of which patients with grade III injuries require a CT urinoma study has not been resolved, but at our institution patients with multiple deep lacerations or deep lacerations close to the renal collecting system undergo this imaging 2 to 3 days after injury.

Urologists at our institution recommend technetium-99m mercaptoacetyltriglycine (MAG3) nuclear medicine scans 8 weeks after injury for patients with severe grade III or grade IV renal injuries to counsel the patient on expected eventual renal function. Although this is not an AUA guideline, they have found it useful for patient education.

URETERAL INJURIES

The ureters run from the ureteropelvic junction through the retroperitoneum to the ureterovesical junction. Acute ureteral injury is rare, comprising less than 1% of all genitourinary injuries from violent trauma. The ureters are well-protected in the retroperitoneum, lying deep within the body and surrounded by fat and other organs. Only 20% of ureteral injuries result from external trauma; 80% occur intraoperatively.[20] The remainder of this section focuses on external trauma, and iatrogenic injuries are not discussed herein.

The vast majority of ureteral injuries (81%–91%) arise from gunshot wounds, with stab wounds (5%–9%) and blunt trauma (4%–10%) accounting for the remainder.[20] High forces are necessary to produce blunt injury, such as a fall from height or high-speed motor vehicle crash. The resulting rapid deceleration tends to disrupt the ureter at fixed points along its course, most commonly at the ureteropelvic junction, followed by the ureterovesical junction.[20] Stab wounds typically damage a short segment of ureter, where it is directly

injured by the penetrating object. In contrast, gunshot injuries can produce a blast effect, injuring the ureter some distance beyond the path of the bullet with vascular damage reported up to 2 cm beyond the grossly visible injury.[20]

Gross or microscopic hematuria is present in many patients with ureteral injury, but up to one-quarter may present without hematuria, and its absence does not exclude an injury.[20] Variability in the presence of hematuria, rarity of ureteral and ureteropelvic junction injuries (in 0.2% in blunt trauma), and difficulty in clinical diagnosis result in delays in diagnosis for the majority of patients with this injury with attendant adverse impact on urologic and overall outcomes.[21] The radiologist can play a critical role in identifying ureteral injuries and improving patient outcomes.

The ureters are seen on the standard imaging for torso trauma. Fluid identified around the ureters on the parenchymal phase should raise concern for a ureteral injury with resultant urinary extravasation, although the fluid more commonly results from renal or perinephric injury or from extension of retroperitoneal hematoma from other injuries, such as pelvic ring fractures or disruptions. Delayed images of the region of interest (and the more distal ureter) are indicated to further evaluate for urine leak (**Fig. 10**). In a stable patient, 10-minute delayed images can be obtained to provide adequate time for contrast-opacified urine to travel down the ureters to the bladder. A full-thickness ureteral injury permits some of this contrast-opacified urine to leak beyond the confines of the ureter (**Fig. 11**). Contrast in the ureter distal to this point differentiates a laceration from a transection, because contrast is only able to pass more distally through a partially intact ureter.

A challenge arises if the ureter distal to the site of injury is not opacified. Absence of distal contrast may be due to ureteral transection, clearance of contrast from the distal ureter by peristalsis, or

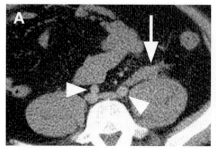 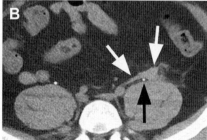

Fig. 10. Periureteral fluid without ureteral injury. (*A*) Axial parenchymal phase CT image demonstrates fluid (*arrow*) around the expected location of the left ureter (which is not clearly visualized). White arrowheads identify the contrast enhancing iliac vessels nearby. (*B*) Axial delayed phase CT image demonstrates contrast in the left ureter (*black arrow*) without contrast extravasation into the adjacent retroperitoneal hematoma (*white arrows*).

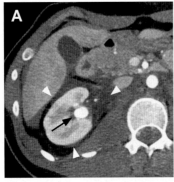 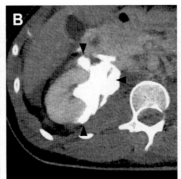 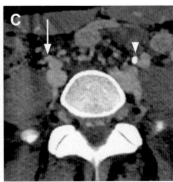

Fig. 11. Ureteropelvic junction (UPJ) avulsion. (*A*) Axial parenchymal phase image demonstrates fluid around the right renal hilum and medial kidney (*white arrowheads*). There is a small amount of contrast in the collecting system (*black arrow*) from earlier injection of contrast. Small foci of high density in the hilum represent enhancing vessels. (*B*) Axial delayed phase CT image demonstrates a large amount of urinary extravasation (*arrowheads*) around the hilum and medial kidney. (*C*) Axial delayed phase CT image more inferiorly demonstrates absence of contrast in the distal right ureter (*arrow*) with expected excreted contrast in the distal left ureter (*arrowhead*). Contrast was absent along the entire course of the right ureter. Although the exact location of the injury is not visualized on this study, findings indicate the presence of a ureteropelvic or proximal right ureteral injury. Absence of contrast in the distal ureter raises concern for complete transection or avulsion, rather than laceration. A ureteral avulsion at the UPJ was identified at surgery.

absence of distal passage of contrast due to poor peristalsis or compression by surrounding hematoma.

If ureteral extravasation is small with symmetric renal enhancement, washout, and excretion of contrast, then it is reasonable to assume that contrast in the bladder is likely from both kidneys and the ureter has not been transected completely (despite the lack of contrast visible in the distal ureter). If, however, ureteral extravasation is large without visible contrast in the distal ureter, then a ureteral transection may be present.

In these situations, distal ureteral contrast could arise theoretically from vesicoureteral reflux of contrast (excreted via the contralateral kidney and ureter) into the ipsilateral ureter, thereby masking a complete ureteral transection. In the absence of findings to suggest asymmetric excretion and reflux, we assume that the distal ureteral contrast represents extension of contrast down the ipsilateral ureter.

If fluid is identified adjacent to the ureter without extravasation on delayed phase images and the kidneys enhance, washout, and excrete normally, then it is reasonable to assume that no ureteral injury is present (even if no contrast is identified in the distal ureter on delayed images).

An AAST grading system exists for ureteral injuries,[22] but is not practical for radiologists, because it requires differentiation of a less than or greater than 50% circumferential laceration and differentiation of less than or greater than 2 cm of devascularization. This distinction usually

cannot be adequately evaluated with CT and may be impossible to evaluate with any imaging technique. It can even be challenging to evaluate with direct visualization intraoperatively. Radiologists should report the presence of a laceration, its location, and any concerns for a transection (if contrast is not seen distally in the normal ureter).

BLADDER INJURIES
Epidemiology

External traumatic bladder injuries are uncommon, occurring in less than 2% of patients undergoing surgery for abdominal trauma.[23,24] The majority of blunt traumatic injuries (up to 90%) result from a motor vehicle or motorcycle crash or a pedestrian struck by a vehicle. The next most common causes include falls, industrial trauma, pelvic crush injuries, and blows to the lower abdomen.[24–26] The percentage of bladder injuries caused by penetrating trauma varies from 0% to 45%, depending on the study patient population.[24] It is present in 3.6% of abdominal gunshot wounds and 20% of penetrating buttock injuries.[24]

Bladder Imaging Technique

Before the widespread use and availability of CT, imaging of the bladder was performed with conventional cystography,[27] using radiographs alone or in conjunction with fluoroscopy. Using this technique, the bladder is filled with contrast via a urethral or suprapubic catheter. At least 2 images are obtained, one with the bladder maximally filled and another after bladder drainage to detect extravasated contrast that may have been obscured by the distended bladder. Additional images of the partially filled bladder or oblique views may also be helpful.

The 2014 AUA guidelines[2] permit the use of either conventional cystography or CT cystography (CTC), because they consider these techniques to have similar sensitivity and specificity.[27–30] Although this may have been true in earlier studies, we would expect CTC to be more sensitive with the use of thinner axial images and multiplanar reformations. In addition, reduced experience in fluoroscopy with the increased use of CT would be expected to decrease sensitivity for smaller lacerations.

We focus on CTC, because this study is the more common method of evaluating the bladder for acute injury after trauma (**Fig. 12**). CTC can be performed without moving the patient from the CT scanner to a fluoroscopy suite some distance away, requires no additional technologists to set up and help perform the examination, and circumvents the radiologist vacating the reading room for an extended time to perform the study.

Box 1 describes the technique for performing a CTC. Although we refer to the use of a urethral catheter elsewhere in this article, a suprapubic catheter provides the same capabilities for filling or draining of the bladder.

The exact quantity of contrast required to distend the bladder adequately has not been clearly demonstrated with many references suggesting 300 to 350 mL or more. If the contrast is freely flowing into the bladder, we continue filling the bladder until the bag of contrast (containing approximately 500 mL) is empty, stops filling the bladder, or the patient becomes uncomfortable. Greater amounts of instilled contrast allow a greater volume of extravasated contrast, likely improving the accurate diagnosis of bladder rupture.[31] Furthermore, a large contrast volume may be necessary in large patulous bladders.

Performing the CTC after the parenchymal phase CT prevents extravasated bladder contrast from obscuring other vascular injuries on the parenchymal phase (and possible arterial phase) CT that may be life threatening and require urgent management, such as pelvic embolization or surgery before evaluation of the bladder. In addition, review of the initial CT scan may demonstrate the presence of unsuspected pelvic fluid and/or pelvic ring injuries that would justify performing a CTC.

Although imaging after draining the bladder is essential in conventional cystography, it is unnecessary in CTC and should be avoided to eliminate needless radiation to the pelvis.[27]

Delayed images with passive antegrade filling of the bladder with contrast excreted by the kidneys are not adequate to exclude bladder injury. These images may demonstrate injuries occasionally, if contrast manages to leak out through the defect. Without retrograde filling, adequate distension and stressing of the bladder cannot be ensured, and injuries will be missed.[27,32,33]

Indications for Imaging

Although most patients with blunt bladder injury have pelvic fractures (85%–89%),[31,32] only a

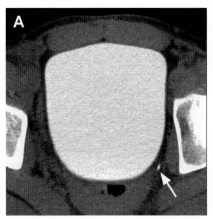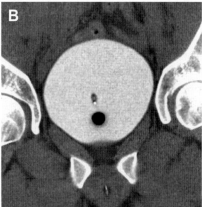

Fig. 12. Normal CT cystogram. Axial (*A*) and coronal (*B*) images from a normal CT cystogram show a bladder filled with contrast instilled through a urethral catheter visualized in (*B*). The bladder is appropriately distended without extravasation of contrast or bladder wall abnormality. Contrast is also seen on the axial images in the distal left ureter (*arrow*) from left renal excretion.

Box 1
CT cystogram (CTC) technique

Drain urine via catheter to remove unopacified urine or extremely dense excreted contrast from the bladder.

Hang container of dilute water soluble contrast (~2–3 g of iodine per 100 mL of volume) 40 cm above bladder to generate adequate pressure. Connect to catheter.

Fill the bladder with contrast until flow of contrast stops, bladder distension is uncomfortable to patient, or ≥350 mL of contrast has been instilled.

Obtain 2.5- to 5-mm low-dose axial images through the pelvis. Coronal and sagittal reformations may help with challenging cases.

If delayed images of the pelvis are not required, obtain the CTC after the parenchymal/venous phase imaging.

If delayed images are being obtained for other reasons, fill the bladder with contrast and obtain CTC images as part of that scan.

Box 2
Indications for obtaining a CT cystogram after blunt abdominal trauma

Gross hematuria and free intraperitoneal fluid or perivesical fluid

or

High levels of hematuria and pelvic ring injury

1. Dipstick UA ≥3+ or microscopic UA >30 RBC/HPF or gross hematuria

   and

2. Pelvic ring injury
   - Fracture disrupting the osseous ring of the pelvis
   - Ligamentous disruption of pelvis (sacro-iliac joint or symphysis pubis disruption)

Abbreviations: HPF, high power field; RBC, red blood cells; UA, urinalysis.

---

minority of patients with blunt pelvic fractures have bladder injuries (6%–8%).[25] Thus, CTC imaging all patients with pelvic fractures is inappropriate. In addition, patients may have bladder injuries without pelvic fractures, and additional criteria are required to select these patients for further imaging.

The exact indications for imaging of blunt bladder injury are not consistently agreed upon in the literature. The 2014 AUA guidelines[2] direct evaluation (CTC or conventional cystography) for patients with pelvic fracture and gross hematuria, because bladder injury is reported in 29% of these patients. It also directs (but with lower strength evidence) that "Clinicians should perform retrograde cystography in stable patients with gross hematuria and a mechanism concerning for bladder injury, or in those with pelvic ring fractures and clinical indicators of bladder rupture." Avey and colleagues[25] demonstrated that bladder rupture only occurred in patients with significant hematuria (>30 red blood cells per high power field) and that no bladder ruptures were found in patients with isolated acetabular fractures. Indications for obtaining CTC are provided in **Box 2** and are based on these references and others.[24,32,34] Although not well-addressed in the literature, we also perform CTC for displaced osseous fragments within or abutting the bladder. Patients with microscopic or gross hematuria after penetrating trauma in the region of the bladder require evaluation of the bladder with CTC or with direct visualization.[2]

Bladder Injuries

Intraperitoneal (IP) bladder ruptures (IPBR) are full-thickness disruptions of the bladder wall and overlying parietal peritoneum, allowing urine to leak from the bladder into the IP space. Extraperitoneal (EP) bladder ruptures (EPBR) are full-thickness disruptions of the bladder wall that allow urine to leak from the bladder into the EP space. Combined bladder ruptures (CBR) are a combination of IPBR and EPBR, with urine leaking into both the IP and EP spaces.

Additional less severe bladder injuries (without complete wall disruption) have also been described, including bladder wall contusions and interstitial ruptures. An interstitial rupture represents a tear of the inner wall of the bladder that does not extend through the full thickness of the bladder wall and thus does not result in the leakage of urine from the bladder. Of these less severe injuries, contusions are most common.

The most common rupture of the bladder is EPBR (60%–90%).[23,35] IPBR are less common (15%–25%),[23,35] and CBR are even less common (5%–12%).[23,35,36] Interstitial ruptures are extremely rare.

IPBR require surgical repair. Blunt IPBR traumatic injuries typically result in a large tear in the dome of the bladder that cannot be treated successfully with catheter drainage alone. Leakage of urine from the bladder into the IP space can result in sepsis and chemical or infectious peritonitis.[1,2,24,31]

Uncomplicated EPBR are managed conservatively with catheter drainage, because 85% resolve within 10 days and almost all resolve within 3 weeks.[26] A follow-up CTC should be obtained at 10 days to evaluate for resolution.[24] However, some patients may undergo surgical repair of the bladder in conjunction with operative management of other regional injuries. Patients with complicated injuries, such as bone spicules in the bladder, rectal or vaginal lacerations, poorly draining bladder, and/or bladder neck injuries, should undergo surgical repair.[2,24]

Computed Tomography Cystography Findings

Bladder wall contusions may present with hematuria. They are often difficult or impossible to visualize on imaging studies and may present as mild bladder wall thickening, irregularity, or differential attenuation. Interstitial ruptures are extremely rare and can also be difficult to identify on imaging studies with imaging features similar to bladder wall contusion.

A full-thickness defect in the bladder wall may be well visualized on CTC. The defect may not be identified, however, if the bladder (partially) collapses as contrast leaks out or due to small defect size. Diagnosis of bladder rupture is made by identifying the administered contrast external to the bladder and determining if the contrast is in the IP or EP space. The contrast administered retrograde into the bladder should be of high enough density that it can be identified clearly leaking from the bladder, even if mixed with unopacified urine, blood, or other fluids. However, it should not be so dense as to cause steak artifacts and limit evaluation of adjacent structures.

Contrast in the IP spaces fills the same locations and has a similar appearance to ascites, except for its greater density. It can accumulate in the pelvic spaces, including the rectovesical space, rectouterine space, or vesicouterine pouch. It can also extend superiorly in the paracolic gutters or between leaves of mesentery and bowel loops to reach the superior abdomen adjacent to the diaphragm, spleen, and liver (**Fig. 13**). IP fluid has well-defined borders that are round, curvilinear, or triangular. This is in contrast with fluid in the EP spaces, which tends to insinuate between EP fat and fascia and produces a more streaky or flame-shaped appearance. EP contrast can also extend beyond the boundaries of the pelvis (**Fig. 14**), penetrating into and through defects in the abdominal wall and pelvic muscles to subcutaneous tissues and dissecting into the scrotum and thigh. Contrast is seen in the IP and EP spaces in a CBR (**Fig. 15**).

The AAST grading system for bladder injuries[19] requires determination of the size of the bladder laceration (<2 or >2 cm) and determination of extension into the bladder neck or ureteral orifice. Although CTC may occasionally identify a laceration longer than 2 cm, it is not reliable in evaluating laceration length. Radiologists should report ruptures near the inferior bladder that might extend

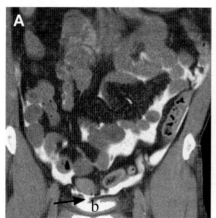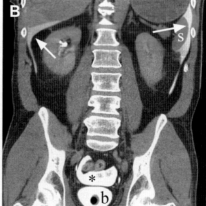

Fig. 13. Intraperitoneal bladder rupture. (*A*) Coronal images from CT cystogram shows contrast leaking from incompletely distended urinary bladder (*b*) through a defect in the bladder dome (*arrow*) and outlining bowel loops in the lower abdomen. (*B*) Coronal image more posteriorly shows upper abdominal contrast (*arrows*) outlining the spleen (*s*) and inferior to the liver in Morison's pouch. Contrast also collects in rectovesical pouch (***) above the bladder (*b*).

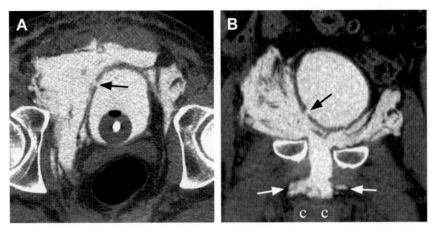

Fig. 14. Extraperitoneal bladder rupture. Axial (*A*) and coronal (*B*) images from a CT cystogram show extraperitoneal contrast collecting anterior and predominantly to the right of bladder. This produces an asymmetric "molar tooth" appearance on the axial image, with the crown anterior to the bladder, and the roots extending posteriorly lateral to the bladder. The bladder wall defect can be seen (*black arrow*). On the coronal image, contrast extends through the diastatic pubic symphysis to the perineum (*white arrows*) above the penile corpora (*c*).

into the bladder neck to prompt further evaluation by a urologist, because CTC cannot reliably confirm or exclude this injury. As a result of these limitations, the AAST system is not generally helpful in reporting of CTC findings.

A radiologic classification also exists,[36] but all of the relevant information can be more simply communicated if the actual injuries (IPBR, EPBR, CBR, contusion) are reported, along with the location of the injury (if visible, especially if near the bladder neck), and extent of contrast spread to the more distal structures, such as the thigh or scrotum.

Awareness of the following pitfalls can help to avoid misdiagnoses. A CBR with a large EPBR component may not demonstrate the IPBR on CTC. This is thought to be secondary to the contrast rapidly leaking out of the EP defect and preventing the bladder from being adequately distended and leaking into the IP space. Thus, an IPBR cannot be excluded if a poorly distended bladder with large EP contrast collection is noted on CTC. Refluxed contrast in the vagina may simulate a bladder rupture, but careful review of the contrast location avoids this error. Osseous fragments from pelvic fractures or extravasated contrast from vessels, bowel, or urethra may also be mistaken for evidence of bladder rupture, but careful windowing of images and comparison with other phases of imaging or prior studies should prevent these errors.[37,38]

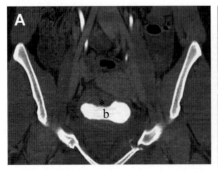
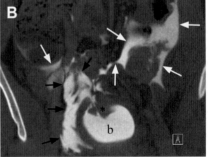

Fig. 15. Combined bladder rupture. (*A*) Coronal image from delayed phase of outside facility CT demonstrates contrast in urinary bladder (*b*) and bilateral ureters. Thickening of the bladder dome (*) likely is clot but no bladder leak was seen. (*B*) Subsequent CT cystogram coronal image shows clot (*) with adjacent defect in bladder dome with both extraperitoneal (*black arrows*) and intraperitoneal (*white arrows*) contrast.

SUMMARY

Urinary system trauma can be diagnosed rapidly and accurately by CT, as a part of the CT imaging of traumatized patients, without the need to transfer patients to fluoroscopy suites. Fluid around the kidneys, ureters, or bladder may represent extravasated urine, and further imaging may be necessary to characterize injuries fully. Real-time review of the initial trauma scan allows determination of the need for delayed images through the kidneys or ureters and can result in radiation savings for patients who do not require delayed images. This review also provides an opportunity to determine if a CTC is required, permitting it to be performed while the patient is still on the scanner. This can reduce radiation exposure if it is performed in conjunction with additional required delayed imaging. Low-dose protocols, such as the CT urinoma study, should be used to follow up on renal extravasation, rather than higher dose studies such as CT IVP.

REFERENCES

1. Avery LL, Scheinfeld MH. Imaging of male pelvic trauma. Radiol Clin North Am 2012;50(6):1201–17.
2. Morey AF, Brandes S, Dugi DD 3rd, et al. Urotrauma: AUA guideline. J Urol 2014;192(2):327–35.
3. Safir MH, McAninch JW. Diagnosis and management of trauma to the kidney. Curr Opin Urol 1999;9(3):227–31.
4. Alonso RC, Nacenta SB, Martinez PD, et al. Kidney in danger: CT findings of blunt and penetrating renal trauma. Radiographics 2009;29(7):2033–53.
5. Lee YJ, Oh SN, Rha SE, et al. Renal trauma. Radiol Clin North Am 2007;45(3):581–92, ix.
6. Morey AF, Bruce JE, McAninch JW. Efficacy of radiographic imaging in pediatric blunt renal trauma. J Urol 1996;156(6):2014–8.
7. Brown SL, Elder JS, Spirnak JP. Are pediatric patients more susceptible to major renal injury from blunt trauma? A comparative study. J Urol 1998;160(1):138–40.
8. Schmidlin FR, Iselin CE, Naimi A, et al. The higher injury risk of abnormal kidneys in blunt renal trauma. Scand J Urol Nephrol 1998;32(6):388–92.
9. Jalli R, Kamalzadeh N, Lotfi M, et al. Accuracy of sonography in detection of renal injuries caused by blunt abdominal trauma: a prospective study. Ulus Travma Acil Cerrahi Derg 2009;15(1):23–7.
10. Johnson PT, Horton KM, Fishman EK. How not to miss or mischaracterize a renal cell carcinoma: protocols, pearls, and pitfalls. AJR Am J Roentgenol 2010;194(4):W307–15.
11. Qin R, Wang P, Qin W, et al. Diagnosis and treatment of renal trauma in 298 patients. Chin J Traumatol 2002;5(1):21–3.
12. Leppaniemi A, Lamminen A, Tervahartiala P, et al. MRI and CT in blunt renal trauma: an update. Semin Ultrasound CT MR 1997;18(2):129–35.
13. Ku JH, Jeon YS, Kim ME, et al. Is there a role for magnetic resonance imaging in renal trauma? Int J Urol 2001;8(6):261–7.
14. Santucci RA, Wessells H, Bartsch G, et al. Evaluation and management of renal injuries: consensus statement of the renal trauma subcommittee. BJU Int 2004;93(7):937–54.
15. Moore EE, Shackford SR, Pachter HL, et al. Organ injury scaling: spleen, liver, and kidney. J Trauma 1989;29(12):1664–6.
16. Kawashima A, Sandler CM, Corl FM, et al. Imaging of renal trauma: a comprehensive review. Radiographics 2001;21(3):557–74.
17. Harris AC, Zwirewich CV, Lyburn ID, et al. CT findings in blunt renal trauma. Radiographics 2001;21(Spec No):S201–14.
18. Buckley JC, McAninch JW. Revision of current American Association for the Surgery of Trauma Renal Injury grading system. J Trauma 2011;70(1):35–7.
19. Moore EE, Cogbill TH, Malangoni MA, et al. Organ injury scaling. Surg Clin North Am 1995;75(2):293–303.
20. Elliott SP, McAninch JW. Ureteral injuries: external and iatrogenic. Urol Clin North Am 2006;33(1):55–66, vi.
21. Ortega SJ, Netto FS, Hamilton P, et al. CT scanning for diagnosing blunt ureteral and ureteropelvic junction injuries. BMC Urol 2008;8:3.
22. Moore EE, Cogbill TH, Jurkovich GJ, et al. Organ injury scaling. III: chest wall, abdominal vascular, ureter, bladder, and urethra. J Trauma 1992;33(3):337–9.
23. Carroll PR, McAninch JW. Major bladder trauma: mechanisms of injury and a unified method of diagnosis and repair. J Urol 1984;132(2):254–7.
24. Gomez RG, Ceballos L, Coburn M, et al. Consensus statement on bladder injuries. BJU Int 2004;94(1):27–32.
25. Avey G, Blackmore CC, Wessells H, et al. Radiographic and clinical predictors of bladder rupture in blunt trauma patients with pelvic fracture. Acad Radiol 2006;13(5):573–9.
26. Corriere JN Jr, Sandler CM. Bladder rupture from external trauma: diagnosis and management. World J Urol 1999;17(2):84–9.
27. Quagliano PV, Delair SM, Malhotra AK. Diagnosis of blunt bladder injury: a prospective comparative study of computed tomography cystography and conventional retrograde cystography. J Trauma 2006;61(2):410–21 [discussion: 421–2].
28. Peng MY, Parisky YR, Cornwell EE 3rd, et al. CT cystography versus conventional cystography in

evaluation of bladder injury. AJR Am J Roentgenol 1999;173(5):1269–72.

29. Chan DP, Abujudeh HH, Cushing GL Jr, et al. CT cystography with multiplanar reformation for suspected bladder rupture: experience in 234 cases. AJR Am J Roentgenol 2006;187(5):1296–302.

30. Deck AJ, Shaves S, Talner L, et al. Computerized tomography cystography for the diagnosis of traumatic bladder rupture. J Urol 2000;164(1):43–6.

31. Corriere JN Jr, Sandler CM. Management of the ruptured bladder: seven years of experience with 111 cases. J Trauma 1986;26(9):830–3.

32. Morey AF, Iverson AJ, Swan A, et al. Bladder rupture after blunt trauma: guidelines for diagnostic imaging. J Trauma 2001;51(4):683–6.

33. Haas CA, Brown SL, Spirnak JP. Limitations of routine spiral computerized tomography in the evaluation of bladder trauma. J Urol 1999;162(1):51–2.

34. Shin SS, Jeong YY, Chung TW, et al. The sentinel clot sign: a useful CT finding for the evaluation of intraperitoneal bladder rupture following blunt trauma. Korean J Radiol 2007;8(6):492–7.

35. Vaccaro JP, Brody JM. CT cystography in the evaluation of major bladder trauma. Radiographics 2000; 20(5):1373–81.

36. Sandler CM, Hall JT, Rodriguez MB, et al. Bladder injury in blunt pelvic trauma. Radiology 1986; 158(3):633–8.

37. Pistoia F, Markowitz SK, Sussman SK. Contrast material in posterior vaginal fornix mimicking bladder rupture: CT features. J Comput Assist Tomogr 1989;13(1):153–5.

38. Power N, Ryan S, Hamilton P. Computed tomographic cystography in bladder trauma: pictorial essay. Can Assoc Radiol J 2004;55(5):304–8.

Negative Computed Tomography for Acute Pulmonary Embolism
Important Differential Diagnosis Considerations for Acute Dyspnea

Daniel B. Green, MD[a], Constantine A. Raptis, MD[a],
Isidro Alvaro Huete Garin, MD[b], Sanjeev Bhalla, MD[a],*

KEYWORDS

- CT pulmonary angiography (CTPA) • Pulmonary embolism (PE) • Dyspnea
- Emergency department (ED) • Alternative diagnosis • Indication creep

KEY POINTS

- Most computed tomography pulmonary angiography (CTPA) performed for the evaluation of acute dyspnea is negative for pulmonary embolism. Many of these examinations provide alternative explanations for dyspnea.
- The most common alternative diagnoses include pneumonia, cardiogenic pulmonary edema, pleural effusion, and atelectasis.
- Nonthrombotic emboli (fat, amniotic fluid, tumor) might be suggested based on a combination of pulmonary and cardiac findings.
- Pleural and pericardial enhancement may not be seen on the arterial phase of CTPA but findings of tension are readily discernible.

INTRODUCTION

Acute pulmonary embolism (PE) is thought to represent the third most common cause of cardiovascular death in the United States after myocardial infarction and stroke, affecting 300,000 to 600,000 patients annually.[1] Most reported deaths from PE are considered to be related to a failure of diagnosis.[2] The potential lethality of this condition makes it a major concern in the emergency department (ED), often prompting diagnostic imaging.

One of the major symptoms of PE, dyspnea, is also one of the most common presenting symptoms to the ED in general. According to the most recent *National Hospital Ambulatory Medical Care Survey: Emergency Department Summary of 2007*, dyspnea was reported in more than 2.5 million patients presenting to United States EDs, making it the eighth most common presenting complaint in patients younger than 65 years and the second most common complaint in patients older than 65 years.[3]

Over the past decade, computed tomography (CT) pulmonary angiography (CTPA) has become recognized as the standard for diagnosis of acute PE.[4] With its increased speed, availability, and

[a] Mallinckrodt Institute of Radiology, Washington University School of Medicine, 510 South Kingshighway, St Louis, MO 63110, USA; [b] Department of Radiology, Catholic University, Marcoleta 367, 2o piso, Santiago, Chile
* Corresponding author.
E-mail address: bhallas@mir.wustl.edu

accuracy, CTPA is now the principal method for imaging PE in the ED, reserving ventilation-perfusion scintigraphy for special patient populations (eg, pregnant women and patients with intravenous contrast allergies) and magnetic resonance for certain centers of expertise.[5,6] The noninvasive nature of CT combined with the proximity of CT scanners to most EDs has resulted in a decreased threshold for imaging patients with dyspnea. Despite the occasional use of D-dimer testing and the application of clinical metrics such as the Wells criteria or Geneva Score, the prevalence of PE on CTPA in most centers is usually between 10% and 20%.[7–9]

Although many CTPA examinations performed for dyspnea provide no explanation for the dyspnea, an alternative explanation may be seen in 25% to 67% of cases.[9–14] These cases usually include congestive heart failure, pneumonia, pleural effusion, or atelectasis. This article focuses on alternative diagnoses of dyspnea that may be diagnosed on CTPA for PE. The goal is to provide a structured approach with examples for practicing radiologists. Diagnoses seen on CT but unlikely to explain the patient's dyspnea are not discussed.[15]

PARENCHYMAL DISEASE AND NONTHROMBOEMBOLIC EMBOLI

Pulmonary edema, pneumonia, pleural effusion, and atelectasis represent the most common alternative diagnoses for dyspnea on CTPA, emphasizing the importance of a thorough investigation of the lung windows before calling a study negative. With routine use of 1-mm to 2-mm thick soft tissue images and frequent use of dedicated 3-mm to 5-mm lung windows, the CTPA has a resolution close to that obtained with high-resolution CT. Analysis of the lung windows should include observation of the predominant pattern (ground glass, consolidation, nodules, or septal line thickening), the predominant location of the abnormality (upper lobe vs lower lobe and central vs peripheral), and any other relevant findings (pleural effusion, lymphadenopathy, and so forth).

Pulmonary edema may be cardiogenic or noncardiogenic. The former tends to present with bilateral pleural effusions and symmetric consolidation or ground glass. When septal lines are present, they tend to be smooth, and the heart is usually enlarged (**Fig. 1**). Although it is tempting to think of cardiogenic edema as progressing through stages from mild bronchiolocentric cuffing to septal line thickening to ground-glass or frank consolidation, many patients present with only 1 of these manifestations. Occasionally, early cardiogenic edema is focal or unilateral. In acute mitral valve regurgitation, such as in papillary muscle rupture following myocardial infarction, only 1 venous territory may be involved or more severely involved; usually the right upper lobe.[16] Unilateral venous edema may also be secondary to an obstructing mass or fibrosing mediastinitis (**Fig. 2**).[17] With underlying emphysema, superimposed pulmonary edema is often asymmetric and can even simulate a cavitary pneumonia or fibrosis.

Noncardiogenic pulmonary edema may also present to the ED with dyspnea. In contrast with cardiogenic edema, pleural effusions should be absent or very small, and the heart is usually of normal size. Septal lines are typically absent, and pulmonary opacities tend to spare the peripheral 1 to 2 cm of lung (**Fig. 3**). A general symmetry of findings creates a bat-wing appearance on coronal imaging. Many causes of noncardiogenic edema force an acute ED presentation, including sepsis, drowning, high-altitude pulmonary edema, drug use, recent pregnancy, inhalation injury, upper airway injury, intracranial hemorrhage, and diffuse alveolar damage (the underlying disorder of the adult respiratory syndrome [acute respiratory distress syndrome]). Findings of diffuse

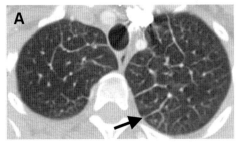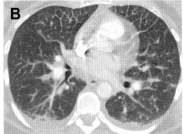

Fig. 1. A 46-year-old woman with cardiogenic pulmonary edema. Lung windows show smooth bilateral interlobular septal thickening extending to the pleural surfaces (*arrow* in *A*). Small bilateral effusions can be seen inferiorly (*B*).

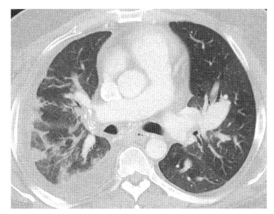

Fig. 2. A 41-year-old man with fibrosing mediastinitis. A partially calcified right hilar mass results in unilateral pulmonary edema and pleural effusion secondary to pulmonary vein stenosis.

alveolar damage consist of areas of secondary lobular sparing, a gradient of increased density of consolidation in the dependent part of the lungs, and traction bronchiectasis in the affected areas.[18] When idiopathic, it indicates acute interstitial pneumonia, which is one of the idiopathic inflammatory pneumonias.

Infectious pneumonia is also a common diagnosis on CTPA that is negative for PE. When the diagnosis is evident on chest radiography, CTPA can be avoided. However, many infectious pneumonias elude detection on conventional radiography. On CT, infectious bacterial pneumonia appears as nonenhancing consolidation. A small pleural effusion is common but not essential for diagnosis. One variation of pneumonia, the so-called round pneumonia, presents as a rounded opacity with enhancing vessels running through it and possibly air bronchograms (Fig. 4).[19] Usually, the clinical history suggests an infection to help differentiate from a malignancy with air bronchograms, such as adenocarcinoma. Another variant of community-acquired pneumonia may present with tiny branching nodules (tree-in-bud pattern), most commonly reported with mycoplasma pneumonia when diffuse (Fig. 5).[20] Viral pneumonias tend to present with ill-defined ground-glass nodules and pleural effusions.[20,21] Septal lines may be present. Pneumocystis pneumonia and fungal pneumonias present with dyspnea in

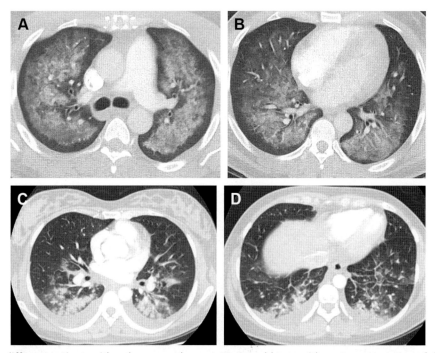

Fig. 3. Two different patients with pulmonary edema. A 40-year-old man with acute presentation of shortness of breath after crack cocaine use (A, B). Diffuse bilateral ground-glass opacities sparing the lung periphery and the absence of pleural effusions are typical of noncardiogenic pulmonary edema. Note the absence of pleural effusions and septal line thickening. A 27-year-old woman with shortness of breath following delivery of twins (C, D). Bilateral and symmetric patchy consolidations with septal line thickening represent findings of pulmonary edema. Postpartum pulmonary edema can be either noncardiogenic or cardiogenic in the setting of postpartum cardiomyopathy.

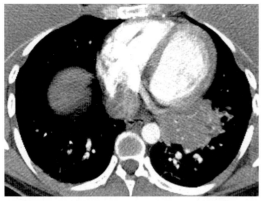

Fig. 4. A 34-year-old woman presented with left-sided chest pain and cough and was diagnosed with round pneumonia. A round, nonenhancing mass with enhancing vessels running through it is consistent with round pneumonia. However, in this scenario follow-up imaging (usually radiography) should be obtained to exclude a neoplasm. The absence of a pleural effusion is typical of round pneumonia.

immunocompromised patients. In patients with acquired immunodeficiency syndrome (AIDS) and a low CD4 count, pneumocystis pneumonia typically has a crazy-paving pattern (ground glass with smooth septal lines), occasionally in an upper lung distribution (**Fig. 6**).[22] The absence of pleural effusions distinguishes this entity from cardiogenic pulmonary edema. Fungal infection frequently affects neutropenic patients and manifests as multiple nodules with surrounding ground-glass halos.[23]

Mycobacterial infection rarely presents to the ED solely with dyspnea. A cavitary airspace process in the upper lungs along with tree-in-bud opacities with an upper lung and midlung predominance should raise suspicion for a post-primary mycobacterial infection.[24]

Aspiration pneumonitis may lead to pneumonia and present with dyspnea. The most important feature suggestive of aspiration is its dependent location; usually in the posterior segments of the upper and lower lobes. Aspiration tends to present as nodules, usually in a centrilobular or tree-in-bud pattern (**Fig. 7**).[25] When severe, it may progress to nonenhancing consolidation or even noncardiogenic edema. Clinically, patients frequently have neuromuscular or gastroesophageal disorders.

Rarely, pulmonary hemorrhage presents to the ED with dyspnea. Hemorrhage may take one of 2 forms: bleeding from a vessel (usually an enlarged collateral bronchial artery) or diffuse hemorrhage (as in the setting of vasculitis or anticoagulation).[26] A gross observation of hemoptysis is usually present and is helpful in making the diagnosis. Depending on the cause, the radiographic pattern varies. Bleeding from a vessel simulates aspiration pneumonitis, because aspirated blood is responsible for most of the parenchymal findings. Extravasated contrast is rarely depicted, and enlarged collateral arteries are instead more commonly seen. Vasculitis and diffuse pulmonary hemorrhage present with a pattern akin to noncardiogenic pulmonary edema (**Fig. 8**). At first, the airspace disease is ground glass in attenuation (possibly with faint septal lines), followed by progression to high-attenuation consolidation, which is best seen on a narrow CT window width (around 200 HU vs the standard 400 HU of a normal soft tissue window width).

Atelectasis represents one of the most common findings in patients presenting to the ED with dyspnea. Occasionally, it is secondary to small

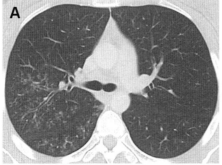
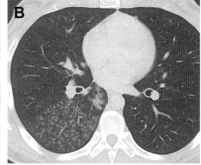

Fig. 5. A 27-year-old woman with mycoplasma pneumonia. Tree-in-bud opacities may be seen in any type of infectious bronchiolitis/pneumonia. When encountered, the location of the tree-in-bud is helpful in suggesting the correct diagnosis. In this case, unilateral diffuse involvement of the right lung (*A, B*) is typical of a bacterial bronchiolitis/pneumonia. Note the absence of a pleural effusion.

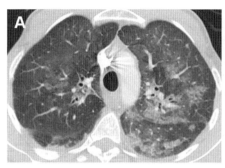
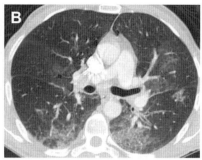

Fig. 6. A 54-year-old man with human immunodeficiency virus/AIDS, cough, and right-sided chest pain. He was diagnosed with pneumocystis pneumonia (PCP), which presented with patchy bilateral ground-glass opacities (A, B). This appearance can be seen in immunosuppressed patients and may be missed on conventional radiography. PCP may have an upper lung predominance. Pleural effusions are characteristically absent.

airways disease, most notably asthma. Whether or not atelectasis is responsible for the acute presentation is difficult to determine, but if substantial, shunting may occur through areas of collapse and result in systemic hypoxemia.[12] On the early arterial phase of a CTPA, atelectasis should enhance, and volume loss should also be seen (**Fig. 9**). Consolidated areas of lung are well delineated by fissures in cases of lobar atelectasis. The bronchi in areas of atelectasis should be examined closely. If air bronchograms are present, treatment may solely consist of vigorous pulmonary toilet. If the bronchi are filled with low-attenuating fluid, bronchoscopy should be considered to potentially diagnose a central obstructing mass or relieve mucous plugging.

In the ED, nonthrombotic emboli may also be diagnosed on CTPA. The best-known example of this phenomenon is septic emboli, which are more easily diagnosed on lung windows. Filling defects are rarely seen in the pulmonary arteries on soft tissue windows caused by septic emboli. Instead, the typical findings are cavitary nodular areas of peripheral consolidation (**Fig. 10**).[27] Although these cavitary nodules are more commonly seen with septic emboli, granulomatosis with polyangiitis (formerly known as Wegener granulomatosis) can have a similar appearance. Blood cultures may be positive with septic emboli, whereas a positive antinuclear cytoplasmic antibody test suggests vasculitis. A vegetation is occasionally seen on the tricuspid valve, or an infected source is suggested by a thrombosed vein or catheter-associated thrombus.

Microembolic disease (fat emboli, amniotic fluid emboli, tumor emboli, and talc emboli) may also be diagnosed on lung windows.[28] This disease presents with tiny centrilobular ground-glass nodules or tree-in-bud opacities (**Fig. 11**).[29] Occasionally tumor emboli may be seen as filling defects in the pulmonary arteries with attenuation similar to the primary lesion (**Fig. 12**). Unlike the airway causes for centrilobular nodules or tree-in-bud opacities described earlier, these vascular causes do not have any associated air trapping, but they should increase pulmonary vascular resistance.

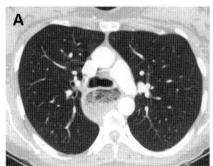
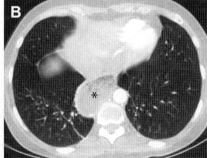

Fig. 7. A 43-year-old woman with aspiration bronchiolitis. Tree-in-bud opacities and centrilobular nodules can be seen in a dependent location (A, B) accompanied by a markedly dilated esophagus (*asterisk* in B) filled with debris. The combination of these findings is typical of achalasia with gastroesophageal reflux and aspiration bronchiolitis.

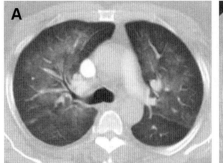
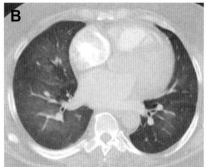

Fig. 8. A 60-year-old man with hemoptysis and pulmonary hemorrhage. Diffuse bilateral ground-glass opacities sparing the lung periphery are seen without pleural effusions (*A, B*). The appearance is similar to noncardiogenic pulmonary edema (see **Fig. 2**) and pneumocystis pneumonia (see **Fig. 6**). The presence of hemoptysis and a competent immune system suggests the diagnosis of hemorrhage.

The net effect may be transient enlargement of the main pulmonary artery and possibly the right ventricle.[29] Iatrogenic emboli (most commonly methylmethacrylate) may be diagnosed on either lung or soft tissue windows. The size of the embolized particles determines their location in the lungs.[30] Rarely, embolized foreign material manifests as a pneumonitis characterized by peripheral (suggesting embolic) airspace disease and no discernible arterial filling defect. One notorious example of this phenomenon is free silicone injection directly into the subcutaneous tissues as a means of achieving inexpensive cosmesis.[31] However, the ensuing pneumonitis can be lethal.

PLEURAL DISEASE

Most pleural processes significant enough to result in dyspnea are large enough to detect on conventional radiography. However, a large pneumothorax, and even one under tension, may be initially diagnosed on CTPA. These large effusions tend to represent hemothorax, empyema, or a malignant effusion. The attenuation of the fluid is helpful in suggesting a hemothorax if greater than 30 HU (**Fig. 13**). The classic split pleura sign of empyema (**Fig. 14**) and the pleural nodularity of a malignancy are better seen on venous phase imaging and therefore may be missed on the arterial phase of CTPA. In an empyema, loculation of the fluid, droplets of gas, or supleural edema may be clues to the diagnosis, whereas typical features of malignant pleural disease are subpleural extension of a nodule or involvement of the mediastinal pleura.

If a pleural effusion causes dyspnea, it should be drained. Clinicians must also look for any signs of tension exerted by the effusion, because this can have a similar clinical significance to a tension pneumothorax. Mediastinal shift is readily

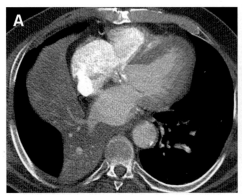
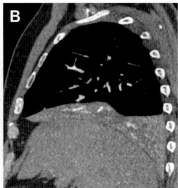

Fig. 9. A 74 year-old man with lung cancer presenting with hemoptysis and dyspnea and right middle lobe/lower lobe collapse. Progression of lung cancer results in obstruction of the bronchus intermedius. Enhancing consolidations with sharply demarcated borders (from the fissures), as seen on the transaxial (*A*) and sagittal (*B*) images, are typical for lobar atelectasis.

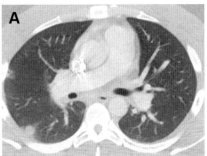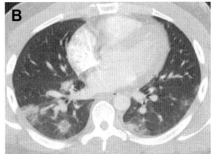

Fig. 10. A 28-year-old man with shortness of breath and leg cellulitis resulting in septic emboli. Peripheral nodules with ground-glass halos and central lucency or cavitation are often seen in septic emboli in the setting of endocarditis. Because these are microemboli, filling defects usually are not seen in the pulmonary arteries. As in this case, diagnosis rests on the lung windows (A, B).

observed, but diaphragmatic inversion can easily be overlooked. Because it results in paradoxic aeration of the affected and unaffected sides, diaphragmatic inversion can be problematic.[32] Review of the coronal images aids detection of this phenomenon.

AIRWAY AND OBSTRUCTIVE DISEASE

Airway diseases explain many of the presentations of dyspnea to the ED and overlap the presentations with other obstructive lung diseases, such as emphysema and bronchitis. Although the CT findings of emphysema and bronchitis are well known, the challenge lies in determining whether they explain the clinical presentation of acute dyspnea. Therefore, the importance of detecting an airway process is that it prompts the clinical team to refocus its history and physical examination to shed more light on the patient's presentation.

On CTPA, the search pattern should include evaluation of the trachea and bronchi for any areas of wall thickening, luminal narrowing, or a focal mass. Most patients who present with tracheal disease as the explanation for dyspnea have an endoluminal mass (usually squamous cell cancer, adenoid cystic carcinoma, or metastasis) or a history of intubation injury (Fig. 15).[33,34]

Small airways diseases are slightly harder to diagnose. CT findings center on the direct signs of tree-in-bud opacities from dilated bronchioles in the setting of a bronchiolitis and the indirect sign of mosaic attenuation secondary to air trapping.[35] Mosaic attenuation can be difficult to detect on CTPA, which usually does not include exhalation images.

CARDIOVASCULAR DISEASE

Most cardiovascular diseases (acute coronary and aortic syndromes) present with chest pain rather than dyspnea. The main exception is congestive heart failure, which typically results in pulmonary edema and pleural effusions. These entities are discussed earlier.

Another important cardiovascular explanation for dyspnea is cardiac tamponade. Cardiac

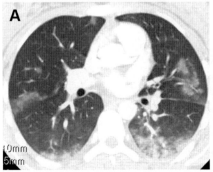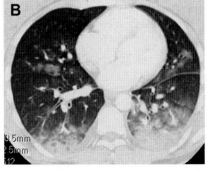

Fig. 11. A 23-year-old woman recently postpartum with amniotic fluid embolism (A, B). Amniotic fluid embolus. The key to making this diagnosis is the clinical history combined with the ground-glass opacities. Amniotic fluid will result in a chemical pneumonitis adjacent to the terminal arteriole.

796

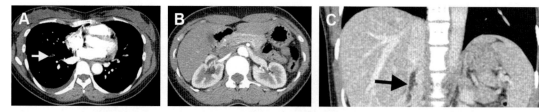

Fig. 12. A 42-year-old woman with right-sided chest pain and tumor emboli from an angiomyolipoma. Fat atten-uation filling defect (*arrow* in *A*) in a segmental pulmonary artery is an embolized portion of the renal angiomyo-lipoma (*B*). Portions of this mass are also seen within the right kidney and inferior vena cava and are best seen in the coronal plane (*arrow* in *C*).

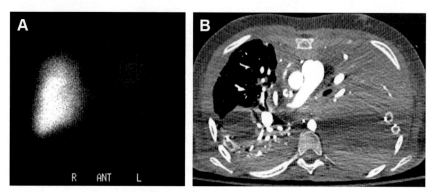

Fig. 13. An 11-year-old girl status post bilateral lung transplant and large left hemothorax. The perfusion scan (*A*) showed marked decrease in the left lung perfusion. Subsequent CT (*B*) showed a large hemothorax despite thor-acostomy tubes. Both tubes had kinked in the immediate perioperative period.

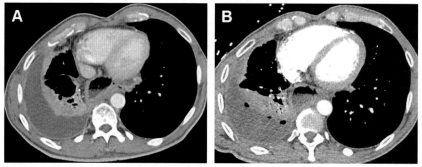

Fig. 14. A 55-year-old man with an empyema following gastric pull-through surgery. Thickened and enhancing pleura is more easily visualized on the venous phase (*A*) compared with the arterial phase PE protocol (*B*). Fluid between the enhancing visceral and parietal pleural layers forms the split pleura sign. Also note the droplets of gas within the empyema.

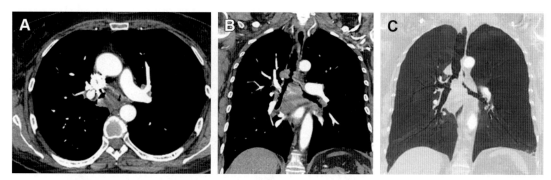

Fig. 15. A 59-year-old woman with hemoptysis and progressive dyspnea from a tracheal neoplasm. Irregular airway wall thickening was seen on the transverse image (*A*) involving the distal trachea, which is better seen on the coronal (*B*) and minimum intensity projection images (*C*) and left main bronchus typical of a malignancy. The histology in this case showed squamous cell carcinoma.

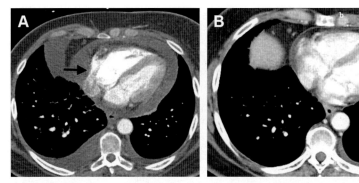

Fig. 16. A 57 year-old woman with metastatic lung cancer. A pericardial effusion causes deformation of the right atrium (*arrow* in *A*) suggestive of tamponade physiology. Pericardial thickening and enhancement is more easily seen on the venous phase of a CT scan performed 1 month earlier (*B*).

tamponade can be a challenging diagnosis on CTPA, which is usually not performed with electrocardiogram (ECG) gating. Tamponade results from acute accumulation of fluid or gas within the pericardial space. The fluid or gas exerts mass effect on the underlying heart and can impede diastolic filling. If untreated by drainage, the condition can be fatal. CT findings of tamponade include notching of the right ventricle in early diastole (when the volume of the right ventricle is low and therefore intracameral pressure is low) and of the right atrium in late diastole (when right atrial volume is at its lowest) (**Fig. 16**). Without ECG gating, the notching on the right heart may be harder to localize to a phase of the cardiac cycle. Other CT findings include a sigmoid-shaped interventricular septum and evidence of increased right heart pressures, including distended cavae and flow of intravenous contrast through collateral pathways.[36] CT is almost never the sole imaging study used to diagnose tamponade, but the features should be recognized in order to expedite echocardiography and guide the echocardiographer. Occasionally,

the features of tamponade are not appreciated by the echocardiographer, particularly in the setting of a tension pneumopericardium.[37]

Care must also be taken in attempting to diagnose the cause of the pericardial effusion based on the CTPA. As with the pleural diseases described earlier, enhancement of the pericardium can be missed on the arterial phase of the CTPA. In diagnosing pericarditis, clinicians should look for pericardial thickening and edema of the pericardial and epicardial fat. Malignancy presents with areas of nodular thickening, occasionally extending into the epicardial fat (**Fig. 17**).

ABDOMINAL AND DIAPHRAGMATIC DISEASE

Most CTPA covers a portion of the abdomen, usually to the level of the adrenal glands. One potential explanation for dyspnea is a large diaphragmatic hernia. When 1 hemidiaphragm is elevated, phrenic nerve palsy should be considered (**Fig. 18**). However, these palsies rarely present with acute dyspnea. Acute accumulation of fluid,

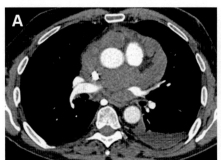
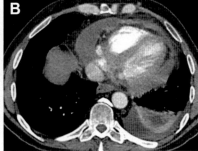

Fig. 17. A 62-year-old man with metastatic melanoma. Nodular pericardial enhancement and fluid accumulation (*A, B*) are typical of a malignant pericardial effusion.

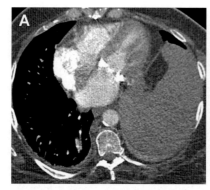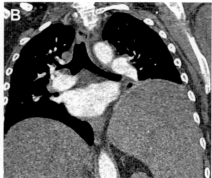

Fig. 18. A 58-year-old woman with left phrenic nerve palsy sustained during recent orthopedic surgery. The left hemidiaphragm is markedly elevated on the transverse image (*A*) but is better appreciated on the coronal image (*B*).

air, or blood within the peritoneum may present with dyspnea from mass effect on the thorax. These patients typically have abdominal pain as well.

SUMMARY

Since its advent in the 1990s, CTPA has become the standard for the evaluation of PE in the ED. As the protocol has gained acceptance, the number of studies positive for PE in patients with acute dyspnea has declined, whereas the number of negative studies has increased. The ability to detect alternative causes for acute dyspnea has driven the increased usage of CTPA, contributing to the indication creep of this examination.

To most effectively approach the CTPA, which is more likely to be negative for PE than positive, radiologists must be familiar with the strengths of this examination (parenchymal disease) and the potential limitations (pleural and pericardial enhancement). They must also understand how to extract the most information from the study (combining parenchymal disease with an evaluation of the right heart) and when to suggest an alternative cause of dyspnea (pulmonary, abdominal, and airway disease).

REFERENCES

1. Naess IA, Christiansen SC, Romundstadt P, et al. Incidence and mortality of venous thrombosis: a population-based study. J Thromb Haemost 2007; 5:692–9.
2. Dalen J. Pulmonary embolism: what have we learned since Virchow? Natural history, pathophysiology, and diagnosis. Chest 2002;122:1440–56.
3. National hospital ambulatory medical care survey: 2007 emergency department summary. 2010. Available at: http://www.cdc.gov/nchs/data/nhsr/nhsr026.pdf. Accessed December 14, 2014.
4. Kuriakose J, Patel S. Acute pulmonary embolism. Radiol Clin North Am 2010;48:31–50.
5. Leung AN, Bull TM, Jaeschke R, et al, ATS/STR Committee on Pulmonary Embolism in Pregnancy. American Thoracic Society documents: an official American Thoracic Society/Society of Thoracic Radiology clinical practice guideline–evaluation of suspected pulmonary embolism in pregnancy. Radiology 2012;262:635–46.
6. Stein PD, Chenevert TL, Fowler SE, et al, (Prospective Investigation of Pulmonary Embolism Diagnosis III) Investigators. Gadolinium-enhanced magnetic resonance angiography for pulmonary embolism: a multicenter prospective study (PIOPED III). Ann Intern Med 2010;152:434–43.
7. Shujaat A, Shapiro JM, Eden E. Utilization of CT pulmonary angiography in suspected PE in a major emergency department. Pulm Med 2013;2013:1–6.
8. Chandra S, Sarkar PK, Chandra D, et al. Finding an alternative diagnosis does not justify increased use of CT-pulmonary angiography. BMC Pulm Med 2013;13:1–8.
9. van Es J, Douma RA, Schreuder SM, et al. Clinical impact of findings supporting an alternative diagnosis on CT pulmonary angiography in patients with suspected pulmonary embolism. Chest 2013; 144:1893–9.
10. Kim KI, Muller NL, Mayo JR. Clinically suspected pulmonary embolism: utility of spiral CT. Radiology 1999;210:693–7.
11. Cross JJ, Kemp PM, Walsh CG. A randomized trial of spiral CT and ventilation perfusion scintigraphy for the diagnosis of pulmonary embolism. Clin Radiol 1998;53:177–82.
12. Tsai KL, Gupta E, Haramati LB. Pulmonary atelectasis: a frequent alternative diagnosis in patients undergoing CTPA for suspected pulmonary embolism. Emerg Radiol 2004;10(5):282–6.

13. Tresoldi S, Kim YH, Baker SP, et al. MDCT of 220 consecutive patients with suspected acute pulmonary embolism: incidence of pulmonary embolism and of other acute or non-acute thoracic findings. Radiol Med 2008;113(3):373–84.

14. Hall WB, Truitt SG, Scheunemann LP, et al. The prevalence of clinically relevant incidental findings on chest computed tomographic angiograms ordered to diagnose pulmonary embolism. Arch Intern Med 2009;169(21):1961–5.

15. Gotway MB, Nagai BK, Reddy GP, et al. Incidentally detected cardiovascular abnormalities on helical CT pulmonary angiography: spectrum of findings. AJR Am J Roentgenol 2001;176:421–7.

16. Attias D, Mansencal N, Auvert B, et al. Prevalence, characteristics, and outcomes of patients presenting with cardiogenic unilateral pulmonary edema. Circulation 2010;122(11):1109–15.

17. Rossi SE, McAdams HP, Rosado-de-Christenson ML, et al. Fibrosing mediastinitis. Radiographics 2001;21(3):737–57.

18. Joynt GM, Antonio GE, Lam P, et al. Late-stage adult respiratory distress syndrome caused by severe acute respiratory syndrome: abnormal findings at thin-section CT. Radiology 2004;230(2):339–46.

19. Wagner AL, Szabunio M, Hazlett KS, et al. Radiologic manifestations of round pneumonia in adults. AJR Am J Roentgenol 1998;170(3):723–6.

20. Tarver RD, Teague SD, Heitkamp DE, et al. Radiology of community-acquired pneumonia. Radiol Clin North Am 2005;43(3):497–512.

21. Kim EA, Lee KS, Primack SL, et al. Viral pneumonias in adults: radiologic and pathologic findings. Radiographics 2002;22(Spec No):S137–49.

22. Kanne JP, Yandow DR, Meyer CA. Pneumocystis jiroveci pneumonia: high-resolution CT findings in patients with and without HIV infection. AJR Am J Roentgenol 2012;198(6):W555–61.

23. Heussel CP, Kauczor HU, Ullmann AJ. Pneumonia in neutropenic patients. Eur Radiol 2004;14(2):256–71.

24. Jeong YJ, Lee KS. Pulmonary tuberculosis: up-to-date imaging and management. AJR Am J Roentgenol 2008;191(3):834–44.

25. Franquet T, Giménez A, Rosón N, et al. Aspiration diseases: findings, pitfalls, and differential diagnosis. Radiographics 2000;20(3):673–85.

26. Bruzzi JF, Rémy-Jardin M, Delhaye D, et al. Multi-detector row CT of hemoptysis. Radiographics 2006; 26(1):3–22.

27. Han D, Lee KS, Franquet T, et al. Thrombotic and nonthrombotic pulmonary arterial embolism: spectrum of imaging findings. Radiographics 2003; 23(6):1521–39.

28. Jorens PG, Van Marck E, Snoeckx A, et al. Non-thrombotic pulmonary embolism. Eur Respir J 2009;34(2):452–74.

29. Franquet T, Giménez A, Prats R, et al. Thrombotic microangiopathy of pulmonary tumors: a vascular cause of tree-in-bud pattern on CT. AJR Am J Roentgenol 2002;179(4):897–9.

30. Habib N, Maniatis T, Ahmed S, et al. Cement pulmonary embolism after percutaneous vertebroplasty and kyphoplasty: an overview. Heart Lung 2012; 41(5):509–11.

31. Restrepo CS, Artunduaga M, Carrillo JA, et al. Silicone pulmonary embolism: report of 10 cases and review of the literature. J Comput Assist Tomogr 2009;33(2):233–7.

32. Wang JS, Tseng CH. Changes in pulmonary mechanics and gas exchange after thoracentesis on patients with inversion of a hemidiaphragm secondary to large pleural effusion. Chest 1995;107(6): 1610–4.

33. Macchiarini P. Primary tracheal tumours. Lancet Oncol 2006;7(1):83–91.

34. Zias N, Chroneou A, Tabba MK, et al. Post tracheostomy and post intubation tracheal stenosis: report of 31 cases and review of the literature. BMC Pulm Med 2008;8:18.

35. Abbott GF, Rosado-de-Christenson ML, Rossi SE, et al. Imaging of small airways disease. J Thorac Imaging 2009;24(4):285–98.

36. Restrepo CS, Lemos DF, Lemos JA, et al. Imaging findings in cardiac tamponade with emphasis on CT. Radiographics 2007;27(6):1595–610.

37. Lee SH, Kim WH, Lee SR, et al. Cardiac tamponade by iatrogenic pneumopericardium. J Cardiovasc Ultrasound 2008;16(1):26–8.

Imaging Patterns and Management Algorithms in Acute Stroke
An Update for the Emergency Radiologist

Behroze A. Vachha, MD, PhD, Pamela W. Schaefer, MD, FACR*

KEYWORDS

• Stroke • Infarct • MR imaging • MRA • Perfusion • Diffusion • CT angiography • CT perfusion

KEY POINTS

- The clinical diagnosis of acute stroke is inaccurate in approximately 10%–30% of cases; other conditions may demonstrate clinical and imaging appearances that mimic acute infarction.
- The emergency radiologist is critical in the evaluation and triage of patients with symptoms of acute ischemic stroke.
- Noncontrast CT (NCCT) and gradient-recalled echo MR imaging show similar accuracy in the diagnosis of acute intracerebral hemorrhage; NCCT is usually the first imaging modality used to assess acute stroke.
- Diffusion-weighted MR imaging is the gold standard for infarct core. CT and MR perfusion are used to detect ischemic penumbra.
- CT angiography is diagnostically superior to MR angiography for evaluation of vasculature; time-of-flight MRA allows for adequate evaluation of vasculature in those who cannot receive contrast.

INTRODUCTION

Stroke is the fourth leading cause of death in the United States and a leading cause of serious, long-term adult disability.[1] Arterial ischemia accounts for 87% of strokes; the remaining strokes are mostly hemorrhagic.[2] Major advances in treatment of acute ischemic stroke over the past decade have markedly improved the outcomes in stroke patients with the potential for remarkable recovery.[3] Current treatment approaches are commonly restricted by the time elapsed since witnessed symptom onset. For intravenous tissue plasminogen activator (IV tPA), the currently approved treatment window is 3 to 4.5 hours from the time of stroke onset.[4,5] For intraarterial therapy, the time window is typically 0 to 6 hours for thrombolytic agents and 0 to 8 hours for mechanical therapies.[6–8] Beyond these traditional time-based treatment approaches, recent clinical trials are evaluating whether or not it is safe to give IV tPA to patients with unwitnessed symptom onset and MR imaging evidence of early ischemic changes (eg, MR WITNESS trial; clinicaltrials.gov/show/NCT0128224).

The clinical diagnosis of acute stroke is inaccurate in approximately 10% to 30% of cases.[9–12] Furthermore, conditions such as encephalitis, mass lesions, seizures, hypoglycemia, drug toxicity, and metabolic disturbances may demonstrate clinical and imaging appearances that mimic acute infarction.[9–11] The emergency

The authors have nothing to disclose.
Neuroradiology, Massachusetts General Hospital, Harvard Medical School, 55 Fruit Street, Boston, MA 02114, USA
* Corresponding author.
E-mail address: pschaefer@mgh.harvard.edu

radiologic.theclinics.com

radiologist, therefore, plays a critical role in the evaluation and triage of patients with symptoms of acute ischemic stroke, particularly with respect to the selection and rapid implementation of proper imaging techniques, recognition of early ischemic changes, and differentiation of stroke from other brain disorders.

This article focuses on the radiologic approach to the evaluation of the patient with acute ischemic stroke, including a brief overview of cerebral vascular territories, practical imaging recommendations for patients presenting with symptoms suggesting acute ischemic stroke, and the imaging appearance of acute infarcts on CT and MR imaging.

NORMAL CEREBROVASCULAR ANATOMY AND DISTRIBUTIONS

The intracranial circulation can be divided conveniently into the anterior and posterior circulations, which anastomose through the circle of Willis in the majority of cases. The anterior circulation consists of the intradural internal carotid artery (ICA) and major branches, namely, the anterior cerebral artery (ACA), the middle cerebral artery (MCA), the ophthalmic artery, and the anterior choroidal artery. The anterior communicating artery connecting the 2 ACAs, and the left and right posterior communicating arteries connecting the ipsilateral ICA to the ipsilateral posterior cerebral artery are also considered part of the anterior circulation.[13] The posterior circulation includes the vertebral arteries, the basilar artery, the cerebellar arteries, and the terminal bifurcation of the basilar artery into the right and left posterior cerebral arteries.[13] Deep penetrating branches of the major intracranial arteries supply the deep gray nuclei and the brainstem. These include the medial lenticulostriate arteries (arising from the A1 segment of the ACA), lateral lenticulostriate arteries (arising from the M1 segment of the MCA), peduncular perforating, thalamogeniculate, and thalamoperforating arteries (arising from the posterior communicating arteries and the P1 segment of the posterior cerebral artery), and the pontine perforating and medullary perforating arteries (arising from the vertebrobasilar system). Approximate vascular territories of the major intracranial arteries are depicted in **Fig. 1**.

IMAGING PROTOCOLS IN ACUTE ISCHEMIC STROKE

Four critical questions should be addressed for appropriate characterization and management of acute stroke.[14–16] (1) Is there intracranial hemorrhage that excludes thrombolytic therapy or a stroke mimic that explains the patient's presentation? (2) Is there thrombus/embolus in a large vessel that can be targeted for endovascular therapy? (3) Is there a nonsalvageable infarct "core" and if so, how large? (4) Is there salvageable "ischemic penumbra" or severely ischemic but potentially viable brain tissue? Imaging protocols vary from institution to institution and are based on access to different imaging modalities, preferences of treating physicians, and the availability of neurointerventional therapy on an emergent basis.[17,18] **Fig. 2** illustrates an experience and evidence-based imaging algorithm to select acute stroke patients for IV tPA and endovascular therapy used at our institution. Eventually, however, the practical challenge for the emergency radiologist is to define a standardized imaging algorithm, taking into account the resources available at his or her local institution that allow for improved patient outcomes without delaying treatment.

IMAGING OF THE BRAIN PARENCHYMA

Both CT and MR imaging can be used to evaluate the cerebral parenchyma in acute stroke. The goals of both modalities are to (1) exclude the presence of intracranial hemorrhage and mimics of stroke that would preclude the patient from receiving thrombolytic therapy[19] and (2) detect and quantify infarcted tissue. The imaging time courses for CT and MR imaging in infarction are summarized in **Table 1**.

Noncontrast Computed Tomography

Noncontrast CT (NCCT) of the head offers several practical advantages over MR imaging in the acute setting (**Table 2**) and is usually the first imaging modality used to assess acute stroke in the majority of emergency departments in the United States.[20,21]

Exclusion of hemorrhage

The presence of intracranial hemorrhage is an absolute contraindication to the administration of IV tPA. NCCT has been considered the accepted standard-of-care imaging modality for exclusion of intracranial hemorrhage based on data from early CT scanners and practical experience[22,23]; however, formal studies that have used a true reference standard, such as surgical or pathologic confirmation to support level I evidence, are lacking and the actual sensitivity and specificity of NCCT in detecting intracranial hemorrhage are unknown.[24] Furthermore, recent studies have suggested that the accuracy of MR imaging techniques for detection of intracranial hemorrhage in the acute stroke setting (within 6 hours) is

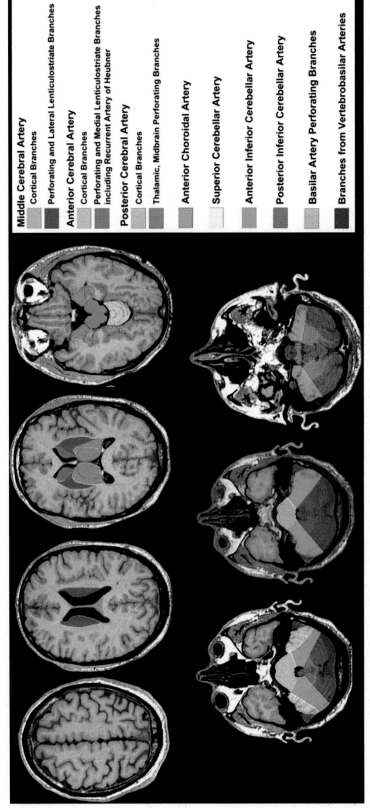

Middle Cerebral Artery
Cortical Branches
Perforating and Lateral Lenticulostriate Branches

Anterior Cerebral Artery
Cortical Branches
Perforating and Medial Lenticulostriate Branches including Recurrent Artery of Heubner

Posterior Cerebral Artery
Cortical Branches
Thalamic, Midbrain Perforating Branches

Anterior Choroidal Artery

Superior Cerebellar Artery

Anterior Inferior Cerebellar Artery

Posterior Inferior Cerebellar Artery

Basilar Artery Perforating Branches

Branches from Vertebrobasilar Arteries

Fig. 1. Approximate vascular territories of the major cerebral arteries and their branches. There is considerable variability in these territories particularly in the basal ganglia, brainstem, and posterior fossa.

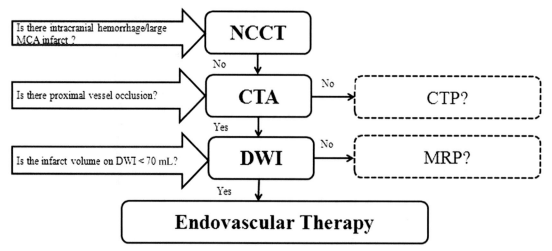

Fig. 2. Massachusetts General Hospital (MGH) acute stroke imaging algorithm for triage of patients with acute ischemic strokes. All patients undergo noncontrast CT (NCCT) followed by CT angiography (CTA). If the patient has severe neurologic deficits (National Institutes of Health Stroke Scale Score ≥8), no intracranial hemorrhage, no evidence of hypodensity greater than one-third of the MCA territory, and the presence of a proximal occlusion, then the patient undergoes diffusion-weighted MR imaging (DWI) if there are no contraindications to MR imaging. If the lesion is less than 70 mL on DWI, then the patient is triaged to endovascular therapy. If the patient is not eligible for endovascular therapy, then the patient may get an MR perfusion scan to assist in patient management. If the patient is not eligible for MR imaging, then a CT perfusion (CTP) study may be obtained after CTA to assist in patient management. (*Modified from* Gonzalez RG, Copen WA, Schaefer PW, et al. The Massachusetts General Hospital acute stroke imaging algorithm: an experience and evidence based approach. J Neurointerv Surg 2013;5(Suppl 1):i7–i12.)

equivalent to NCCT.[25,26] Despite these findings, the presence of clinical trials that have demonstrated the benefit of IV thrombolysis in patients selected by NCCT in the emergent setting[20,21,24] and the more practical considerations, such as the wide availability of CT scanners in most emergency departments, have led to its continued popularity as the preferred modality to exclude intracranial hemorrhage in acute stroke imaging.

Detection of infarcted tissue

NCCT findings of acute stroke syndrome are typically subtle in the first 6 hours and include loss of differentiation between cortical, basal ganglia, and insular gray matter and adjacent white matter; loss of cortical sulci as well as reduced sylvian fissure and basal cistern size owing to mild swelling; parenchymal hypodensity; and hyperdensity within an intracranial vessel from acute thrombus (**Fig. 3**).[12,21,27] Detection of these early signs of infarction varies based on levels of experience of the emergency radiologist, the size of the infarct, time since stroke onset, and the use of narrow window levels.[28]

The hyperdense vessel sign is seen in approximately 30% of patients with an M1 occlusion (see **Fig. 3**) and less commonly in patients with an MCA insular branch, ICA, or basilar artery occlusion.[29,30] Riedel and colleagues[31]

demonstrated that a thrombus length exceeding 8 mm on NCCT predicts that a vessel is unlikely to recanalize with IV therapy. Loss of the hyperdense vessel on NCCT after recanalization is an indicator of a favorable outcome after IV therapy.[32]

Hypodensity on NCCT is thought to represent infarct core, or tissue that is destined to progress to infarction. CT hypodensity is thought to be owing to an increase in tissue water content with a resultant reduction in x-ray attenuation.[33] Shortly after vascular occlusion, cell hypoxia leads to depletion of cellular ATP, failure of the Na^+–K^+–ATPase and other ionic pumps, a net migration of ions from the extracellular to the intracellular space with water following by osmosis, and the development of cytotoxic edema. Because there is no overall increase in tissue water, NCCT is insensitive for the detection of acute ischemia at very early time points. Within a few hours, there is breakdown of the blood–brain barrier and vasogenic edema begins develop. The progressive increase in total tissue water results in increasing hypodensity on NCCT and the increased sensitivity of NCCT to detect acute ischemia. The sensitivity for detection of acute ischemia within the first 3 hours after stroke onset is reported as 67% or less in most trials, but improved to 71% by using narrow window width and center level settings.[34–37] Reported specificities for detection of

Table 1
Time course of infarction on CT and MR imaging

Stage	CT	MR-DWI	MR-ADC	MR-FLAIR
Hyperacute (0–6 h)	Hyperdense artery sign; subtle decreased attenuation	Hyperintense	Hypointense	Hyperintense clot, hyperintense collateral vessels, isointense to mildly hyperintense parenchyma
Acute (6–24 h)	Decreased attenuation	Hyperintense	Hypointense	Hyperintense
Early subacute (1–7 d)	Decreased attenuation, progressive swelling	Hyperintense	Hypointense	Hyperintense
Late Subacute (1–4 wk)	Decreased attenuation and progressive swelling up to 1–2 wk, after which edema progressively resolves	Hyperintense (owing to T2 shine through)	Progressive increase of ADC - Isointense at 1–2 wk (pseudonormalization) then hyperintense	Hyperintense
Chronic	Hypodense encephalomalacia	Hypointense	Hyperintense	Hyperintense in periphery, centrally hypointense owing to cavitation

Abbreviations: ADC, apparent diffusion coefficient; DWI, diffusion-weighted image; FLAIR, fluid-attenuated inversion recovery.

Table 2
Advantages and limitations of CT and MR imaging in acute stroke

Characteristics	NCCT	MR Imaging
Wide availability in emergency settings	++	−
Rapid image acquisition	++	+
Safety for patients with metallic implants	++	−
Easy accessibility for unstable patients, patients with monitors/ventilators	++	−
Sensitivity for detection of hemorrhage	++	++ (GRE, SWI)
Sensitivity of detecting acute infarction	−	++ (DWI)
Differentiation between infarction and stroke mimics	+	++
Ionizing radiation	+	−

Abbreviations: DWI, diffusion-weighted imaging; GRE, gradient echo; NCCT, noncontrast CT; SWI, susceptibility weighted imaging.

acute ischemia on NCCT are high, ranging from 89% to 95%.[37]

Hypodensity on NCCT has important clinical applications. If the NCCT demonstrates hypodensity involving more than one-third of the MCA territory, the risks of "malignant MCA infarction," hemorrhagic transformation with attempted revascularization, or both are increased and IV thrombolytic therapy is not administered.[15,38]

The Alberta Stroke Program Early CT Score (AS-PECTS) was developed to provide a systematic and standardized approach of assessing early ischemic changes in regions of the MCA territory.[39] In ASPECTS, 10 regions in the MCA territory are assigned a binary score of 0 or 1 depending on the presence (1) or absence (0) of hypodensity; the total number of ischemic regions is subtracted from 10 such that a normal CT receives an ASPECTS score of 10 points, and a score of 0 indicates diffuse involvement throughout the MCA territory (**Fig. 4**). In general, ASPECTS has substantial interreader agreement.[39] Patients with an ASPECTS score of 7 or less have a substantially increased risk of thrombolysis-related parenchymal hemorrhage, have a trend toward poorer outcomes, and are less likely to benefit from IV tPA.[39–41] Although the decision to treat patients with intraarterial therapy varies between institutions, in general, patients with ASPECTS scores of 8 to 10 are considered good candidates and those with a score of less than 5 are typically not treated.

MR Imaging

MR imaging is increasingly becoming available in the emergency departments of large tertiary hospitals and offers superior evaluation of the brain parenchyma for early ischemic changes and stroke mimics.

Exclusion of hemorrhage

The sensitivity of MR imaging for the detection of hemorrhage depends on the age of the hemorrhage as well as the MR imaging sequence used (**Table 3**). The accuracy of MR imaging techniques for the detection of acute intracranial hemorrhage

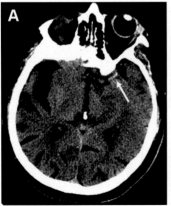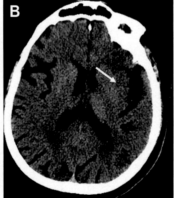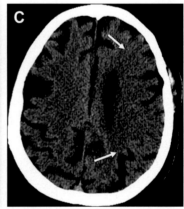

Fig. 3. Early signs (<6 hours) of cerebral infarction on noncontrast head CT. Hyperdensity in the proximal left middle cerebral artery (MCA) represents an acute thrombus in the MCA and is referred to as the "hyperdense MCA sign" (*arrow* in *A*). There is loss of the normal gray white matter differentiation between the insular cortex and the external capsule, referred to as the "insular ribbon sign" (*arrow* in *B*). There is loss of gray-white matter differentiation in the left frontal lobe and minimal sulcal effacement (region between 2 *arrows* in *C*).

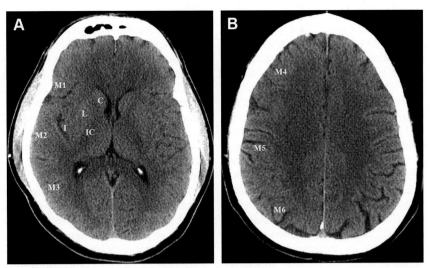

Fig. 4. The Alberta Stroke Program Early CT Score (ASPECTS) system is based on assessing 10 topographic regions of the middle cerebral artery (MCA) distribution on 2 axial slices. One slice is centered at the level of the basal ganglia and thalami (*A*) and the second slice is adjacent to the most superior margin of the ganglionic structures such that both slices do not overlap (*B*). Each demarcated region (M1, M2, M3, M4, M5, M6, the insula [I], the caudate [C], the lentiform nucleus [L], and the internal capsule [IC]) accounts for 1 point in the ASPECTS system. For each area involved by ischemia, 1 point is subtracted from a total of 10 points in each cerebral hemisphere.

has been reported as likely equivalent to NCCT, while T2*-weighted sequences (gradient-recalled echo [GRE] and susceptibility weighted imaging [SWI]) are noted to be better than NCCT in the detection of subacute and chronic microhemorrhages.[25,26,42,43] Although any prior known intracranial hemorrhage is deemed an absolute contraindication to IV tPA, recent studies have found no increased risk of hemorrhagic conversion of acute ischemic stroke treated with thrombolytic therapy in patients with up to 5 microhemorrhages detected on conventional GRE sequences.[44,45]

Detection of infarcted tissue

MR sequences typically used in the evaluation of acute stroke include diffusion-weighted imaging (DWI) with apparent diffusion coefficient (ADC) maps, fluid-attenuated inversion recovery (FLAIR), and T2*-weighted gradient-echo or SWI.

DWI is an MR sequence with image contrast dependent on the magnitude of the relative motion or diffusion of water molecules. DWI is the gold standard and provides level I evidence for identifying infarct core.[24] Unlike NCCT, it is highly sensitive and specific (approaching 100%) for the

Table 3
Stages of hemorrhage on MR and CT

Stage	Predominant Component[a]	CT	MR-T1	MR-T2	T2*
Hyperacute (<24 h)	Oxyhemoglobin	Hyperdense	Isointense	Hyperintense	No susceptibility
Acute (1–3 d)	Deoxyhemoglobin	Hyperdense	Isointense	Hypointense	Susceptibility
Early subacute (>3 d–1 wk)	Intracellular methemoglobin	Mildly hyperdense to isodense	Hyperintense	Hypointense	Susceptibility
Late subacute (1 wk–mo)	Extracellular methemoglobin	Isodense to hypodense	Hyperintense	Hyperintense	No susceptibility
Chronic	Hemosiderin	Hypodense	Hypointense	Hypointense	Susceptibility

[a] Frequently, hematomas contain >1 component. For simplicity, we delineate the predominant component at a particular stage of evolution of intracranial hemorrhage.

detection of restricted diffusion as early as 30 minutes after an ischemic event.[46] The biophysical basis is complex. With the onset of cytotoxic edema in acute stroke, there is an increased fraction of water molecules in the intracellular compared with the extracellular space. Water movement is more restricted in the intracellular compartment compared with the extracellular compartment because cellular organelles, cytoskeletal macromolecules, and other subcellular structures serve as barriers to the random motion of water molecules.[47,48] Furthermore, increased intracellular viscosity owing to microtubule dissociation, fragmentation of cellular components owing to breakdown of the energy-dependent cytoskeleton, and decreased cytoplasmic mobility have been suggested as explanations for the reduction of intracellular metabolite ADCs in ischemic brain.[49,50] With cellular swelling, there is also reduced extracellular space volume and a decrease in the diffusion of low-molecular-weight molecules, likely owing to increased tortuosity of extracellular space pathways.[51,52]

DWI images have both T2 and diffusion components. Therefore, it is important to view the ADC maps (whose signal intensity is equal to the magnitude of the ADC) in conjunction with the DWI images. An acute infarct, with restricted diffusion, is hyperintense on DWI images and hypointense on ADC maps (Fig. 5). Lesions with elevated diffusion (such as vasogenic edema) can be hypointense, isointense, or hyperintense on DWI images depending on the strength of the T2 and diffusion components, but is always hyperintense on ADC maps.

Multiple studies have demonstrated that initial DWI infarct volumes of greater than 70 mL are highly predictive of poor clinical outcomes irrespective of time of presentation and treatment in most patients.[53–56] As a consequence, most interventionalists who incorporate DWI into their decision process will not treat patients with anterior circulation infarcts measuring greater than 70 mL. However, younger patients and patients with right hemisphere strokes can have good outcomes with substantially larger lesion volumes and exceptions are, at times, made in those circumstances.[55–58] The "ABC/2" method has been used to rapidly and accurately calculate the volume of infarcted tissue (Fig. 6). This technique measures lesions in 3 orthogonal axes and has high intrarater and interrater reliability (71%–99%).[59]

Similar to NCCT, FLAIR requires disruption of the blood–brain barrier and development of vasogenic edema to detect acute ischemia. Edema associated with infarction presents earliest on FLAIR sequences, but still has a sensitivity of only 29% in the first 6 hours from stroke onset.[46,60,61] Hyperintense signal on T2-weighted images begins is not usually identified in the first 8 hours and hypointense signal signifying edema on T1-weighted images in the first 16 hours.[62] With this approximate guideline in mind, for those patients in whom the time of stroke onset is unknown ("wake-up" strokes), an infarct on DWI and ADC without matching hyperintensity on FLAIR suggests that the stroke likely occurred less than 6 hours previously (see Fig. 5). Several studies and clinical trials (eg, MR Witness: A Study of Intravenous Thrombolysis with Alteplase in MR

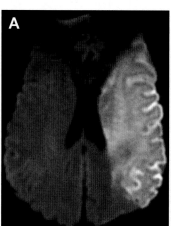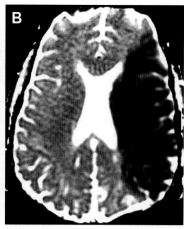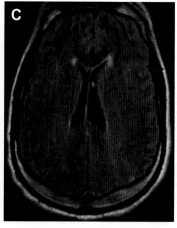

Fig. 5. Hyperacute infarction on MR imaging. A 74-year-old man presented approximately 5 hours after onset of right-sided hemiplegia and aphasia. Hyperintense signal within the majority of the left middle cerebral artery territory infarction on diffusion-weighted imaging sequences (A) with corresponding hypointensity on apparent diffusion coefficient maps (B) and only minimal hyperintensity on fluid-attenuated inversion recovery (C) is consistent with a hyperacute (<6 hours) infarction.

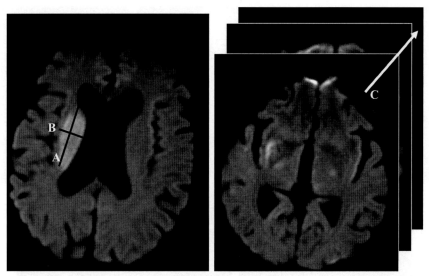

Fig. 6. The ABC/2 formula provides a rapid and easy method of assessing the volume of an infarct. The region of the abnormal signal intensity on diffusion-weighted imaging (DWI) can be measured by 3 orthogonal axes. A and B are measured on the axial slice with the largest region of DWI signal involvement (DWI image, *left*). C is calculated from the number of axial slices on which the abnormality appears multiplied by the slice thickness (DWI images, *right*). A, B, and C are then multiplied and the product divided by 2 for the volume of infarcted tissue. A lesion greater than 70 mL implies a poor prognosis.

Imaging-Selected Patients, ClinicalTrials.gov Identifier: NCT01282242) have used the presence of a DWI–FLAIR mismatch to guide thrombolysis in patients with unknown stroke onset time.[61,63–67]

Hyperintense vessel sign (HVS) on FLAIR images is observed frequently in the hemisphere with arterial occlusion.[68] The clinical implications of HVS remain uncertain. A recent study evaluating patients with MCA territory strokes categorized hyperintense vessels on FLAIR as proximal and distal.[69] According to the authors of that study, proximal HVS is a marker for arterial occlusion, presumably the result of the thrombus inside the arterial lumen, whereas distal HVS in patients with MCA occlusion results from pial collateral blood flow from the anterior and posterior cerebral arteries. Furthermore, patients with more prominent distal HVS had smaller initial, 24-hour, and subacute ischemic lesion volumes and lower initial National Institute of Health Stroke Scale scores, suggesting that prominent distal HVS may provide a mechanism for discriminating tissue kept viable for extended periods by way of a well-developed collateral network.[69] Other authors have shown that a greater extent of FLAIR hyperintense vessels is associated with a larger initial infarct volume, a greater perfusion deficit, a greater final infarct volume and hemorrhagic transformation; these findings suggest that FLAIR HVS may represent inadequate collaterals.[70]

After evaluating the DWI and FLAIR sequences, the radiologist should evaluate T2*-weighted MR imaging sequences (GRE and SWI). Intraarterial thrombus can be detected as "blooming" hypointensity on T2*-weighted MR imaging sequences (**Fig. 7**) and is the correlate of the CT "hyperdense vessel sign." In a recent study, SWI identified clot in 93% of proximal MCA occlusions.[71] GRE is less sensitive, with the susceptibility vessel sign on this sequence being more common in patients with cardioembolic strokes (with fibrin-rich clots) than with other stroke subtypes.[72] Prominent asymmetric hypointense cortical veins have been identified within the ischemic region using SWI and are likely owing to an increase in the deoxyhemoglobin to oxyhemoglobin ratio caused by hypoperfusion-induced increases in the oxygen extraction fraction.[73,74] It has been hypothesized that, because SWI is sensitive to oxygen extraction fraction–associated changes in deoxygenated hemoglobin seen in hypoperfused tissue, it may be used to provide metabolic information similar to mean transit time (MTT) on perfusion-weighted images (PWI).[75] Several recent studies have reported that the DWI–SWI mismatch in acute stroke is similar to the DWI–PWI mismatch, suggesting that the DWI–SWI mismatch may demarcate the ischemic penumbra and have a similar ability to predict stroke evolution as the DWI–PWI mismatch.[73,75–77]

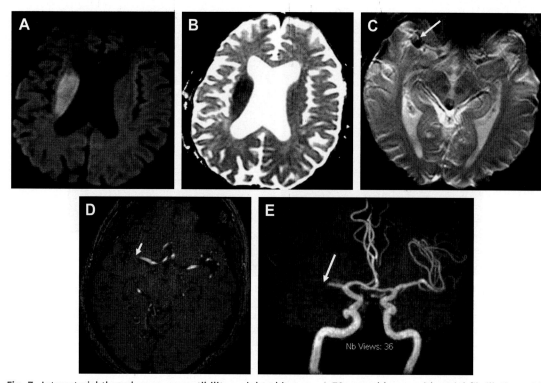

Fig. 7. Intraarterial thrombus on susceptibility weighted images. A 70-year-old man with atrial fibrillation with sudden onset of left-sided weakness approximately 3 hours before MR imaging. There is an acute infarction in the right caudate body and corona radiata, with restricted diffusion characterized by hyperintensity on the diffusion-weighted imaging (DWI) sequence (*A*) and hypointensity on the apparent diffusion coefficient map (*B*). Gradient-recalled echo T2* susceptibility weighted image (*C*) demonstrates blooming hypointense signal (*arrow*) consistent with right middle cerebral artery thrombus. Three-dimensional MR imaging time of flight source images (*D*) and MR imaging maximal intensity projection images (*E*) demonstrate an abrupt cutoff of flow related enhancement within the M1 segment of the right middle cerebral artery (*arrow*).

IMAGING OF THE CEREBRAL VASCULATURE

Vascular imaging in acute stroke extends from the aortic arch to the cranial vertex. The intracranial circulation is evaluated to identify and characterize the vascular lesion and to quantify the extent of collateral flow. Evaluation of the extracranial circulation is performed mainly to identify and characterize a potentially thrombotic or embolic source and to assist in determining whether therapy should be medical or surgical; occlusions are usually treated pharmacologically, whereas endarterectomy or stent placement is indicated for symptomatic patients with greater than 70% stenosis of the common or ICA. Digital subtraction angiography (DSA) remains the gold standard for vascular imaging, but is an invasive procedure with inherent risks and is time consuming. Advantages of CT versus MR techniques in general are outlined in **Table 2**. The following sections describe advantages and limitations specific to CT angiography (CTA) and MR angiography (MRA).

Computed Tomography Angiography

The main practical benefit of CTA over MRA is that most CT scanners are capable of performing CTA immediately after NCCT. Once hemorrhage has been excluded, IV tPA can be initiated while the patient is undergoing CT vascular imaging without any time lost in screening the patient and equipment for MR compatibility.

At the authors' institution, CTA is typically performed by injecting 80 mL of IV contrast at 3.5 to 5 mL/s with a power injector followed by saline. A technologist performs 3-plane, orthogonal, maximal intensity projection images of the head at the scanner in a few minutes. The combination of these maximal intensity projections and the source axial images allows rapid localization and definition of extent of intravascular thrombus and nearly always allows adequate evaluation of the arterial vasculature for the purposes of triage for thrombolytic therapy (**Fig. 8**). For the neck, a technologist typically performs 2-plane orthogonal maximal intensity projection images. These, in

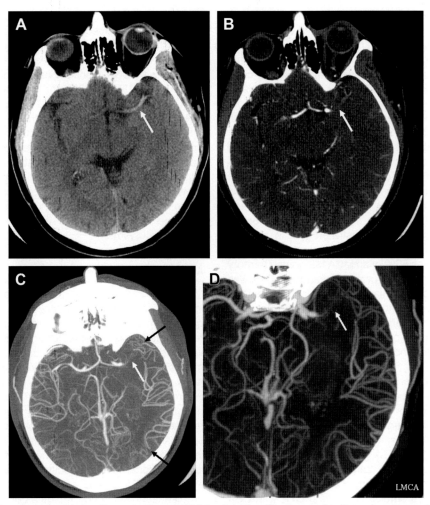

Fig. 8. Utility of maximal intensity projections (MIPs) in clot identification and collateral assessment. A 71-year-old man presented 3 hours after sudden onset of aphasia. Axial noncontrast head CT demonstrates hyperdensity within the proximal left middle cerebral artery (MCA) consistent with clot (*arrow* in *A*). Occlusion of a short segment of the proximal left MCA by intravascular thrombus on CTA source images (*arrow* in *B*) is better defined on the axial MIP (*white arrow* in *C*) and axial 3-dimensional reformats (*arrow* in *D*) as a short segment without contrast opacification. There is robust collateral flow seen between the black arrows on the axial MIP images (*C*).

combination with the source images (SI), allow definition of dissection, atherosclerotic plaque, degree of stenosis, and detection of intraluminal thrombus within the carotid and vertebral arteries. In the acute stroke setting, additional delayed-phase CTA may also be necessary to differentiate between true occlusion and delayed opacification owing to slow flow.

CTA of the head has very high sensitivity (97%–100%) and specificity (98%–100%) for detecting proximal intracranial occlusions and stenosis compared with DSA, and can be acquired more rapidly than with MRA.[78–80] Identification of proximal occlusions is critical to patient management because vascular lesions that involve the proximal intracranial vessels result in the largest infarcts with the greatest likelihood of hemorrhagic transformation, but also allow the greatest potential benefit from intraarterial thrombolysis or mechanical thrombectomy. By using a true intravascular contrast agent, CTA of the head is not susceptible to artifactual vessel narrowing caused by turbulent flow on time-of-flight (TOF) MRA images, and is not susceptible to the phase and susceptibility artifacts that affect gadolinium contrast-enhanced MRA images.[23] In addition, the spatial resolution of CTA is twice that of MRA. Consequently, although both MRA and CTA are accurate for identifying proximal occlusions, CTA of the head is superior to MRA for detecting occlusions in more distal vessels.[78,79]

In the head, CTA-SI greatly improves the detection of subtle, early parenchymal ischemic changes compared with NCCT alone. In the early days of CTA, a steady-state level of contrast was reached during scanning and the CTA-SI could be considered whole brain perfused blood volume images and an approximation of the infarct core. However, with current, faster CTA protocols, a steady state is not reached, the CTA-SI are more blood flow weighted, and they frequently overestimate infarct core size.

CTA is also useful for assessing the extent of leptomeningeal collateral circulation.[81] The presence (see Fig. 8) or absence (Fig. 9) of a robust collateral circulation on CTA can predict the final infarct volume after endovascular therapy and the clinical response to treatment.[82–84] Souza and colleagues[85] demonstrated that in patients with ICA and/or M1 occlusions, absent collaterals in greater than 50% of an MCA M2 branch territory (malignant collateral profile) detected by CTA was highly specific for larger admission DWI infarct core and poor outcome. Furthermore, Puetz and colleagues[86] demonstrated that a malignant collateral profile on CTA predicted poor prognosis despite IV thrombolysis within 3 hours from symptom onset.

For evaluation of the extracranial circulation, CTA of the neck is also superior to MRA of the neck owing to better spatial resolution and absence of flow artifacts, allowing accurate evaluation of vascular narrowing and luminal surface irregularities.[87–91] CTA is an accurate modality for detection of severe carotid artery disease and especially for the detection of occlusions. A meta-analysis of 28 studies comparing CTA with DSA found CTA to have a pooled sensitivity of 85% and a pooled specificity of 93% for detection of 70% to 99% stenosis, whereas the sensitivity and specificity for detection of an occlusion were 97% and 99%, respectively.[92] Studies comparing CTA with MRA for carotid and vertebral artery dissection found both modalities have similar correlation with DSA (sensitivities and specificities range from 51% to 100% and 67% to 100% for CTA, and 50% to 100% and 29% to 100% for MRA, respectively); however, the limitations of MRA in detecting dissection, including obscuration of mural hematoma by hyperintense signal from an adjacent occlusive thrombus and lack of hyperintense signal within mural hematoma on T1-weighted images in early dissection, are overcome by CTA.[93,94] In addition, CTA may be more sensitive for identifying intimal flaps and pseudoaneurysms.[95]

Magnetic Resonance Angiography

MRA techniques utilized in acute stroke imaging include non–contrast-enhanced TOF and gadolinium-enhanced MRA, with 3-dimensional reformatted images generated to assist further in vessel evaluation (see Fig. 7). Briefly, TOF techniques use a gradient echo sequence that saturates out signal from the stationary spins within a volume of tissue. This is accomplished by multiple radiofrequency pulses, followed by dephasing and rephasing gradients. Thus, the only unsaturated spins (signal) are within blood flowing from outside into the volume of interest. Generally, the contrast is proportional to the velocity of flow. Contrast-enhanced MRA techniques, based on a short rapid gradient echo sequence, image a bolus of IV gadolinium contrast in the arterial phase. The contrast agent shortens the T1 of opacified vessels compared with the longer T1 relaxation times of

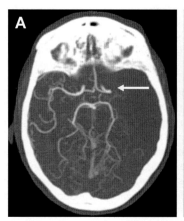 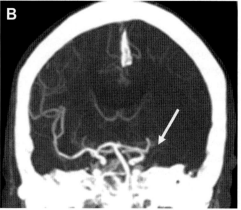

Fig. 9. Assessment of collateral flow on CT angiography (CTA) maximal intensity projections (MIPs). An 80-year-old woman with atrial fibrillation and right-sided hemiparesis 2 hours before imaging. Axial CTA MIP image (A) and coronal CTA MIP image (B) demonstrate occlusion of the left M1 segment of the MCA (arrow) with absence of collateral vasculature, consistent with a malignant collateral profile.

the surrounding soft tissues. This allows for good separation of vessels from surrounding soft tissues on image acquisition. Compared with TOF-MRA, gadolinium-enhanced MRA allows coverage of a greater volume with a shorter acquisition time, is less affected by motion artifact, provides better signal-to-noise ratio, and has fewer artifacts related to dephasing from turbulence and saturation effects. However, gadolinium-enhanced MRA has poorer spatial resolution compared with 3-dimensional TOF MRA and is subject to venous contamination. For these reasons, gadolinium-enhanced MRA is often used to image the large vessels of the neck, whereas 3-dimensional–TOF–MRA is used to image the small vessels of the head.

Gadolinium-enhanced MRA is highly accurate in differentiating surgical from nonsurgical carotid stenosis.[96] TOF MRA is sensitive for detecting proximal intracranial occlusions.[97] However, from a practical standpoint, MRA images of the head and neck are generally inferior to CTA images for scanning acute stroke patients on an emergency basis; they take longer and motion artifact is a common problem. Additionally, when compared with CTA, gadolinium-enhanced MRA images have a narrower window for acquiring images during peak contrast enhancement and, consequently, inadequate arterial enhancement and venous contamination are common problems. Given these findings, most institutions prefer CTA to MRA for evaluation of vessels, limiting the use of MRA techniques to evaluation of patients with allergies to CT contrast agents, patients with renal failure, and patients vulnerable to radiation effects, such as children and pregnant women.

EVALUATING TISSUE VIABILITY/PERFUSION IMAGING
Computed Tomography and Magnetic Resonance Perfusion Imaging

In the acute stroke setting, CT and MR perfusion imaging are generally performed with a bolus tracking technique in which a contrast agent is injected rapidly (5–7 cc/s) into a peripheral IV catheter and images are obtained repeatedly as the contrast agent passes through the brain. The images obtained are then converted by a computer to contrast agent concentration versus time curves. Various parameters are calculated: (1) cerebral blood volume (CBV) is a measure of the total volume of blood within an imaging voxel including blood in the tissues and blood vessels; (2) cerebral blood flow (CBF) is a measure of the total volume of blood moving through a voxel in a given unit of time; (3) MTT is the time difference between the arterial inflow and venous outflow; (4) time to peak enhancement is the time from the beginning of contrast material injection to the maximum concentration of contrast material within a region of interest, and (5) T_{max} is the time at which the convolved residue function reaches its maximum.[98–101] The evaluation of brain perfusion is based on the central volume principle, according to which, MTT = CBV/CBF. These parameters are derived from perfusion source data using deconvolution analyses and color-coded perfusion maps can be generated automatically at the scanner.[98–102]

CT perfusion imaging can be performed on any standard helical CT scanner immediately after the NCCT. Briefly, brain tissue increases and then decreases again in density as an iodine-based contrast agent passes through the brain. The technique uses a standard cine protocol that obtains approximately 60 sequential images for each scan location over a given volume of coverage (slab). The slab is up to 16 cm for the latest 256 and 320 detector scanners. The volume of tissue imaged is typically divided into 5-mm-thick slices. The arterial input function is usually chosen from the ACA or the top of the ICA, or may be automatically chosen by the vendor software using a summation of large vessels. The venous output function is usually chosen from the superior sagittal sinus.

Perfusion-weighted MR imaging (PWI) either achieves perfusion contrast by an exogenous method, such as the administration of gadolinium contrast, or by an endogenous method, such as the labeling of hydrogen-1 protons in water, also known as arterial spin labeling.[103] The primary method is a dynamic susceptibility (T2*) contrast sequence that relies on the decrease in signal caused by magnetic susceptibility effects of gadolinium as it passes through the intracranial vasculature.[104] Because blood passes through the brain parenchyma rapidly, the most commonly used sequence is a single shot gradient echo echo-planar sequence capable of multiple slice acquisition from a single repetition time. Approximately 60 images are obtained for each 5-mm brain slice, and the whole brain is covered. The arterial input is typically chosen automatically using cluster analysis.[105] In contrast, the arterial spin labeling technique does not require the use of IV contrast and exploits the spins of labeled endogenous water protons to measure perfusion with 2 sets of images obtained, one that is sensitive to flow and one that is not sensitive to flow. A subtracted image is then generated by subtracting the flow-sensitive image from the flow-insensitive image to create a CBF map.

A number of studies have demonstrated that lesion volumes on CT perfusion maps (CBV, CBF, and MTT) correlate highly with those obtained from similar MR perfusion maps.[106] Operationally, for MR imaging, the volume of the lesion on DWI is thought to represent the infarct core or nonsalvageable tissue. For CT, definition of the infarct core is more controversial; some investigators use thresholded CT–CBV, whereas others use thresholded CT–CBF to identify infarct core.[107–109] Still other investigators believe that CT perfusion maps cannot identify reliably infarct core owing to poor contrast-to-noise ratios and large measurement error.[110] Tissue that seems to be normal on DWI or thresholded CT CBV/CBF images and abnormal on MTT and other transit images such as T_{max} is thought to represent the ischemic penumbra. The penumbra represents tissue that may progress to infarction or may recover, depending on the timing of reperfusion and the degree of collateralization. It is tissue that can potentially be salvaged with reperfusion therapy.

Interpretation of perfusion maps is often done through direct visual inspection, which allows for speed and simplicity, but has the disadvantage of being dependent on subjective user interpretation.[98] Currently, most centers advocate using quantitative perfusion parameters to identify areas

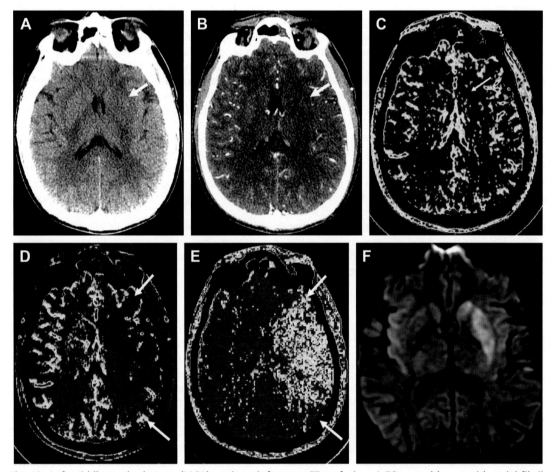

Fig. 10. Left middle cerebral artery (MCA) territory infarct on CT perfusion. A 76-year-old man with atrial fibrillation presenting 3 hours after onset of right leg weakness. Noncontrast CT (*A*) demonstrates subtle hypodensity within the left basal ganglia (*arrow*). CT angiography source image (*B*) increases the conspicuity of ischemia in the left basal ganglia (*arrow*). Cerebral blood volume (CBV) map (*C*) demonstrates focal decreased cerebral blood volume in the left anterior basal ganglia (*arrow*) with more normal CBV in the remainder of the left basal ganglia. Cerebral blood flow (CBF) map (*D*) demonstrates severely decreased blood flow in the left basal ganglia with a much larger region of less severely decreased cerebral blood flow conforming to the left MCA vascular territory (*arrows*). There is corresponding prolonged mean transit time (MTT) abnormality on MTT map (denoted by *arrows* on *E*). Diffusion-weighted image (DWI; *F*) obtained 20 minutes after the CT perfusion scan demonstrates acute infarction in the left basal ganglia, corresponding with the region with severely decreased CBF. The region characterized by normal DWI but abnormal CBF and MTT represents the imaging-defined ischemic penumbra.

of infarct core and penumbra. Unfortunately, there is no standardization or validation of CT perfusion acquisition or postprocessing techniques, and quantitative perfusion parameter map values vary widely across different vendor platforms.[102] For example, Dani and colleagues[111] reviewed 20 CT perfusion and 49 MR perfusion studies. They noted that published thresholds of infarct core on CT perfusion were as follows: CT–CBV ranging from 2.0 to 2.3 mL/100 g; CT-MTT of 6 seconds; and CT relative CBF of 0.34.[111] CT perfusion parameter thresholds for penumbra were CT–MTT ranging from 6.53 to 7.0 seconds; relative CT–MTT from 1.45 to 2.2; CT–CBF of 27.9 mL/

100 g/min; relative CT–CBF ranging from 0.50 to 0.63; and CT–CBV of 1.69 mL/100 g.[111] MR perfusion parameter thresholds for penumbra were MR–MTT ranging from 1.78 to 8.1 seconds, MR time to peak enhancement from 4 to 7 seconds, MR–CBF from 18 to 37.2 mL/100 g/min, and relative MR–CBF from 0.58 to 0.61.[111]

The timing of reperfusion therapy is another source of variability. A study found lower CBF thresholds for infarction in tissue that was reperfused earlier,[112] confirming a primate model demonstrating that the CBF threshold for tissue infarction with reperfusion at 2 to 3 hours was 10 to 12 mL/100 g/min, whereas the threshold for

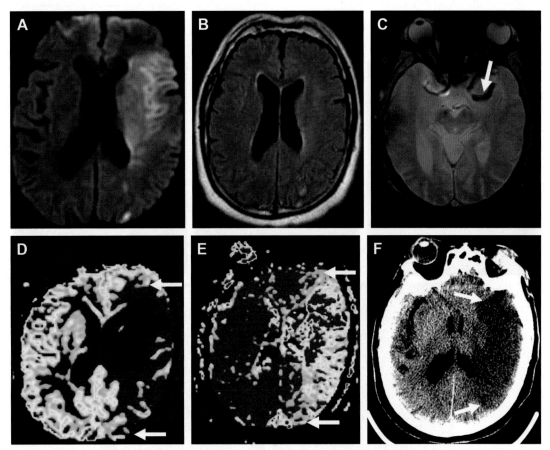

Fig. 11. Left middle cerebral artery (MCA) territory infarct on MR perfusion: diffusion-weighted image (DWI)–mean transit time (MTT)/cerebral blood flow (CBF) perfusion mismatch. A 79-year-old woman with atrial fibrillation presenting 4 hours after developing right-sided weakness. (*A*) DWI image reveals a region of restricted diffusion in the left basal ganglia, deep white matter, insular ribbon, and inferior frontal lobe. There are also small foci with restricted diffusion in the left parietal region. These findings are in the vascular territory of the left MCA. (*B*) Fluid-attenuated inversion recovery (FLAIR) image demonstrates no significant increased signal, suggesting acute infarction. (*C*) Susceptibility weighted image demonstrates blooming artifact within the left M1 segment (*arrow*), consistent with acute thrombus. There is decreased CBF (*arrows, D*) and increased MTT (*arrows, E*) throughout most of the visualized left MCA territory in a region much larger than the DWI abnormality. These findings are consistent with a DWI–MTT and DWI–CBF mismatch of approximately 50%. The DWI normal but CBF or MTT abnormal tissue represents the imaging-defined ischemic penumbra. Noncontrast head CT (*F*) obtained 2 days later demonstrates extension of the left MCA infarct (*arrows*) into the ischemic penumbra.

tissue infarction with permanent occlusion was 17 to 18 mL/100 g/min. Furthermore, normal CBF in human parenchyma varies by 3-fold, depending on age and location.[113,114] Schaefer and colleagues[115] demonstrated different CT–CBF thresholds for penumbra progressing to infarction in gray versus white matter. Payabvash and colleagues[116] demonstrated variable regional ischemic vulnerability of the brain to hypoperfusion on CT perfusion, suggesting that location-specific rather than whole-brain thresholds may provide more accurate assessment of infarct core and penumbra. Variability in initial and follow-up imaging times and variability in postischemic tissue responses further complicate interpretation of perfusion maps.

The assumption that the thresholded CT CBV/CBF–MTT/T_{max} mismatch and the DWI-MTT/T_{max} mismatch represent the ischemic penumbra on CT perfusion and MR PWI, respectively, suggests that patients with a large mismatch would be most likely to benefit from reperfusion therapy. Conversely, it is suggested that patients with little or no mismatch should not receive aggressive therapies because their infarctions are unlikely to increase in size and they should be spared the associated risk of hemorrhage. The concept that the mismatch should be used as selection criteria for IV thrombolysis or endovascular procedures is supported by some recent studies. For example, in the Diffusion and Perfusion Imaging Evaluation for Understanding Stroke Evolution (DEFUSE) trial

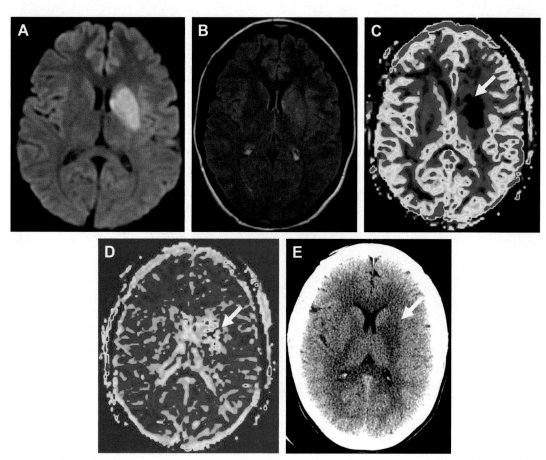

Fig. 12. Left middle cerebral artery (MCA) territory infarct on MR perfusion: diffusion-weighted image (DWI)–mean transit time (MTT)/cerebral blood flow (CBF) perfusion match. A 25-year-old woman presented 8 hours after onset of right-sided weakness and aphasia. (*A*) DWI demonstrates restricted diffusion within the left basal ganglia and deep white matter, consistent with acute left MCA territory infarction. (*B*) Fluid-attenuated inversion recovery (FLAIR) images demonstrate mild associated hyperintensity. Perfusion maps demonstrate an area of decreased CBF (denoted by *arrow* in *C*) and an area of increased MTT (denoted by *arrow* in *D*), which is matched with the DWI infarct volume. A noncontrast head CT (*E*) obtained 2 days later demonstrates no significant progression of the left basal ganglia infarct (*arrow*).

Table 4
Nonischemic conditions that may mimic stroke clinically and show restricted diffusion on MR imaging

Condition	Imaging Characteristics Differentiating It from Acute Stroke
Venous infarct	Nonarterial distribution on CT and MR imaging. Venous occlusion seen as hyperdensity within dural venous sinuses or cortical veins on NCCT, lack of opacification on CTV, lack of normal flow voids on T2-weighted images, susceptibility on SWI, and lack of normal flow related enhancement on MRV. Mixed areas of restricted and elevated diffusion on DWI/ADC. More commonly hemorrhagic than arterial infarct and primarily affects white matter instead of cortex. May present with seizures, which is uncommon for acute stroke.
Seizures	DWI signal abnormality does not conform to a vascular distribution and is typically confined to the cortex. DWI abnormalities are usually reversible over the course of a few days and typically do not progress to encephalomalacia. Acute vascular imaging demonstrates hyperemia rather than the vascular occlusion or stenosis typically seen with acute stroke. Acute stroke patients rarely present with a seizure.
Hypoglycemia	T2 hyperintensity and restricted diffusion within the basal ganglia, internal capsules, hippocampi, occipital lobes, middle cerebellar peduncles and brainstem. Diagnosis is based on distribution and low blood glucose.
Herpes simplex encephalitis	Restricted diffusion and FLAIR hyperintensity within the cortical and subcortical regions of the medial temporal lobes, inferior frontal lobes, the insula and the cingulate gyri. Presentation with seizure and fever. Diagnosis based on PCR.
Low-grade glial neoplasm	Regional hypodensity that seems to be similar to stroke on NCCT. Has elevated diffusion. Frequently presents with a seizure. Does not conform to a vascular distribution.
Demyelinative lesion	Acute lesions can have restricted diffusion. Enhancement is common, and not seen with acute ischemic lesions. Associated white matter lesions. Young patients.

Abbreviations: ADC, apparent diffusion coefficient; CTV, CT venography; DWI, diffusion-weighted imaging; FLAIR, fluid-attenuated inversion recovery; MRV, MR venography; NCCT, noncontrast CT; PCR, polymerase chain reaction; SWI, susceptibility weighted imaging.

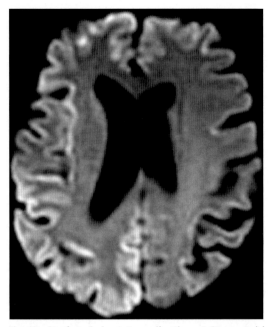

Fig. 13. Stroke mimic: status epilepticus. A 71-year-old woman with witnessed seizure. Axial diffusion-weighted image demonstrates restricted diffusion involving the cortical ribbon of the right cerebral hemisphere.

the patients with "target mismatch" that had early reperfusion relative to those with "no mismatch" or "malignant" profiles.[56,117] In the more recent DEFUSE-2 trial, a "target mismatch" profile was defined as (1) a ratio between the volumes of critically hypoperfused tissue (T_{max} >6 s) and ischemic core (ADC <600 × 10^{-6} mm^2/s) of 1.8 or more, with an absolute difference of 15 mL or more; (2) ischemic core volume of less than 70 mL; and (3) less than 100 mL of tissue with severe delay in bolus arrival (T_{max} >10 s). Early reperfusion was defined as greater than 50% reduction in volume of the perfusion lesion (T_{max} >6 s) between baseline and early follow-up. The study demonstrated favorable clinical response associated with reperfusion in the target mismatch group, but not in the group without a target mismatch. Similarly, when large vessel occlusion and a CT perfusion–defined penumbra to core mismatch of greater than 20% (with core defined as relative CT–CBF of <40% involving less than one-third of the MCA territory and penumbra defined as relative MTT of >145%) were used as selection criteria, IV tenecteplase was associated with better reperfusion and clinical outcomes compared with IV alteplase for the treatment of acute ischemic stroke within 6 hours of symptom onset.[118]

Even when an acute stroke patient is not a candidate for IV thrombolytic or endovascular therapy, PWI should be performed. For patients who cannot undergo evaluation of infarct by

and the DEFUSE-2 trial, patients receiving reperfusion therapy between 3 and 6 hours were stratified based on predefined DWI–PWI imaging profiles, and both showed favorable clinical response in

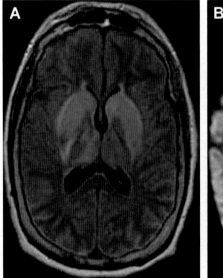

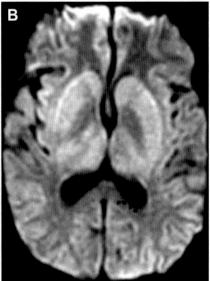

Fig. 14. Stroke mimic: hypoglycemia. A 69-year-old woman with altered mental status found to have low blood sugar. (*A*) Axial fluid-attenuated inversion recovery (FLAIR) image demonstrates relatively symmetric FLAIR signal abnormality involving bilateral caudate nuclei, putamina, and thalami with relative sparing of the globus pallidi. (*B*) Axial diffusion-weighted images show associated restricted diffusion involving these areas.

Table 5
Summary of CT and MR imaging techniques for evaluating infarct core, infarct penumbra, and vasculature

Modality	Infarct Core	Penumbra	Vasculature
CT	Hypodensity defines the infarct core Specific but not sensitive Hypodensity involving one-third of the MCA territory is a contraindication to thrombolysis	Not seen	Hyperdense vessel denotes site of intravascular thrombus
MR imaging (DWI, FLAIR, T2, GRE)	DWI/ADC hyperintensity/hypointensity is the most sensitive and specific imaging marker of infarct core - level 1 evidence DWI core >70 mL suggests poor patient prognosis and is a contraindication to IA therapy at many centers FLAIR - little to hyperintensity in first 6 h; used to determine time of stroke onset and treatment in patients with wake up strokes GRE/SWI detects hemorrhagic conversion	SWI - Asymmetric cortical veins with increased deoxyhemoglobin may define the penumbra	FLAIR - hyperintensity in clot and in collateral vessels T2 - loss of normal flow void GRE/SWI - susceptibility artifact in clot
CTA	CTA source images improve detection of ischemia but tend to overestimate infarct core	Cannot define	Highly sensitive and specific for the detection of proximal vessel occlusions CTA MIPS increase conspicuity of vascular stenosis and occlusion CTA MIPS - reliable for quantifying degree of collateral circulation
MRA	Cannot define	Cannot define	Overall, less sensitive and specific for detecting intracranial stenosis and occlusions compared with CTA Relatively accurate for detecting proximal vessel occlusions. TOF MRA is invaluable alternative for patients with renal insufficiency or IV contrast allergy
CTP	Estimated by thresholded CBV or CBF, but large variability in absolute and relative values because techniques and postprocessing methods are not standardized and there is large measurement error. Less sensitive and specific than DWI	Estimated by tissue that is normal on thresholded CBV or CBF but abnormal on thresholded CBF or MTT maps, but large variability in values because techniques and postprocessing methods are not standardized and there is large measurement error.	CTA and CTP can be acquired simultaneously on some scanners
MRP	Not used to define infarct core because DWI is far more sensitive and specific	Estimated by CBF reduction and MTT/T_{max}/TTP prolongation, but large variability in relative values because techniques and postprocessing methods are not standardized and there is large measurement error. DWI volume - T_{max} >6 volume mismatch has been shown to be useful in some clinical trials	Cannot define

Abbreviations: ADC, apparent diffusion coefficient; CBF, cerebral blood flow; CBV, cerebral blood volume; CTA, CT angiography; CTP, CT perfusion; DWI, diffusion-weighted imaging; FLAIR, fluid-attenuated inversion recovery; GRE, gradient-recalled echo; IA, intraarterial; IV, intravenous; MCA, middle cerebral artery; MIPS, maximal intensity projections; MRP, MR perfusion; MTT, mean transit time; SWI, susceptibility weighted imaging; T_{max}, time at which the convolved residue function reaches its maximum; TOF, time of flight; TTP, time to peak enhancement.

DWI, CT perfusion increases the detection of acute ischemia. In 1 study, CT perfusion increased the sensitivity of detecting acute stroke by 18% compared with NCCT alone, and by 12% compared with NCCT and CTA-SI.[119] Patients with a DWI–PWI mismatch should receive more rigorous blood pressure management so that the penumbral tissue does not progress to infarction. Furthermore, in patients with focal neurologic deficits but normal DWI, perfusion imaging can help to determine whether or not the acute deficit is ischemic; a wedge-shaped perfusion deficit suggests that the patient has ischemic but viable tissue, and normal perfusion suggests a nonvascular etiology for the patient's symptoms.

In a patient with a DWI abnormality in 1 vascular territory, perfusion imaging can help to determine stroke etiology; for example, PWI demonstrating abnormalities in multiple vascular territories suggests a cardioembolic or vasculitic etiology. Perfusion imaging can also help to predict the development of malignant MCA infarction[120] and improve stroke patient outcome prediction models.[57,58] **Figs. 10–12** provide examples of CT and MR perfusion.

STROKE MIMICS

Many conditions can clinically present as focal neurologic deficits and can be misdiagnosed as

---

Box 1
What the physician needs to know: key facts

- Imaging is urgently required to rule out intracranial hemorrhage and stroke mimics, as well as quantify the extent of infarcted tissue so as to appropriately select patients for IV thrombolytic therapy.

- NCCT and GRE MR imaging show similar accuracy in the diagnosis of acute intracerebral hemorrhage, but NCCT is typically used to make the decision of whether or not to treat with IV tPA.

- Diffusion-weighted MR imaging is the gold standard for infarct core and is markedly more sensitive than NCCT (which is specific but not sensitive).

- Intraarterial thrombus can be detected as a hyperdense vessel sign on NCCT and "blooming" hypointensity on T2*-weighted MR imaging sequences (GRE and SWI)

- For those patients in whom the time of stroke onset is unknown ("wake-up" strokes), an infarct on DWI and ADC with little to no hyperintensity on FLAIR suggests that the stroke occurred <6 hours previously.

- CTA is diagnostically superior to MRA for evaluation of vasculature; it allows for better identification of dissection, identification of intraluminal thrombus and differentiation of occlusion from critical stenosis in the neck, and better identification of proximal and distal emboli as well as collateral vessel assessment. However, TOF MRA allows for adequate evaluation of vasculature in those patients who cannot receive contrast. TOF MRA of the circle of Willis is sensitive for identifying proximal vessel occlusions. Contrast-enhanced MRA of the neck is accurate for identifying surgical carotid stenosis.

- CTA is the best method for evaluating collateral vessels. CTA collateral assessment may be important in treatment decisions. The extent of FLAIR hyperintense vessels also provides information collateral vessel status.

- CTP increases the detection of ischemia compared with NCCT and CTA-SI. Some investigators believe that thresholded CT-CBV or CT-CBF are useful for identifying infarct core, whereas others believe that the large measurement error and lack of standardization render it unreliable.

- CTP and MRP can be used to define the ischemic penumbra. Lack of standardization prevents the acceptance of universal thresholds. A $T_{max} > 6$ has been used to define the penumbra in a number of trials. Combined multimodal parenchymal, perfusion and vascular imaging with CT or MR imaging can identify patients with an ischemic penumbra who may benefit from acute reperfusion therapies

- Even when patients are not candidates for IV or IA therapy, perfusion imaging may be used to guide blood pressure management, predict malignant MCA infarction, predict outcome, determine stroke etiology, and differentiate stroke from stroke mimics.

Abbreviations: ADC, apparent diffusion coefficient; CBF, cerebral blood flow; CBV, cerebral blood volume; CTA, CT angiography; CTP, CT perfusion; DWI, diffusion-weighted imaging; FLAIR, fluid-attenuated inversion recovery; GRE, gradient-recalled echo; IA, intraarterial; IV, intravenous; IV tPA, intravenous tissue plasminogen activator; MCA, middle cerebral artery; MRA, MR angiography; MRP, MR perfusion; NCCT, noncontrast CT; SWI, susceptibility weighted imaging; T_{max}, time at which the convolved residue function reaches its maximum; TOF, time of flight.

acute stroke. Furthermore, many of these conditions may have imaging appearances that can mimic acute infarction. In **Table 4**, we briefly delineate a few of these conditions and provide imaging characteristics that help distinguish them from acute infarction. **Figs. 13** and **14** demonstrate examples of stroke mimics.

PEARLS AND PITFALLS IN ACUTE STROKE IMAGING

If hemorrhage is identified on the NCCT in a patient with acute stroke symptoms, then this may represent intraparenchymal hemorrhage from a number of underlying etiologies or hemorrhagic transformation of ischemic infarct. A CTA should be performed to search for an underlying arterial lesion or venous sinus thrombosis. Initial or delayed imaging on CTA may demonstrate a "spot sign" which is indicative of active bleeding and is associated with an increased risk of continued bleeding and poor outcomes.[19] The presence of a large region of hypoattenuation on NCCT increases the risk of hemorrhagic transformation after thrombolytic therapy and is a relative contraindication for IV tPA.[19] A hyperdense vessel sign on NCCT does not always correspond with clot on CTA[121] and can be seen with beam hardening, increased hematocrit, arterial wall microcalcifications, and hypodense brain parenchyma in the setting of diffuse cerebral edema.[12]

If there is a lack of apparent contrast opacification of vasculature on initial images of CTA, then delayed images should be obtained to determine whether there is critical vascular narrowing versus occlusion.[121] CTA-SI increase the detection of acute ischemia compared with NCCT alone.

A pitfall of some CT perfusion acquisitions is their relatively limited z-direction coverage compared with MR PWI, which is capable of providing information about the whole brain.[102] Most centers are able to achieve at least 8 mm of coverage by using a double contrast injection or table toggling technique. Postprocessing of CT perfusion and PWI images is not standardized. Improper placement of arterial and venous regions of interest, truncation of the time course curves, and use of different vendor software packages can affect both visual and quantitative assessment of CT perfusion and MR perfusion metrics.[98] Automated postprocessing software, training of technologists, and quality control measures are becoming more easily available, thus simplifying this process.[98]

Brainstem and deep gray nuclei lacunes may not be identified on early DWI images. If a brainstem lesion is suspected, then coronal DWI with higher resolution can often elucidate small infarcts that may have been missed on traditional axial DWI images. Restricted diffusion may be caused by a number of other entities, such as hypoglycemia, a single demyelinative lesion, and seizures that should not be confused with acute ischemic stroke. On T2*-weighted sequences, the presence of fewer than 5 chronic microhemorrhages in the absence of hemorrhage on NCCT is not a contraindication to thrombolysis; however, the risk of hemorrhage with greater than 5 chronic microhemorrhages is unknown.[19]

WHAT THE REFERRING PHYSICIAN NEEDS TO KNOW: KEY POINTS

A summary of CT and MR techniques for identifying the infarct core, determining infarct penumbra, and evaluating vasculature is provided in **Table 5**. **Box 1** provides key facts regarding what the referring physician needs to know regarding imaging in acute stroke.

SUMMARY

Neuroimaging plays a key role in the initial workup of patients with symptoms of acute stroke, especially before initiating treatment. Understanding the advantages and limitations of available CT and MR imaging techniques and how to use them optimally in the emergency setting has direct implications on expected prognoses and therapeutic interventions aimed at improving clinical outcomes in patients with acute ischemic strokes.

REFERENCES

1. Go AS, Mozaffarian D, Roger VL, et al. Heart disease and stroke statistics–2014 update: a report from the American Heart Association. Circulation 2014;129(3):e28–292.
2. Grysiewicz RA, Thomas K, Pandey DK. Epidemiology of ischemic and hemorrhagic stroke: incidence, prevalence, mortality, and risk factors. Neurol Clin 2008;26(4):871–95, vii.
3. Mair G, Wardlaw JM. Imaging of acute stroke prior to treatment: current practice and evolving techniques. Br J Radiol 2014;87(1040):20140216.
4. Del Zoppo GJ, Saver JL, Jauch EC, et al. Expansion of the time window for treatment of acute ischemic stroke with intravenous tissue plasminogen activator: a science advisory from the American Heart Association/American Stroke Association. Stroke 2009;40(8):2945–8.
5. Lees KR, Bluhmki E, von Kummer R, et al. Time to treatment with intravenous alteplase and outcome in stroke: an updated pooled analysis of ECASS, ATLANTIS, NINDS, and EPITHET trials. Lancet 2010;375(9727):1695–703.

6. Penumbra Pivotal Stroke Trial Investigators. The penumbra pivotal stroke trial: safety and effectiveness of a new generation of mechanical devices for clot removal in intracranial large vessel occlusive disease. Stroke 2009;40(8):2761–8.

7. Adams HP Jr, del Zoppo G, Alberts MJ, et al. Guidelines for the early management of adults with ischemic stroke: a guideline from the American Heart Association/American stroke association stroke council, clinical cardiology council, cardiovascular radiology and intervention council, and the atherosclerotic peripheral vascular disease and quality of care outcomes in research interdisciplinary working groups: the American academy of neurology affirms the value of this guideline as an educational tool for neurologists. Stroke 2007; 38(5):1655–711.

8. Smith WS, Sung G, Starkman S, et al. Safety and efficacy of mechanical embolectomy in acute ischemic stroke: results of the MERCI trial. Stroke 2005;36(7):1432–8.

9. Kose A, Inal T, Armagan E, et al. Conditions that mimic stroke in elderly patients admitted to the emergency department. J Stroke Cerebrovasc Dis 2013;22(8):e522–7.

10. Liu X, Almast J, Ekholm S. Lesions masquerading as acute stroke. J Magn Reson Imaging 2013; 37(1):15–34.

11. Merino JG, Luby M, Benson RT, et al. Predictors of acute stroke mimics in 8187 patients referred to a stroke service. J Stroke Cerebrovasc Dis 2013; 22(8):e397–403.

12. Osborn A. Osborn's brain: imaging, pathology, and anatomy. Manitoba (Canada): Amirsys, Inc; 2013.

13. Osborn A. Diagnostic cerebral angiography. Philadelphia: Lippincott Williams & Wilkins; 1999.

14. Lev MH, Nichols SJ. Computed tomographic angiography and computed tomographic perfusion imaging of hyperacute stroke. Top Magn Reson Imaging 2000;11(5):273–87.

15. Schellinger PD, Fiebach JB, Hacke W. Imaging-based decision making in thrombolytic therapy for ischemic stroke: present status. Stroke 2003; 34(2):575–83.

16. Warach S. Tissue viability thresholds in acute stroke: the 4-factor model. Stroke 2001;32(11): 2460–1.

17. Wintermark M, Albers GW, Broderick JP, et al. Acute Stroke Imaging Research Roadmap II. Stroke 2013;44(9):2628–39.

18. Gonzalez RG, Copen WA, Schaefer PW, et al. The Massachusetts General Hospital acute stroke imaging algorithm: an experience and evidence based approach. J Neurointerv Surg 2013; 5(Suppl 1):i7–12.

19. Wintermark M, Sanelli PC, Albers GW, et al. Imaging recommendations for acute stroke and transient ischemic attack patients: a joint statement by the American society of neuroradiology, the American college of radiology and the society of neurointerventional surgery. J Am Coll Radiol 2013;10(11):828–32.

20. DeLaPaz RL, Wippold FJ 2nd, Cornelius RS, et al. ACR Appropriateness criteria(R) on cerebrovascular disease. J Am Coll Radiol 2011; 8(8):532–8.

21. von Kummer R, Bourquain H, Bastianello S, et al. Early prediction of irreversible brain damage after ischemic stroke at CT. Radiology 2001;219(1):95–100.

22. Paxton R, Ambrose J. The EMI scanner. A brief review of the first 650 patients. Br J Radiol 1974; 47(561):530–65.

23. Kunst MM, Schaefer PW. Ischemic stroke. Radiol Clin North Am 2011;49(1):1–26.

24. Wintermark M, Sanelli PC, Albers GW, et al. Imaging recommendations for acute stroke and transient ischemic attack patients: a joint statement by the American society of neuroradiology, the American college of radiology, and the society of neurointerventional surgery. AJNR Am J Neuroradiol 2013;34(11):E117–27.

25. Fiebach JB, Schellinger PD, Gass A, et al. Stroke magnetic resonance imaging is accurate in hyperacute intracerebral hemorrhage: a multicenter study on the validity of stroke imaging. Stroke 2004;35(2):502–6.

26. Kidwell CS, Chalela JA, Saver JL, et al. Comparison of MRI and CT for detection of acute intracerebral hemorrhage. JAMA 2004;292(15):1823–30.

27. Wardlaw JM, Mielke O. Early signs of brain infarction at CT: observer reliability and outcome after thrombolytic treatment–systematic review. Radiology 2005;235(2):444–53.

28. Kalafut MA, Schriger DL, Saver JL, et al. Detection of early CT signs of >1/3 middle cerebral artery infarctions: interrater reliability and sensitivity of CT interpretation by physicians involved in acute stroke care. Stroke 2000;31(7):1667–71.

29. Goldmakher GV, Camargo EC, Furie KL, et al. Hyperdense basilar artery sign on unenhanced CT predicts thrombus and outcome in acute posterior circulation stroke. Stroke 2009;40(1):134–9.

30. Leys D, Pruvo JP, Godefroy O, et al. Prevalence and significance of hyperdense middle cerebral artery in acute stroke. Stroke 1992;23(3):317–24.

31. Riedel CH, Zimmermann P, Jensen-Kondering U, et al. The importance of size: successful recanalization by intravenous thrombolysis in acute anterior stroke depends on thrombus length. Stroke 2011; 42(6):1775–7.

32. Kharitonova T, Thoren M, Ahmed N, et al. Disappearing hyperdense middle cerebral artery sign in ischaemic stroke patients treated with intravenous thrombolysis: clinical course and prognostic

significance. J Neurol Neurosurg Psychiatry 2009; 80(3):273–8.

33. Jaillard A, Hommel M, Baird AE, et al. Significance of early CT signs in acute stroke. A CT scan-diffusion MRI study. Cerebrovasc Dis 2002;13(1): 47–56.

34. von Kummer R, Meyding-Lamade U, Forsting M, et al. Sensitivity and prognostic value of early CT in occlusion of the middle cerebral artery trunk. AJNR Am J Neuroradiol 1994;15(1):9–15 [discussion: 16–8].

35. Grotta JC, Chiu D, Lu M, et al. Agreement and variability in the interpretation of early CT changes in stroke patients qualifying for intravenous rtPA therapy. Stroke 1999;30(8):1528–33.

36. Roberts HC, Dillon WP, Furlan AJ, et al. Computed tomographic findings in patients undergoing intra-arterial thrombolysis for acute ischemic stroke due to middle cerebral artery occlusion: results from the PROACT II trial. Stroke 2002;33(6): 1557–65.

37. Lev MH, Farkas J, Gemmete JJ, et al. Acute stroke: improved nonenhanced CT detection–benefits of soft-copy interpretation by using variable window width and center level settings. Radiology 1999; 213(1):150–5.

38. Hacke W, Kaste M, Fieschi C, et al. Randomised double-blind placebo-controlled trial of thrombolytic therapy with intravenous alteplase in acute ischaemic stroke (ECASS II). second European-Australasian acute stroke study investigators. Lancet 1998;352(9136):1245–51.

39. Barber PA, Demchuk AM, Zhang J, et al. Validity and reliability of a quantitative computed tomography score in predicting outcome of hyperacute stroke before thrombolytic therapy. ASPECTS study group. Alberta stroke programme early CT score. Lancet 2000;355(9216):1670–4.

40. Demchuk AM, Hill MD, Barber PA, et al. Importance of early ischemic computed tomography changes using ASPECTS in NINDS rtPA Stroke Study. Stroke 2005;36(10):2110–5.

41. Dzialowski I, Hill MD, Coutts SB, et al. Extent of early ischemic changes on computed tomography (CT) before thrombolysis: prognostic value of the Alberta stroke program early CT score in ECASS II. Stroke 2006;37(4):973–8.

42. Kakuda W, Thijs VN, Lansberg MG, et al. Clinical importance of microbleeds in patients receiving IV thrombolysis. Neurology 2005;65(8):1175–8.

43. Lee SH, Kang BS, Kim N, et al. Does microbleed predict haemorrhagic transformation after acute atherothrombotic or cardioembolic stroke? J Neurol Neurosurg Psychiatry 2008;79(8):913–6.

44. Boulanger JM, Coutts SB, Eliasziw M, et al. Cerebral microhemorrhages predict new disabling or fatal strokes in patients with acute ischemic stroke

or transient ischemic attack. Stroke 2006;37(3): 911–4.

45. Fiehler J, Albers GW, Boulanger JM, et al. Bleeding risk analysis in stroke imaging before thromboLysis (BRASIL): pooled analysis of T2*-weighted magnetic resonance imaging data from 570 patients. Stroke 2007;38(10):2738–44.

46. Mullins ME, Schaefer PW, Sorensen AG, et al. CT and conventional and diffusion-weighted MR imaging in acute stroke: study in 691 patients at presentation to the emergency department. Radiology 2002;224(2):353–60.

47. Benveniste H, Hedlund LW, Johnson GA. Mechanism of detection of acute cerebral ischemia in rats by diffusion-weighted magnetic resonance microscopy. Stroke 1992;23(5):746–54.

48. Mintorovitch J, Yang GY, Shimizu H, et al. Diffusion-weighted magnetic resonance imaging of acute focal cerebral ischemia: comparison of signal intensity with changes in brain water and Na+, K(+)-ATPase activity. J Cereb Blood Flow Metab 1994;14(2):332–6.

49. Wick M, Nagatomo Y, Prielmeier F, et al. Alteration of intracellular metabolite diffusion in rat brain in vivo during ischemia and reperfusion. Stroke 1995;26(10):1930–3 [discussion: 1934].

50. Duong TQ, Ackerman JJ, Ying HS, et al. Evaluation of extra- and intracellular apparent diffusion in normal and globally ischemic rat brain via 19F NMR. Magn Reson Med 1998;40(1):1–13.

51. Niendorf T, Dijkhuizen RM, Norris DG, et al. Biexponential diffusion attenuation in various states of brain tissue: implications for diffusion-weighted imaging. Magn Reson Med 1996;36(6):847–57.

52. Sykova E, Svoboda J, Polak J, et al. Extracellular volume fraction and diffusion characteristics during progressive ischemia and terminal anoxia in the spinal cord of the rat. J Cereb Blood Flow Metab 1994;14(2):301–11.

53. Yoo AJ, Chaudhry ZA, Nogueira RG, et al. Infarct volume is a pivotal biomarker after intra-arterial stroke therapy. Stroke 2012;43(5):1323–30.

54. Yoo AJ, Verduzco LA, Schaefer PW, et al. MRI-based selection for intra-arterial stroke therapy: value of pretreatment diffusion-weighted imaging lesion volume in selecting patients with acute stroke who will benefit from early recanalization. Stroke 2009;40(6):2046–54.

55. Sanak D, Nosal V, Horak D, et al. Impact of diffusion-weighted MRI-measured initial cerebral infarction volume on clinical outcome in acute stroke patients with middle cerebral artery occlusion treated by thrombolysis. Neuroradiology 2006;48(9):632–9.

56. Lansberg MG, Straka M, Kemp S, et al. MRI profile and response to endovascular reperfusion after stroke (DEFUSE 2): a prospective cohort study. Lancet Neurol 2012;11(10):860–7.

57. Schaefer PW, Pulli B, Copen WA, et al. Combining MRI with NIHSS thresholds to predict outcome in acute ischemic stroke: value for patient selection. AJNR Am J Neuroradiol 2015;36:259–64.

58. Yoo AJ, Barak ER, Copen WA, et al. Combining acute diffusion-weighted imaging and mean transmit time lesion volumes with National Institutes of Health Stroke Scale Score improves the prediction of acute stroke outcome. Stroke 2010;41(8): 1728–35.

59. Sims JR, Gharai LR, Schaefer PW, et al. ABC/2 for rapid clinical estimate of infarct, perfusion, and mismatch volumes. Neurology 2009;72(24):2104–10.

60. Cheng B, Brinkmann M, Forkert ND, et al. Quantitative measurements of relative fluid-attenuated inversion recovery (FLAIR) signal intensities in acute stroke for the prediction of time from symptom onset. J Cereb Blood Flow Metab 2013;33(1): 76–84.

61. Thomalla G, Cheng B, Ebinger M, et al. DWI-FLAIR mismatch for the identification of patients with acute ischaemic stroke within 4.5 h of symptom onset (PRE-FLAIR): a multicentre observational study. Lancet Neurol 2011;10(11):978–86.

62. Yuh WT, Crain MR, Loes DJ, et al. MR imaging of cerebral ischemia: findings in the first 24 hours. AJNR Am J Neuroradiol 1991;12(4):621–9.

63. Thomalla G, Rossbach P, Rosenkranz M, et al. Negative fluid-attenuated inversion recovery imaging identifies acute ischemic stroke at 3 hours or less. Ann Neurol 2009;65(6):724–32.

64. Aoki J, Kimura K, Iguchi Y, et al. Intravenous thrombolysis based on diffusion-weighted imaging and fluid-attenuated inversion recovery mismatch in acute stroke patients with unknown onset time. Cerebrovasc Dis 2011;31(5):435–41.

65. Aoki J, Kimura K, Iguchi Y, et al. FLAIR can estimate the onset time in acute ischemic stroke patients. J Neurol Sci 2010;293(1–2):39–44.

66. Thomalla G, Fiebach JB, Ostergaard L, et al. A multicenter, randomized, double-blind, placebo-controlled trial to test efficacy and safety of magnetic resonance imaging-based thrombolysis in wake-up stroke (WAKE-UP). Int J Stroke 2014; 9(6):829–36.

67. Rimmele DL, Thomalla G. Wake-up stroke: clinical characteristics, imaging findings, and treatment option - an update. Front Neurol 2014;5:35.

68. Kamran S, Bates V, Bakshi R, et al. Significance of hyperintense vessels on FLAIR MRI in acute stroke. Neurology 2000;55(2):265–9.

69. Lee KY, Latour LL, Luby M, et al. Distal hyperintense vessels on FLAIR: an MRI marker for collateral circulation in acute stroke? Neurology 2009; 72(13):1134–9.

70. Hohenhaus M, Schmidt WU, Brunecker P, et al. FLAIR vascular hyperintensities in acute ICA and MCA infarction: a marker for mismatch and stroke severity? Cerebrovasc Dis 2012;34(1): 63–9.

71. Radbruch A, Mucke J, Schweser F, et al. Comparison of susceptibility weighted imaging and TOF-angiography for the detection of Thrombi in acute stroke. PLoS One 2013;8(5):e63459.

72. Cho KH, Kim JS, Kwon SU, et al. Significance of susceptibility vessel sign on T2*-weighted gradient echo imaging for identification of stroke subtypes. Stroke 2005;36(11):2379–83.

73. Viallon M, Altrichter S, Pereira VM, et al. Combined use of pulsed arterial spin-labeling and susceptibility-weighted imaging in stroke at 3T. Eur Neurol 2010;64(5):286–96.

74. Mittal S, Wu Z, Neelavalli J, et al. Susceptibility-weighted imaging: technical aspects and clinical applications, part 2. AJNR Am J Neuroradiol 2009;30(2):232–52.

75. Luo S, Yang L, Wang L. Comparison of susceptibility-weighted and perfusion-weighted magnetic resonance imaging in the detection of penumbra in acute ischemic stroke. J Neuroradiol 2014. http://dx.doi.org/10.1016/j.neurad.2014.07.002.

76. Park MG, Yang TI, Oh SJ, et al. Multiple hypointense vessels on susceptibility-weighted imaging in acute ischemic stroke: surrogate marker of oxygen extraction fraction in penumbra? Cerebrovasc Dis 2014;38(4):254–61.

77. Kao HW, Tsai FY, Hasso AN. Predicting stroke evolution: comparison of susceptibility-weighted MR imaging with MR perfusion. Eur Radiol 2012; 22(7):1397–403.

78. Hirai T, Korogi Y, Ono K, et al. Prospective evaluation of suspected stenocclusive disease of the intracranial artery: combined MR angiography and CT angiography compared with digital subtraction angiography. AJNR Am J Neuroradiol 2002;23(1):93–101.

79. Katz DA, Marks MP, Napel SA, et al. Circle of Willis: evaluation with spiral CT angiography, MR angiography, and conventional angiography. Radiology 1995;195(2):445–9.

80. Nguyen-Huynh MN, Wintermark M, English J, et al. How accurate is CT angiography in evaluating intracranial atherosclerotic disease? Stroke 2008; 39(4):1184–8.

81. Lima FO, Furie KL, Silva GS, et al. The pattern of leptomeningeal collaterals on CT angiography is a strong predictor of long-term functional outcome in stroke patients with large vessel intracranial occlusion. Stroke 2010;41(10):2316–22.

82. Angermaier A, Langner S, Kirsch M, et al. CT-angiographic collateralization predicts final infarct volume after intra-arterial thrombolysis for acute anterior circulation ischemic stroke. Cerebrovasc Dis 2011;31(2):177–84.

83. Bang OY, Saver JL, Kim SJ, et al. Collateral flow averts hemorrhagic transformation after endovascular therapy for acute ischemic stroke. Stroke 2011;42(8):2235–9.

84. Bang OY, Saver JL, Kim SJ, et al. Collateral flow predicts response to endovascular therapy for acute ischemic stroke. Stroke 2011;42(3):693–9.

85. Souza LC, Yoo AJ, Chaudhry ZA, et al. Malignant CTA collateral profile is highly specific for large admission DWI infarct core and poor outcome in acute stroke. AJNR Am J Neuroradiol 2012;33(7): 1331–6.

86. Puetz V, Dzialowski I, Hill MD, et al. Malignant profile detected by CT angiographic information predicts poor prognosis despite thrombolysis within three hours from symptom onset. Cerebrovasc Dis 2010;29(6):584–91.

87. Saba L, Mallarini G. MDCTA of carotid plaque degree of stenosis: evaluation of interobserver agreement. AJR Am J Roentgenol 2008;190(1):W41–6.

88. Bartlett ES, Walters TD, Symons SP, et al. Carotid stenosis index revisited with direct CT angiography measurement of carotid arteries to quantify carotid stenosis. Stroke 2007;38(2):286–91.

89. Bartlett ES, Walters TD, Symons SP, et al. Diagnosing carotid stenosis near-occlusion by using CT angiography. AJNR Am J Neuroradiol 2006; 27(3):632–7.

90. Bartlett ES, Walters TD, Symons SP, et al. Quantification of carotid stenosis on CT angiography. AJNR Am J Neuroradiol 2006;27(1):13–9.

91. Randoux B, Marro B, Koskas F, et al. Carotid artery stenosis: prospective comparison of CT, three-dimensional gadolinium-enhanced MR, and conventional angiography. Radiology 2001;220(1): 179–85.

92. Koelemay MJ, Nederkoorn PJ, Reitsma JB, et al. Systematic review of computed tomographic angiography for assessment of carotid artery disease. Stroke 2004;35(10):2306–12.

93. Provenzale JM, Sarikaya B. Comparison of test performance characteristics of MRI, MR angiography, and CT angiography in the diagnosis of carotid and vertebral artery dissection: a review of the medical literature. AJR Am J Roentgenol 2009; 193(4):1167–74.

94. Elijovich L, Kazmi K, Gauvrit JY, et al. The emerging role of multidetector row CT angiography in the diagnosis of cervical arterial dissection: preliminary study. Neuroradiology 2006;48(9):606–12.

95. Vertinsky AT, Schwartz NE, Fischbein NJ, et al. Comparison of multidetector CT angiography and MR imaging of cervical artery dissection. AJNR Am J Neuroradiol 2008;29(9):1753–60.

96. Alvarez-Linera J, Benito-Leon J, Escribano J, et al. Prospective evaluation of carotid artery stenosis: elliptic centric contrast-enhanced MR angiography and spiral CT angiography compared with digital subtraction angiography. AJNR Am J Neuroradiol 2003;24(5):1012–9.

97. Stock KW, Radue EW, Jacob AL, et al. Intracranial arteries: prospective blinded comparative study of MR angiography and DSA in 50 patients. Radiology 1995;195(2):451–6.

98. Allmendinger AM, Tang ER, Lui YW, et al. Imaging of stroke: part 1, perfusion CT–overview of imaging technique, interpretation pearls, and common pitfalls. AJR Am J Roentgenol 2012;198(1):52–62.

99. Lui YW, Tang ER, Allmendinger AM, et al. Evaluation of CT perfusion in the setting of cerebral ischemia: patterns and pitfalls. AJNR Am J Neuroradiol 2010;31(9):1552–63.

100. Schaefer PW, Ozsunar Y, He J, et al. Assessing tissue viability with MR diffusion and perfusion imaging. AJNR Am J Neuroradiol 2003;24(3):436–43.

101. Sorensen AG, Buonanno FS, Gonzalez RG, et al. Hyperacute stroke: evaluation with combined multisection diffusion-weighted and hemodynamically weighted echo-planar MR imaging. Radiology 1996;199(2):391–401.

102. Konstas AA, Wintermark M, Lev MH. CT perfusion imaging in acute stroke. Neuroimaging Clin N Am 2011;21(2):215–38, ix.

103. Srinivasan A, Goyal M, Al Azri F, et al. State-of-the-art imaging of acute stroke. Radiographics 2006; 26(Suppl 1):S75–95.

104. Rosen BR, Belliveau JW, Vevea JM, et al. Perfusion imaging with NMR contrast agents. Magn Reson Med 1990;14(2):249–65.

105. Mouridsen K, Christensen S, Gyldensted L, et al. Automatic selection of arterial input function using cluster analysis. Magn Reson Med 2006;55(3): 524–31.

106. Schramm P, Schellinger PD, Klotz E, et al. Comparison of perfusion computed tomography and computed tomography angiography source images with perfusion-weighted imaging and diffusion-weighted imaging in patients with acute stroke of less than 6 hours' duration. Stroke 2004; 35(7):1652–8.

107. Kamalian S, Maas MB, Goldmacher GV, et al. CT cerebral blood flow maps optimally correlate with admission diffusion-weighted imaging in acute stroke but thresholds vary by postprocessing platform. Stroke 2011;42(7):1923–8.

108. Campbell BC, Christensen S, Levi CR, et al. Cerebral blood flow is the optimal CT perfusion parameter for assessing infarct core. Stroke 2011;42(12): 3435–40.

109. Wintermark M, Flanders AE, Velthuis B, et al. Perfusion-CT assessment of infarct core and penumbra: receiver operating characteristic curve analysis in 130 patients suspected of acute hemispheric stroke. Stroke 2006;37(4):979–85.

110. Gonzalez RG. Current state of acute stroke imaging. Stroke 2013;44(11):3260–4.

111. Dani KA, Thomas RG, Chappell FM, et al. Computed tomography and magnetic resonance perfusion imaging in ischemic stroke: definitions and thresholds. Ann Neurol 2011;70(3):384–401.

112. Mui K, Yoo AJ, Verduzco L, et al. Cerebral blood flow thresholds for tissue infarction in patients with acute ischemic stroke treated with intra-arterial revascularization therapy depend on timing of reperfusion. AJNR Am J Neuroradiol 2011;32(5): 846–51.

113. Lassen NA. Normal average value of cerebral blood flow in younger adults is 50 ml/100 g/min. J Cereb Blood Flow Metab 1985;5(3):347–9.

114. Frackowiak RS, Lenzi GL, Jones T, et al. Quantitative measurement of regional cerebral blood flow and oxygen metabolism in man using 15O and positron emission tomography: theory, procedure, and normal values. J Comput Assist Tomogr 1980;4(6):727–36.

115. Schaefer PW, Roccatagliata L, Ledezma C, et al. First-pass quantitative CT perfusion identifies thresholds for salvageable penumbra in acute stroke patients treated with intra-arterial therapy. AJNR Am J Neuroradiol 2006;27(1):20–5.

116. Payabvash S, Souza LC, Wang Y, et al. Regional ischemic vulnerability of the brain to hypoperfusion: the need for location specific computed tomography perfusion thresholds in acute stroke patients. Stroke 2011;42(5):1255–60.

117. Albers GW, Thijs VN, Wechsler L, et al. Magnetic resonance imaging profiles predict clinical response to early reperfusion: the diffusion and perfusion imaging evaluation for understanding stroke evolution (DEFUSE) study. Ann Neurol 2006;60(5):508–17.

118. Parsons M, Spratt N, Bivard A, et al. A randomized trial of tenecteplase versus alteplase for acute ischemic stroke. N Engl J Med 2012;366(12): 1099–107.

119. Hopyan J, Ciarallo A, Dowlatshahi D, et al. Certainty of stroke diagnosis: incremental benefit with CT perfusion over noncontrast CT and CT angiography. Radiology 2010;255(1):142–53.

120. Bektas H, Wu TC, Kasam M, et al. Increased blood-brain barrier permeability on perfusion CT might predict malignant middle cerebral artery infarction. Stroke 2010;41(11):2539–44.

121. Mullins ME. Modern emergent stroke imaging: pearls, protocols, and pitfalls. Radiol Clin North Am 2006;44(1):41–62, vii–viii.

Face and Neck Infections
What the Emergency Radiologist Needs to Know

Wayne Scott Kubal, MD

KEYWORDS

- Face infection • Neck infection • Computed tomography (CT)

KEY POINTS

- Knowledge of normal anatomy, such as fat within the pterygopalatine fossa and fat within the retro-antral area, can aid in the diagnosis of a deep facial infection.
- Awareness of the normal computed tomographic appearance of the head and neck structures is also vital to diagnose symmetric diseases such as diagnosing bilateral viral parotitis.
- Differentiation of abscess from cellulitis is important because the therapeutic options differ.
- The localization of the infection is important, not only to identify its space of origin but also to interrogate common routes of spread to other spaces, such as spread of neck infections to the mediastinum, spread of sinus infections to the orbit, and spread of mastoid infections intracranially.
- The radiologist should appreciate the complications that may result from an infection.

INTRODUCTION

A wide variety of infectious disorders of the face and neck may manifest emergently. There are many common sources for head and neck infection, including pharyngitis, dental infection, mastoiditis, penetrating trauma, and sinusitis. Despite widespread access to antibiotics, face and neck infections can still lead to significant morbidity and even mortality. In approximately 10% to 20% of deep neck infections, potentially life-threatening complications are reported.[1] These complications include airway obstruction, mediastinitis, septic emboli, venous sinus thrombosis, intracranial empyema, and intracranial abscess. "As the number of patients who use the emergency room as an initial point of access to healthcare increases, the number of acute neoplastic and nonneoplastic conditions involving the head and neck that are encountered in the emergency room also will increase. Computed tomography (CT) is the first-line imaging modality in the acute setting."[2]

Clinical localization of head and neck infections, especially those that involve the deep neck, is limited. In one series of patients with deep neck involvement, the clinical examination localized the infection in only 42.9% of cases.[3] The treating head and neck surgeons think that "The presentation, spread, and management of neck infection are based on the anatomy of the cervical fascia."[4] The interpreting radiologist, therefore, must have a good understanding of the anatomy of the spaces of the neck. Although the spaces are defined by the cervical fascia, their planes are not easily visualized on a contrast-enhanced CT. Imagers learn the anatomy based on the contents of the space rather than the anatomy based on the fascial planes.

THE PHARYNGEAL MUCOSAL SPACE

The pharyngeal mucosal space contains both mucosa and lymphoid tissues. The lymphoid tissues consist of tonsils and adenoids (Fig. 1). This space is important because many of the upper aerodigestive tract infections start in the pharyngeal

University of Arizona, 1501 Campbell Avenue, PO Box 245067, Tucson, AZ 85724, USA
E-mail address: wkubal@email.arizona.edu

Radiol Clin N Am 53 (2015) 827–846
http://dx.doi.org/10.1016/j.rcl.2015.02.007
0033-8389/15/$ – see front matter © 2015 Elsevier Inc. All rights reserved.

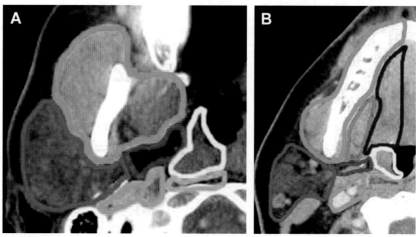

Fig. 1. Spaces of the neck are outlined on axial contrast-enhanced CTs. (*A*) The pharyngeal mucosal space is outlined in yellow. The retropharyngeal space is outlined in orange. The masticator space is outlined in light green. The parotid space is outlined in magenta. The parapharyngeal space is outlined in red. The carotid space is outlined in light blue. (*B*) Two additional spaces are added. The sublingual space is outlined in blue. The submandibular space is outlined in dark green.

mucosal space. Infections in this space can take many forms, including pharyngitis, tonsillitis, suppuration, and tonsillar abscess. These infections may also spread to other spaces. After the infection has cleared, irregular calcifications often remain (**Fig. 2**). Acute tonsillitis is characterized by increased size of the tonsils and increased density as seen on a contrast-enhanced CT. The increased density reflects contrast enhancement

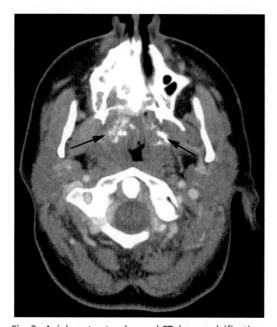

Fig. 2. Axial contrast-enhanced CT shows calcifications within the pharyngeal mucosal spaces bilaterally (*arrows*). These calcifications are secondary to remote infection most commonly tonsillitis.

of the inflamed tissue. In the acute phase of uncomplicated tonsillitis, no areas of hypodensity or fluid collections should be visualized. Enlargement and inflammation of the uvula is often an associated finding (**Fig. 3**A). As the infection progresses, a poorly defined, low-density focus may become apparent. This finding indicates a focal area of cellulitis and edema within the infected tonsil (see **Fig. 3**B). As the infection progresses toward early suppuration, a poorly defined low-density collection is identified, surrounded by an enhancing wall. At this stage, there is early liquefaction in the center of the collection. A true abscess is characterized by a well-defined low-density fluid collection and an enhancing wall. The density of the fluid is typically similar to that of cerebrospinal fluid (see **Fig. 3**C). The distinction between tonsillar cellulitis and tonsillar abscess is important because the therapy is different. If a drainable fluid collection is present, an aspiration of the collection is the standard of care. When the imaging criteria of a fluid density collection with an enhancing wall are applied, the accuracy for the detection of a drainable abscess ranges from 63% to 77% in both pediatric and adult populations.[5,6] Applying an additional imaging criterion of an irregular or scalloped abscess wall increases specificity, but decreases sensitivity. Scalloping of the abscess wall is thought to be a late finding in the evolution of a neck infection, consistent with greater specificity for the presence of pus (see **Fig. 3**D).[7] Clinical examination readily identifies the induration of the overlying mucosa, but has a low sensitivity for differentiating cellulitis from abscess. Clinical examination also tends to

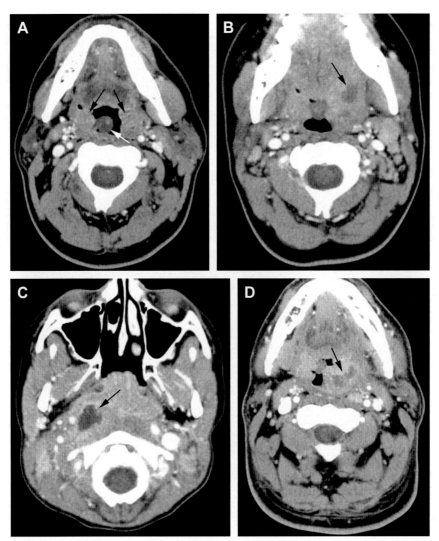

Fig. 3. Axial contrast-enhanced CTs in 4 different patients show infections within the pharyngeal mucosal space. (*A*) The tonsils are enlarged and show increased enhancement bilaterally (*black arrows*). The uvula appears enlarged and edematous (*white arrow*). These findings are compatible with acute tonsillitis. (*B*) There is an area of decreased density within the left tonsillar region (*arrow*). This finding is compatible with cellulitis. (*C*) There is an area of decreased density with an enhancing rim in the right tonsil (*arrow*). This finding is compatible with a tonsillar abscess. (*D*) There is an area of decreased density with an enhancing, scalloped rim in the left tonsil (*arrow*). This finding is compatible with later phase abscess.

underestimate the extent of the infection. In one series of patients with a deep neck infection, physical examination underestimated the extent of the infection in 70% of the patients.[8]

THE RETROPHARYNGEAL SPACE

In adults, the retropharyngeal space contains predominantly fat (see **Fig. 1**). In young children, retropharyngeal nodes are present in the suprahyoid retropharyngeal space. These nodes begin to fibrosis and atrophy after age 4 and completely regress by age 6.[9] The retropharyngeal space has

a bowtie configuration because it is divided by a median raphe. Involvement of this space by an infection is important to appreciate because the retropharyngeal space extends caudally to the level of the mediastinum, most often between T1 and T6.[10] A common pathway for spread is from the pharyngeal mucosal space to the upper retropharyngeal space via the lymphatic channels. When edema or frank fluid is detected within the retropharyngeal space, it is one's duty to follow the retropharyngeal space caudally until it becomes normal or until one is able to evaluate the superior mediastinum for potential mediastinitis (**Fig. 4**).

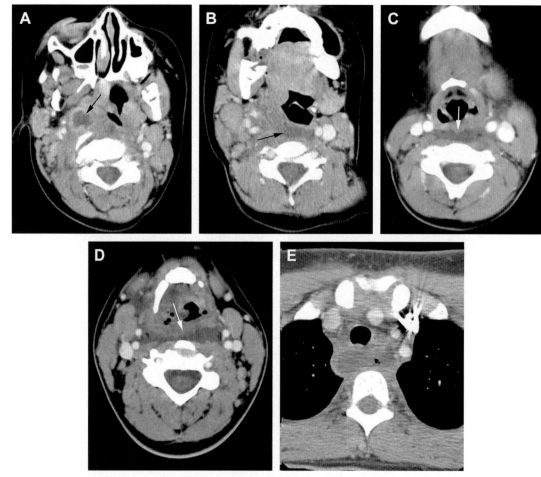

Fig. 4. Axial contrast-enhanced CTs show infection within the pharyngeal mucosal space spreading to the retropharyngeal space and extending to the mediastinum. (*A*) There is a well-defined low-density collection within the right tonsil consistent with a tonsillar abscess (*arrow*). (*B*) There is low-density edema within the retropharyngeal space (*arrow*). (*C*) There is persistent edema within the retropharyngeal space at a lower level in the neck. This image demonstrates the bowtie configuration characteristic of the retropharyngeal space (*arrow*). (*D*) Edema within the retropharyngeal space persists at the level of the hyoid bone (*arrow*). (*E*) The infection extends into the superior mediastinum. Findings on this section are compatible with mediastinitis.

A potential pitfall is the inflammatory condition of calcific tendinitis. Calcific tendinitis patients present with pain and fever. They demonstrate edema and/or fluid within the retropharyngeal space. Typically, the pharyngeal mucosal space in these patients is normal, but the most important key to making an accurate diagnosis is to note the calcifications adjacent to the superior insertion of the longus coli muscle, typically at the C1–C2 level. Other findings worth noting are the absence of cervical lymphadenopathy and the absence of wall enhancement adjacent to the fluid collection (**Fig. 5**).[11,12] The appropriate treatment of calcific tendinitis is with anti-inflammatory medications as opposed to antibiotic therapy. The radiologists can help identify the abnormality and direct the clinicians toward the appropriate treatment.

THE MASTICATOR SPACE

The masticator space contains the muscles of mastication as well as the mandible (see **Fig. 1**). Given its contents, masticator space infections are most often odontogenic in origin and may present following a dental procedure. Masticator space infections may be characterized by swelling and fat stranding adjacent to the affected muscles of mastication. Once the masticator space infection is identified or suspected, careful examination of the bone windows will often help to identify a dental infection or a site of a recent dental procedure (**Fig. 6**). Evaluation of the bone windows may also show evidence of osteomyelitis. This finding is of clinical importance because the osteomyelitis requires aggressive therapy (**Fig. 7**). It is important

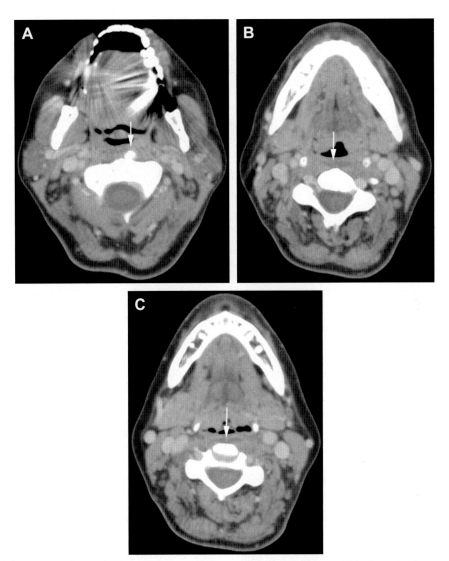

Fig. 5. Axial contrast-enhanced CTs demonstrate calcific tendinitis with edema within the retropharyngeal space. (*A*) Calcification is noted anterior to the C2 vertebral body (*arrow*). This calcification lies at the superior insertion of the longus coli muscle. (*B, C*) A small amount of fluid/edema is present within the retropharyngeal space (*arrow*). The fluid is secondary to calcific tendinitis.

to remember that the masticator space extends along the face and the lateral head above the level of the zygomatic arch to the superior attachment of the temporalis muscle on the parietal bone. Depending on the imaging protocol selected, the examination may not include the entire suprazygomatic masticator space; thus, it is important to extend the range of imaging to include it.

Masticator space infections involving the deep face such as those that involve the medial insertions of the pterygoid muscles may be difficult to detect. They may be associated with minimal paranasal sinus disease within the ipsilateral maxillary sinus. An anatomic pearl for helping to identify these infections in their early stage is to evaluate the pterygopalatine

fossa and the retroantral fat pad. The pterygopalatine fossa should always contain at least some fat. The lateral extent of the pterygopalatine fat becomes contiguous with the retroantral fat (**Fig. 8**).

THE PAROTID SPACE

The parotid space contains the parotid gland (see **Fig. 1**). The deep lobe of the parotid gland extends medial and posterior to the mandible. It is important to have good imaging criteria for the normal density of the parotid gland. The parotid should be of low density compared with muscles and of high density compared with subcutaneous fat on either a contrast-enhanced or noncontrast CT.

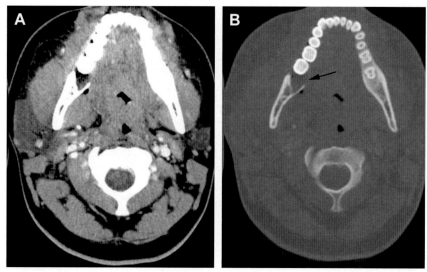

Fig. 6. Axial contrast-enhanced CTs at soft tissue and bone windows demonstrate right masticator space infection. (A) There is enlargement of the right masseter muscle and a small amount of fat stranding surrounding the muscle. (B) Bone window demonstrates a missing posterior mandibular molar on the right (arrow). This finding is secondary to a recent dental extraction.

Infections involving this space may be bacterial, secondary to obstruction of parotid secretions, or viral, such as mumps. Bacterial infections are most often unilateral. Unilateral infections are relatively easy to identify. They are characterized by increased density of the affected gland as well as stranding of the overlying fat. Comparison with

the normal side aids greatly in making the diagnosis (Fig. 9). Bacterial infections of the parotid gland may evolve into a small abscess characterized by an internal area of low attenuation (Fig. 10). Infections associated with sialolithiasis are also most often unilateral (Fig. 11).

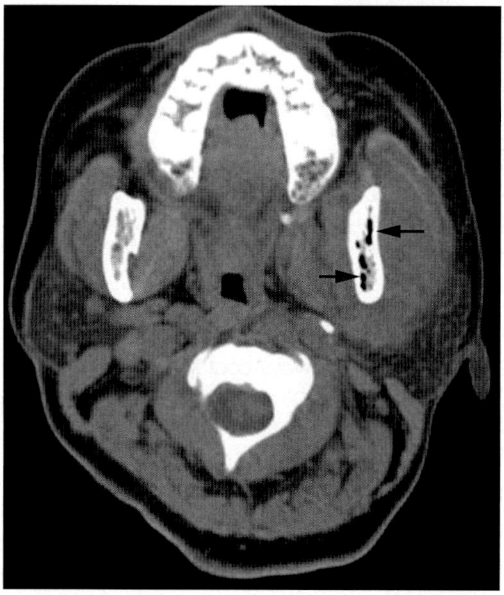

Bilateral parotitis may be overlooked when there is symmetric involvement of the parotid glands with little or no associated fat stranding (Fig. 12). Careful application of the density criteria helps to diagnose the bilateral parotitis. Viral parotitis is bilateral in approximately 75% of cases.[2]

THE CAROTID SPACE

The carotid space contains the internal jugular vein and the carotid artery. Normally, the vessels fill completely with contrast and are easy to identify on a contrast-enhanced examination (see Fig. 1). The carotid space also contains portions of cranial nerves IX–XII and may also contain lymph nodes. When evaluating the carotid space, it is important to identify both the carotid artery and the internal jugular vein. Typically, the common carotid artery lies medial and anterior to the internal jugular vein. A small amount of fat should be seen surrounding these vessels; infiltration of the fat may occur secondary to infection within the carotid space.

In 1936, André Lemierre reported a series of 20 cases where infections were followed by septicemia and septic emboli. Currently, Lemierre syndrome (LS) is understood to mean cases of oropharyngeal infection leading to thrombophlebitis in the neck and associated septic emboli,

Fig. 7. Axial contrast-enhanced CT demonstrates a left masticator space infection with enlargement of the left masseter muscle and considerable fat stranding surrounding the muscle. Careful examination of the left mandible demonstrates gas within the bone consistent with osteomyelitis (arrows).

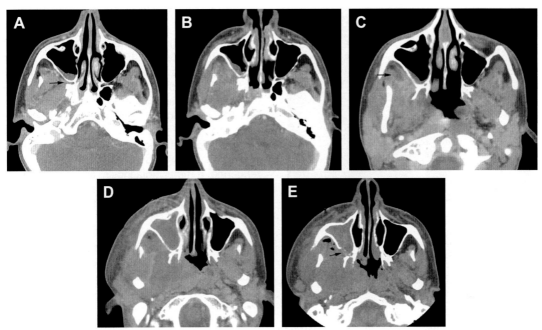

Fig. 8. A series of contrast-enhanced axial CTs in the same patient demonstrate the progression of a right masticator space infection. (*A*) The patient initially presents with right facial pain. A small amount of sinus disease is noted within the right maxillary sinus. An important, but more subtle, finding that was not initially appreciated is infiltration of the fat within the right pterygopalatine fossa (*arrow*). (*B*) Approximately 3 weeks later, the patient returns with increased right facial pain. Swelling and patchy areas of abnormal enhancement within the right masticator space are now easily appreciated. (*C*) Despite intravenous antibiotic therapy, the patient continues to worsen. CT now demonstrates early suppuration just anterior to the mandible (*arrow*). (*D*) The infection has now spread to adjacent spaces with involvement of the superficial face, opacification of the right maxillary sinus, and extension to the right pharyngeal mucosal space. (*E*) There is now bone destruction involving the posterior wall of the maxillary sinus (*arrow*) consistent with osteomyelitis.

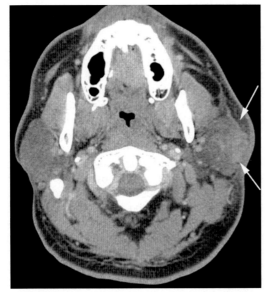

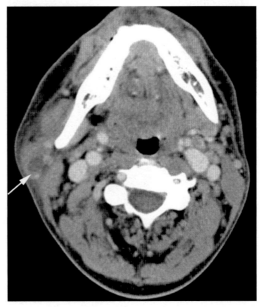

Fig. 9. Contrast-enhanced axial CT demonstrates abnormal contrast enhancement of the left parotid gland (*arrows*). There is also infiltration of the subcutaneous fat adjacent to the gland.

Fig. 10. Contrast-enhanced axial CT demonstrates a low-density area within the right parotid gland (*arrow*). This finding is compatible with an intraparotid abscess.

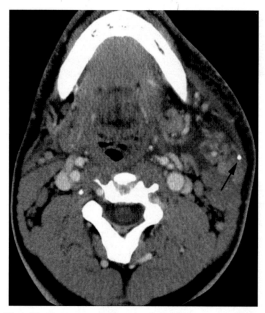

Fig. 11. Contrast-enhanced axial CT demonstrates a small calcific density within the infected left parotid gland (*arrow*). This finding is compatible with sialolithiasis.

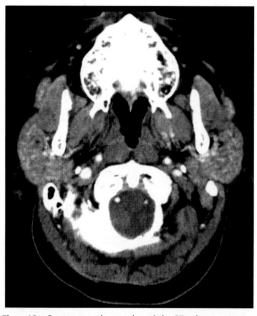

Fig. 12. Contrast-enhanced axial CT demonstrates abnormal increased density secondary to contrast enhancement involving both parotid glands symmetrically. Note that there is no infiltration of the adjacent fat.

typically to the lungs.[13] On contrast-enhanced CT, nonopacification of a vessel indicates thrombosis and fat stranding within the carotid space, which suggests an infection (**Fig. 13**A). When septic thrombophlebitis of the jugular vein is identified, evaluation of the lungs is important to evaluate for possible septic embolic disease (see **Fig. 13**B). "Given the relatively low incidence of LS and its potentially confusing clinical manifestations, recognition of imaging findings consistent with the diagnosis may be crucial to rendering a timely diagnosis and institution of appropriate therapy, and the radiologist may be the initial physician to suggest or establish the diagnosis."[13]

Infection involving the cervical course of the carotid artery can lead to dire consequences. These infections are often associated with comorbidities such as prior surgery and/or prior radiation for a head and neck neoplasm. Infections may cause vasa vasorum thrombosis leading to necrosis of carotid walls. Proteolytic enzymes associated with abscess or cellulitis may also weaken the vessel wall. The weakened vessel wall may progress to pseudoaneurysm formation (**Fig. 14**) or even carotid rupture. Infection involving the carotid artery, especially when a pseudoaneurysm is identified, should be emergently communicated to the referring physician because of the risk of carotid rupture. Treatment options include surgery, permanent endovascular occlusion, or stent reconstruction.[14]

THE SUBLINGUAL SPACE

The sublingual space lies inferior to the mobile portion of the tongue but superior and medial to the mylohyoid muscle (see **Fig. 1**B). It contains the sublingual gland and a small portion of the superior aspect of the submandibular gland. Because the mylohyoid muscle attaches along the medial surface of the mandible, infections in this space may be odontogenic in origin. "Infections of the second or third molar teeth likely involve the submandibular space because the roots of these teeth extend below the insertion of the mylohyoid muscle. If the more anterior teeth are involved, the infection typically is confined to the sublingual space because the roots of these teeth extend above the mylohyoid muscle."[2] Fluid collections or infections within the sublingual space may be localized by noting their position inferior to the mobile tongue and medial and superior to the mylohyoid muscle. Coronal and/or sagittal reformatted images can be very useful in this determination (**Figs. 15 and 16**).

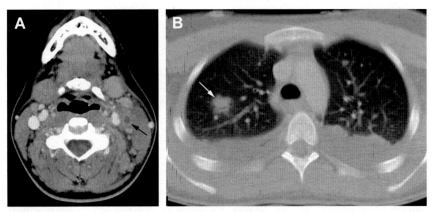

Fig. 13. Contrast-enhanced axial CTs of the neck (*A*) and chest (*B*) demonstrate findings in LS. (*A*) The right carotid artery and internal jugular vein appear normal. On the left there is nonfilling of the lumen of the internal jugular vein, abnormal enhancement of the wall of the jugular vein, and fat infiltration surrounding the jugular vein (*arrow*). These findings are compatible with septic thrombophlebitis involving the left internal jugular vein. (*B*) There are bilateral pleural effusions as well as a right lung opacity (*arrow*). The right lung opacity represents a septic embolus.

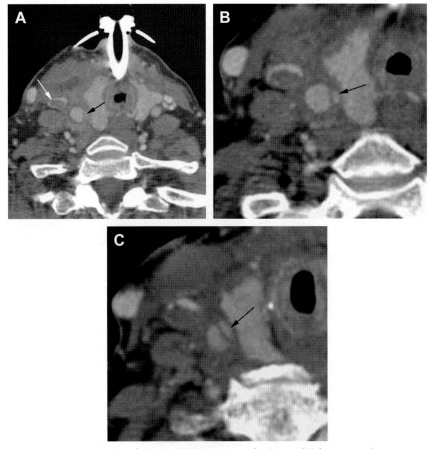

Fig. 14. Contrast-enhanced axial CTs of the neck demonstrate findings of infection and common carotid artery pseudoaneurysm. (*A*) Postoperative changes are present; there is a fluid collection within the right neck and infiltration of the fat within the right carotid space. Thrombus is present within the right internal jugular vein (*white arrow*). The right common carotid artery appears abnormal with a small collection of contrast seen at its medial margin (*black arrow*). (*B*, *C*) Magnified views of the right common carotid demonstrate a contrast filling structure medial to the vessel (*black arrows*). This finding is compatible with a carotid pseudoaneurysm.

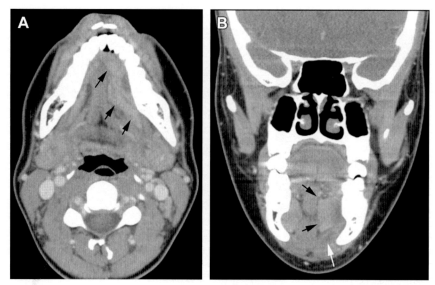

Fig. 15. Contrast-enhanced CTs of the neck demonstrate findings of left sublingual gland infection. (*A*) Axial image demonstrates enlargement and abnormal contrast enhancement of the left sublingual gland (*black arrows*). (*B*) Coronal image also shows the enlarged gland (*black arrows*) and clearly shows its relationship to the mylohyoid muscle (*white arrow*).

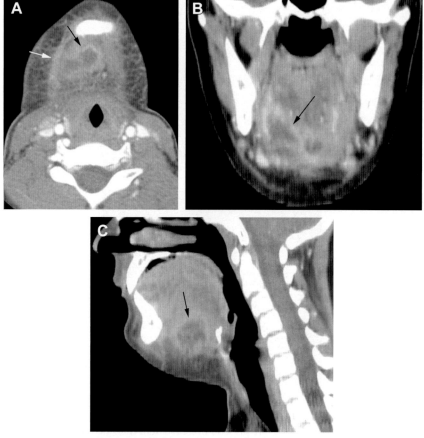

Fig. 16. Contrast-enhanced axial (*A*), coronal (*B*), and sagittal (*C*) CTs of the neck demonstrate findings of a sublingual abscess. (*A*) Axial image demonstrates an irregular rim-enhancing collection within the sublingual space (*black arrow*). Note that the collection lies medial to the mylohyoid muscle (*white arrow*). (*B, C*) Coronal and sagittal images also show the abscess (*black arrow*).

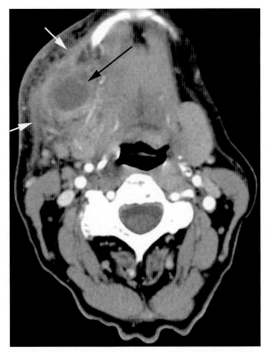

Fig. 17. Contrast-enhanced axial CT demonstrates an abscess within the right submandibular space (*black arrow*). Note the marketed swelling and irregular enhancement of the right platysma muscle (*white arrows*).

THE SUBMANDIBULAR SPACE

The submandibular space lies inferior and lateral to the mylohyoid muscle (see **Fig. 1B**). It is posterior to the free edge of the mylohyoid muscle and communicates with the sublingual space. It contains the submandibular gland, lymph nodes, and, in some cases, a second branchial cleft cyst. Infections involving the second and third mandibular molars can extend to the submandibular space because the roots of these teeth extend below the attachment of the mylohyoid muscle. Abscesses within the submandibular space have an appearance similar to the abscesses within the other spaces of the head and neck. They may result from the suppuration of submandibular lymph nodes (**Fig. 17**). Infections involving the submandibular gland appear similar to parotid gland infections. They are characterized by enlargement and hyperdensity of the gland as well as the infiltration of fat adjacent to the affected gland. When an infected gland is detected, the next step is to perform a careful examination of the glands and along the course of Wharton duct to search for an obstructing calculus (**Fig. 18**).

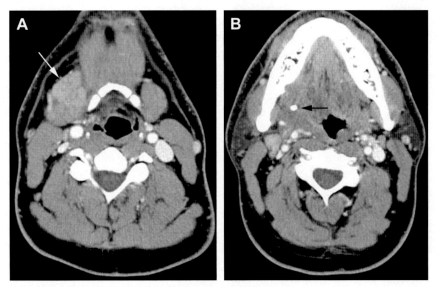

Fig. 18. Contrast-enhanced axial CTs demonstrate right submandibular gland infection secondary to obstruction. (*A*) The right submandibular gland is enlarged and shows increased density secondary to abnormal contrast enhancement (*white arrow*) compared with the normal left submandibular gland. (*B*) Examination of the course of the submandibular duct (ie, Wharton duct) shows a small calcific density consistent with an obstructing sialolith (*black arrow*).

CONGENITAL LESIONS

Second branchial cleft cysts are congenital lesions lying within the submandibular space. They may be clinically occult until they become secondarily infected. They are best defined on imaging by their characteristic location of anterior and deep to the sternocleidomastoid muscle (**Fig. 19**).

Cystic hygromas are congenital, transspatial, cystic malformations involving lymphatics. Like second branchial cleft cysts, they may present when they become secondarily infected. Given their transspatial and often multicystic appearance, these lesions may be difficult to differentiate from a complex abscess (**Fig. 20**).

LUDWIG ANGINA

Wilhelm Friedrich von Ludwig described Ludwig angina in 1836. He reported 5 patients with swelling of the neck that progressed rapidly to involve the soft tissues between the larynx and the floor of the mouth. The pain experienced by these patients helps to account for the name, "Ludwig angina." Currently, the term is used to describe an infection typically involving the floor of the mouth and both the submandibular and the sublingual spaces with potential involvement of the masticator space as well. Ludwig angina is

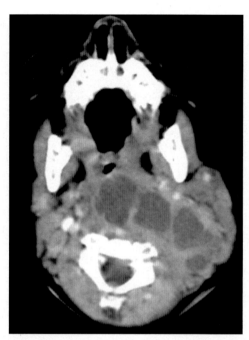

Fig. 20. Contrast-enhanced axial CT demonstrates a complex multispatial fluid collection with mild rim enhancement. This finding represents a congenital venolymphatic malformation (ie, cystic hygroma) that has become secondarily infected.

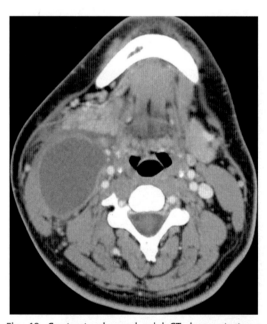

Fig. 19. Contrast-enhanced axial CT demonstrates a fluid collection with mild rim-enhancement lying just deep to the anterior right sternocleidomastoid muscle. This finding represents a congenital second branchial cleft cyst that has become secondarily infected.

a variety of multispatial cellulitis rather than a focal abscess (**Fig. 21**).[2] The infection causes elevation and posterior displacement of the tongue and tense induration between the hyoid bone and the mandible. Displacement of the tongue can occur rapidly, so establishing a secure airway is a treatment priority.[15]

COMPLICATIONS OF DENTAL DISEASE

Patients presenting with lower facial swelling should be evaluated for potential infection arising from pre-existing dental disease. Imaging typically shows infiltration and stranding of the subcutaneous fat typical of facial cellulitis (**Fig. 22**A). The goal of the emergency radiologist is to attempt to identify the source of the infection. Evaluation of the axial CT images through the mandible and the maxilla may show dental roots with surrounding lucency. This radiographic sign is often described as "floating roots" (see **Fig. 22**B). This sign indicates endodontal disease. Endodontal disease typically begins when bacteria infiltrate the tooth and penetrate the enamel (ie, "dental caries"). From the carious lesion, the infection may reach the pulp chamber. The infection spreads to the dental roots and exits at the root apex. The infection then affects the surrounding bone of the

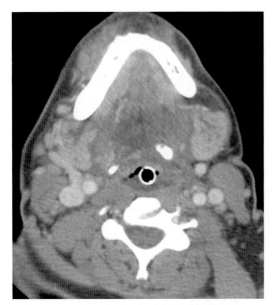

Fig. 21. Contrast-enhanced axial CT demonstrates an extensive infection in involving both the sublingual and submandibular spaces consistent with Ludwig angina. Notice that the airway has been secured with an endotracheal tube.

alveolar ridge, forming a radiologically lucent area of localized osteomyelitis (see **Fig. 22**C). The osteomyelitis may spread to the superficial soft tissues (see **Fig. 22**A) or may develop a confined collection such as a subperiosteal abscess (**Fig. 23**).

COMPLICATIONS OF PARANASAL SINUS DISEASE

Soft tissue swelling of the upper face and/or forehead prompts a radiologic search for the source of infection. It is important to evaluate the paranasal sinuses. The veins draining the sinuses are without valves. When pressure increases within an infected sinus, infection may spread via retrograde thrombophlebitis to the overlying soft tissues of the forehead, forming an area of localized cellulitis (**Fig. 24**A) or a frontal subperiosteal abscess (**Fig. 25**A). This syndrome was described by Percivall Pott in 1760 as Pott puffy tumor. Venous spread of the sinus infection may also extend intracranially to form an empyema. It is important for the radiologist to evaluate the brain using a narrow brain window to enable detection of a small empyema (see **Fig. 24**B). Paranasal sinus infection can also spread to the orbit. Most commonly, ethmoid sinus infection spreads to the medial extraconal space of the orbit forming a subperiosteal abscess (**Fig. 26**). An aggressive infection in the ethmoid sinus might cause osteitis of the thin lamina papyracea, but this route of spread is rare. Most orbital and intracranial complications of sinusitis are due to retrograde thrombophlebitis involving the valveless venous system.[16] Less commonly, paranasal sinus infection can spread to other portions of the orbit, such as the superior orbit with displacement of the globe (see **Fig. 25**B).

ORBITAL INFECTIONS

Orbital infections can arise from a pre-existing sinus infection. When infection of the medial orbit is identified, it is important to evaluate for possible involvement of the nasolacrimal duct. The nasolacrimal duct extends from the medial epicanthus to the nasal cavity. Patency of the nasolacrimal duct is important to maintain normal flow of tears from the lacrimal gland across the surface of the globe to the medial epicanthus and then into the nasal cavity. When infection involves the nasolacrimal duct, more aggressive therapy, including probing of the duct, is probably indicated (**Fig. 27**).

Orbital infections may also result from penetrating trauma, particularly if there is a retained foreign body. Metallic foreign bodies are easy to identify on CT. Nonmetallic foreign bodies, such as wood, are more difficult to identify, and their density may vary over time as their water content changes.[17] Once a metallic foreign body has been excluded, magnetic resonance (MR) may be useful to help to identify a subtle nonmetallic intraorbital foreign body (**Fig. 28**).

COMPLICATIONS OF MASTOID DISEASE

Mastoid disease is easy to identify on CT images as opacification of mastoid air cells. Most mastoid disease is uncomplicated, but when pressure increases within an infected mastoid air space, the infection can spread intracranially. The intracranial infection may cause a venous sinus thrombosis, most commonly affecting the sigmoid and/or transverse sinus. The venous sinus thrombosis may then present clinically as a venous infarction or even an intracranial hemorrhage (**Fig. 29**). The intracranial spread of the infection may also take the form of an empyema (**Fig. 30**) or a brain abscess (**Fig. 31**). Mastoid disease may cause necrosis of the mastoid tip and spread into the adjacent soft tissues to form an abscess (ie, Bezold abscess) (**Fig. 32**). The infection may spread to the lower neck along the plane of the sternocleidomastoid muscle.[15]

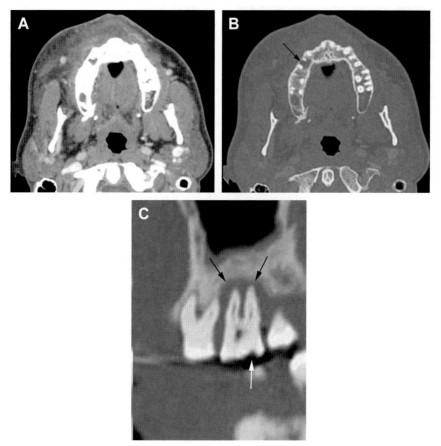

Fig. 22. Contrast-enhanced axial (*A, B*) and sagittal (*C*) CTs demonstrate facial infection secondary to endodontal disease. (*A*) There is extensive right facial infection. (*B*) Examination of the bone window demonstrates abnormal dental roots on the right. The dental roots do not appear to be surrounded by bone but rather they are "floating roots" surrounded by lucency (*black arrow*). (*C*) Magnified sagittal CT shows a break in the dental enamel (ie, dental caries) (*white arrow*). From there infection can migrate into the pulp chamber and dental roots until exiting at the root apex. The infection then causes a localized alveolar ridge osteomyelitis, which is seen on CT as lucency surrounding the roots of the affected tooth (*black arrows*).

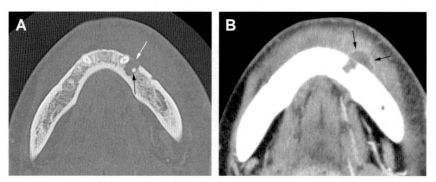

Fig. 23. Contrast-enhanced axial CTs demonstrate a subperiosteal abscess of the mandible secondary to endodontal disease. (*A*) There is a floating dental root in the left mandible (*black arrow*). There is also a break in the outer cortex of the mandible (*white arrow*). (*B*) The endodontal infection has broken through the mandibular cortex and formed a subperiosteal abscess (*black arrows*).

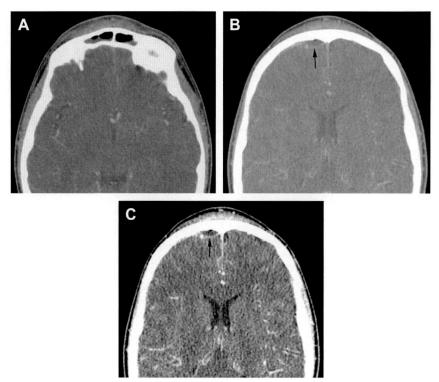

Fig. 24. Contrast-enhanced axial CTs demonstrate frontal sinusitis, soft tissue swelling overlying the forehead, and a frontal empyema. (*A*) Soft tissue swelling is noted over the forehead; there is also a small amount of frontal sinusitis. (*B, C*) There is a small extra-axial fluid collection in the right frontal region (*black arrows*). This collection is much more easily identified using the narrower brain window.

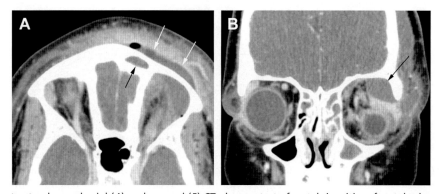

Fig. 25. Contrast-enhanced axial (*A*) and coronal (*B*) CTs demonstrate frontal sinusitis, a frontal subperiosteal abscess, and a subperiosteal abscess of the orbit. (*A*) The visualized portion of the left frontal sinus is opacified (*black arrow*). There is extensive soft tissue swelling overlying the forehead and a subperiosteal fluid collection (*white arrows*) consistent with a subperiosteal abscess. (*B*) Coronal image demonstrates an extraconal fluid collection involving the upper outer quadrant of the left orbit (*black arrow*). This collection represents a subperiosteal orbital abscess.

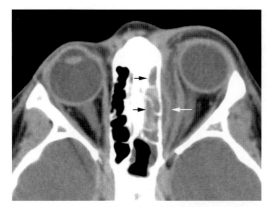

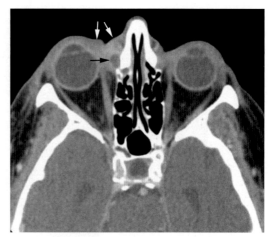

Fig. 26. Contrast-enhanced axial CT demonstrates ethmoid sinusitis and an orbital subperiosteal abscess. The left ethmoid sinus is opacified consistent with ethmoid sinusitis (*black arrows*). Within the left orbit, there is an extraconal medial fluid collection (*white arrow*), which displaces the medial rectus muscle. This finding is consistent with an orbital subperiosteal abscess.

Fig. 27. Contrast-enhanced axial CT demonstrates orbital cellulitis with nasolacrimal duct involvement. There is soft tissue prominence near the right medial epicanthus (*white arrows*) and enlargement with abnormal enhancement of the proximal nasolacrimal duct (*black arrow*).

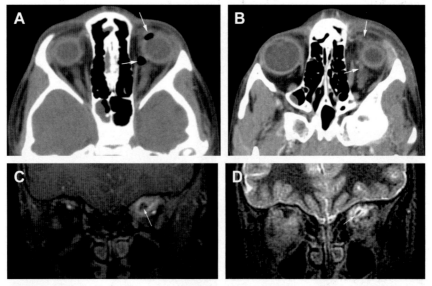

Fig. 28. CT (*A, B*) and MR (*C, D*) demonstrate penetrating orbital trauma with a retained nonmetallic foreign body. (*A*) The initial CT demonstrates evidence for orbital injury with gas both anterior and posterior to the globe (*white arrows*). No foreign body was identified on this study. (*B*) Three days later, a follow-up CT demonstrated orbital infection with stranding identified both anterior and posterior to the abnormal globe (*white arrows*). Because a metallic foreign body had been ruled out by multiple CTs, an MR was performed. (*C*) Coronal contrast-enhanced T1-weighted image with fat saturation demonstrated infection with a small abscess (*white arrow*) in the superior orbit. (*D*) Coronal T2-weighted MR demonstrates a linear foreign body within the area of infection (*white arrow*). Surgical debridement removed a small wooden foreign body.

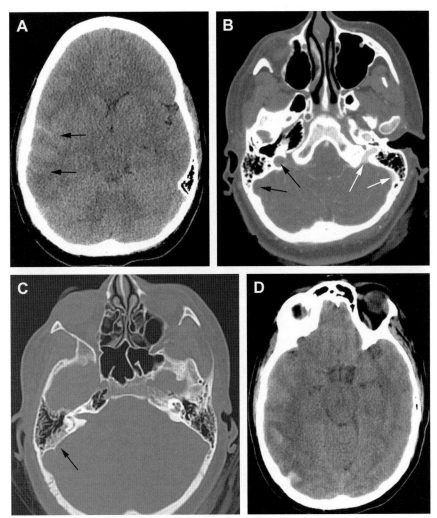

Fig. 29. CTs demonstrate mastoid disease causing venous sinus thrombosis, which progresses to a venous infarct. (*A*) Initial noncontrast CT, obtained in a patient complaining of headache, shows a small amount of right-sided subarachnoid hemorrhage (*black arrows*). CT angiogram was requested to evaluate for the cause of the subarachnoid hemorrhage. (*B*) A single axial image from the CT angiogram shows nonopacification of the right sigmoid sinus (*black arrows*) and normal opacification of the left sigmoid sinus (*white arrows*). (*C*) Evaluation of the initial CT shows fluid within the right mastoid air cells (*black arrow*). (*D*) A few days later, a follow-up CT shows a right-sided hemorrhagic venous infarct.

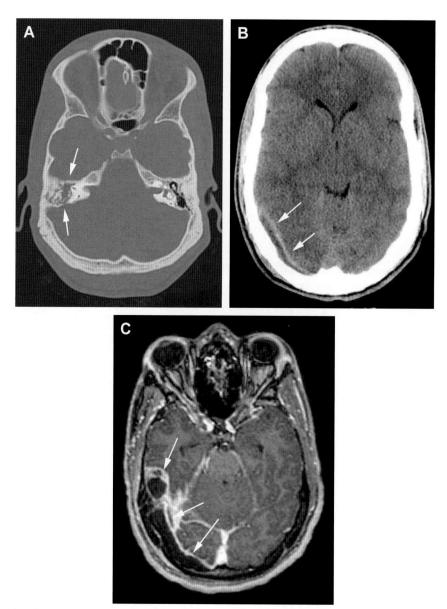

Fig. 30. CT (*A, B*) and MR (*C*) demonstrate mastoiditis progressing to an empyema. (*A*) CT demonstrates fluid within the right mastoid air cells (*white arrows*). This finding is consistent with mastoiditis. (*B*) Contrast-enhanced CT demonstrates a right-sided extra-axial fluid collection with an enhancing rim (*white arrows*). This finding is consistent with an empyema. (*C*) The empyema has increased in volume as shown on a follow-up contrast-enhanced T1-weighted MR (*white arrows*).

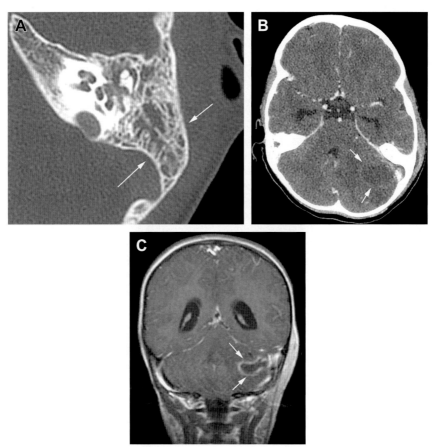

Fig. 31. CT (*A, B*) and MR (*C*) demonstrate mastoiditis progressing to a brain abscess. (*A*) Magnified CT demonstrates fluid within the left mastoid air cells (*white arrows*). This finding is consistent with mastoiditis. (*B*) Contrast-enhanced CT demonstrates a left-sided intra-axial fluid collection with an enhancing rim (*white arrows*). This finding is consistent with a brain abscess. (*C*) The brain abscess is more clearly delineated on a follow-up contrast-enhanced T1-weighted MR (*white arrows*).

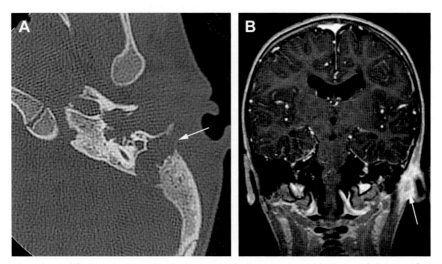

Fig. 32. CT (*A*) and MR (*B*) demonstrate mastoiditis progressing to a Bezold abscess. (*A*) Magnified CT demonstrates fluid within the left mastoid air cells with bony dehiscence (*white arrow*). (*B*) Contrast-enhanced T1-weighted MR demonstrates a left-sided extracranial fluid collection with surrounding enhancement (*white arrow*). This finding adjacent to the mastoid tip is consistent with a Bezold abscess.

SUMMARY

The first key emphasis was to be able to identify potentially subtle infections on CT images. Knowledge of normal anatomy, such as fat within the pterygopalatine fossa and fat within the retroantral area, can aid in the diagnosis of a deep facial infection. Awareness of the normal CT appearance of the head and neck structures is also vital to diagnose symmetric diseases such as diagnosing bilateral viral parotitis.

The next key point of emphasis was to characterize the infection. Differentiation of abscess from cellulitis is important because the therapeutic options differ. The imaging criteria and their accuracy for making this distinction have been discussed earlier.

The localization of the infection is important, not only to identify its space of origin but also to interrogate common routes of spread to other spaces, such as spread of neck infections to the mediastinum, spread of sinus infections to the orbit, and spread of mastoid infections intracranially.

An additional key point of emphasis was to appreciate the complications that may result from an infection. Examples of osteomyelitis, arterial pseudoaneurysm, and venous thrombosis with septic embolization to the lungs were discussed and illustrated.

Through examples, underlying abnormalities were illustrated, which may predispose to infection such as an obstructing salivary calculus, a prior dental procedure, evidence of endodontal disease, or pre-existing congenital structures, such as a second branchial cleft cyst or cystic hygroma, which may become secondarily infected.

The information provided should help the radiologist "to provide an accurate and prompt diagnosis, assess the extent of disease, evaluate for potential complications, and recommend definitive subspecialty evaluation."[2]

REFERENCES

1. Maroldi R, Farina D, Ravanelli M, et al. Emergency imaging assessment of deep neck space infections. Semin Ultrasound CT MR 2012;33(5):432–42.

2. Capps EF, Kinsella JJ, Gupta M, et al. Emergency imaging assessment of acute, nontraumatic conditions of the head and neck. Radiographics 2010; 30(5):1335–52.

3. Wang B, Gao BL, Xu GP, et al. Images of deep neck space infection and the clinical significance. Acta Radiol 2014;55(8):945–51.

4. Scott BA, Stiernberg CM, Driscoll BP. Deep neck space infections. In: Bailey BJ, editor. Head and neck surgery - otolaryngology. 2nd edition. Philadelphia: Lippincott-Raven Publications; 1998. p. 819–35.

5. Vural C, Gungor A, Comerci S. Accuracy of computerized tomography in deep neck infections in the pediatric population. Am J Otolaryngol 2003;24(3): 143–8.

6. Miller WD, Furst IM, Sàndor GK, et al. A prospective, blinded comparison of clinical examination and computed tomography in deep neck infections. Laryngoscope 1999;109:1873–9.

7. Kirse DJ, Roberson DW. Surgical management of retropharyngeal space infections in children. Laryngoscope 2001;111(8):1413–22.

8. Crespo AN, Chone CT, Fonseca AS, et al. Clinical versus computed tomography evaluation in the diagnosis and management of deep neck infection. Sao Paulo Med J 2004;122(6):259–63.

9. Virk JS, Pang J, Okhovat S, et al. Analysing lateral soft tissue neck radiographs. Emerg Radiol 2012; 19(3):255–60.

10. Debnam JM, Guha-Thakurta N. Retropharyngeal and prevertebral spaces: anatomic imaging and diagnosis. Otolaryngol Clin North Am 2012;45(6): 1293–310.

11. Eastwood JD, Hudgins PA, Malone D. Retropharyngeal effusion in acute calcific prevertebral tendinitis: diagnosis with CT and MR imaging. AJNR Am J Neuroradiol 1998;19(9):1789–92.

12. Chung T, Rebello R, Gooden EA. Retropharyngeal calcific tendinitis: case report and review of literature. Emerg Radiol 2005;11(6):375–80.

13. Weeks DF, Katz DS, Saxon P, et al. Lemierre syndrome: report of five new cases and literature review. Emerg Radiol 2010;17(4):323–8.

14. Hirai T, Korogi Y, Sakamoto Y, et al. Emergency balloon embolization for carotid artery rupture secondary to postoperative infection. Cardiovasc Intervent Radiol 1996;19(1):50–2.

15. McKellop JA, Bou-Assaly W, Mukherji SK. Emergency head & neck imaging: infections and inflammatory processes. Neuroimaging Clin N Am 2010; 20(4):651–61.

16. Hoxworth JM, Glastonbury CM. Orbital and intracranial complications of acute sinusitis. Neuroimaging Clin N Am 2010;20(4):511–26.

17. Yamashita K, Noguchi T, Mihara F, et al. An intraorbital wooden foreign body: description of a case and a variety of CT appearances. Emerg Radiol 2007; 14(1):41–3.

Imaging of Ischemia, Obstruction and Infection in the Abdomen

Kevin P. Murphy, MB[a,b], Maria Twomey, MB[a],
Patrick D. McLaughlin, MB BCh BAO, FFR RCSI, FRCPC[c],
Owen J. O'Connor, MD[a,b], Michael M. Maher, MD[a,b,*]

KEYWORDS

- Intestinal obstruction • Intestinal ischemia • Computed tomography • Acute abdomen • Bowel
- Colon

KEY POINTS

- Computed tomography (CT) is the modality of choice in investigation of the acute abdomen in nonpregnant adults but ultrasonography and MR imaging in particular are increasing being used.
- In suspected bowel ischemia, multiphase CT imaging with the use of negative oral contrast in place of positive oral contrast, where possible, is recommended.
- Complete mesenteric arterial occlusion without reperfusion results in bowel thinning and minimal mural enhancement, whereas other causes of intestinal ischemia lead to bowel wall thickening, intramural hemorrhage, and mural hyperenhancement.
- Key findings to interpret regarding bowel obstruction are the location and cause of transition, grade of obstruction, the presence of closed-loop obstruction, and the presence of ischemia.

INTRODUCTION

Intestinal obstruction and intra-abdominal infection associated with the gastrointestinal tract account for a huge proportion of emergency surgical admissions with abdominal symptoms. The former alone accounts for approximately 20% of admissions in this category.[1-3] Intestinal ischemia is uncommon but still carries a mortality in excess of 70%.[4] As a result of the frequency and gravity of the conditions, timely diagnosis of these entities by emergency radiologists is of key importance. This article examines the imaging approach in patients suspected of having the aforementioned conditions, shows key findings, and discusses potential complications.

NORMAL ANATOMY AND IMAGING TECHNIQUES
Important Anatomic Considerations

Knowledge of the vascular supply and drainage of the gastrointestinal tract is of key importance in understanding intestinal ischemia. The celiac trunk, superior mesenteric artery, (SMA) and smaller infraduodenal inferior mesenteric artery (IMA) must be scrutinized routinely on abdominal imaging studies. The celiac trunk supplies the foregut, from the distal esophagus to the midpart of the descending duodenum. The SMA, the artery of the midgut, supplies the gastrointestinal tract from the middle of the second part of the duodenum to the junction of the middle and distal

a Department of Radiology, University College Cork, Cork University Hospital, Wilton, Cork, Ireland; b Department of Radiology, Mercy University Hospital, Grenville Place, Cork, Ireland; c Department of Emergency and Trauma Radiology, Vancouver General Hospital, 899 West 12th Avenue, Vancouver, BC V5Z 1M9, Canada
* Corresponding author. Department of Radiology, University College Cork, Cork University Hospital, Wilton, Cork, Ireland.
E-mail address: m.maher@ucc.ie

Radiol Clin N Am 53 (2015) 847–869
http://dx.doi.org/10.1016/j.rcl.2015.02.008
0033-8389/15/$ – see front matter © 2015 Elsevier Inc. All rights reserved.

thirds of the transverse colon, with the IMA, the hindgut artery, supplying the remainder. Collateralization between the SMA and IMA via the marginal artery of Drummond is variable. In contrast, there is a rich plexus of collaterals between the celiac trunk and SMA. The bowel receives approximately 20% of cardiac output with the mucosa receiving two-thirds of this,[5,6] thus explaining why the mucosa and submucosa are most sensitive to changes in supply in the setting of ischemia.

The relative locations of small and large bowel loops are of significance in assessing for internal hernia, a challenging diagnosis that is frequently a closed-loop obstruction. It is important to carefully evaluate the anatomic relationships of the small bowel loops in relation to the ascending/descending colon or transverse colon respectively. In addition, the paraduodenal spaces should be devoid of extra bowel loops. Intestinal malrotation, which is associated with midgut volvulus and internal herniation, may occur when the small bowel mesentery is short, as signified by finding that the third part of the duodenum does not cross the midline. In such cases the small bowel is characteristically located on the right side of the abdomen and the colon principally left sided. In addition, the SMA and superior mesenteric vein relationship may be reversed.[7]

Malrotation with nonrotation also results in an appendix that lies to the left of midline, a finding that is also present in situs inversus.

The vermiform appendix measures a mean of 11 cm and the tip is most commonly retrocecal (74%), although the remainder have a variable location.[8] Meckel diverticulum is an anatomic variant that results from persistence of part of the omphalomesenteric duct, is present in 2% of the population, and is located approximately 60 cm (2 feet) from the ileocecal valve on the antimesenteric border.[9]

Normal bowel diameter may measure 2.5 cm for the small intestine, 9 cm for the cecum, and 6 cm for the remainder of the colon.[10,11]

Imaging Techniques

Radiography

Abdominal radiography is frequently used in assessment of the acute abdomen. It has a reported sensitivity of 69% to 80% for bowel obstruction[12–15] but is insensitive in assessing for complications or cause. In addition, abdominal radiographs are neither sensitive nor specific for detection of intestinal ischemia or infectious/inflammatory conditions such as diverticulitis, colitis, or appendicitis. The erect chest radiograph remains an essential part of assessment and detection of pneumoperitoneum in suspected hollow viscus perforation.

Computed tomography

Multidetector (MD) computed tomography (CT) is the main modality for the diagnosis of bowel obstruction and ischemia because of its availability, speed, sensitivity, and specificity.[1,2,5,16–24] MD CT has a sensitivity in excess of 80% for intestinal ischemia detection.[5] MD CT accuracy of 95% is reported for detection of high-grade small bowel obstruction, although accuracy is decreased for low-grade obstruction.[25] Sensitivity in excess of 90% is reported for large bowel obstruction.[26,27] Sensitivity and specificity for appendicitis are also in excess of 90%.[20,28]

MR imaging

MR imaging is being increasingly used in detection of bowel obstruction, ischemia, and infection. MR imaging has a sensitivity that is similar to CT in assessing bowel obstruction[29,30] and ischemia.[31,32] In addition, MR imaging is comparable with CT in infectious/inflammatory conditions such as appendicitis and diverticulitis.[20,33,34]

Ultrasonography

In children and pregnancy, ultrasonography is the first-choice modality in assessment of suspected appendicitis. Ultrasonography has a complimentary role to CT and MR imaging in assessing small bowel obstruction and suspected ischemia; however, its main strengths include ready availability in most hospitals, avoidance of exposure to ionizing radiation, and the portable nature of the modality, which means that it can be performed at the bedside in critically ill patients.[30,35,36]

Fluoroscopy

Angiography is rarely used currently for diagnosis in intestinal ischemia but is used during endovascular therapy. In the past, contrast enemas and barium follow-through studies were used as part of large and small bowel obstruction evaluation but current practice means that use has been superseded.

Many investigators advocate a 3-phase protocol for assessing suspected acute mesenteric ischemia. The unenhanced phase can be valuable if mural hyperdensity related to intramural hemorrhage is identified. This finding is a specific indicator of ischemia but is not required in all cases for the diagnosis of bowel ischemia.[37] The absence of positive oral contrast is essential for detection of bowel wall enhancement in suspected ischemia. Intraluminal fluid acts as a good negative oral contrast agent in cases of bowel obstruction. Positive oral contrast in the setting of

Imaging protocols		
	Suspected Ischemia	**Suspected Obstruction or Bowel Infection**
CT phases	Unenhanced Angiographic phase (30–35 s) Portovenous phase (60–65 s)	— — Portovenous phase (60–65 s)
Positive oral contrast	500–600 mL water preferred	Optional in obstruction Preferred in infection
Intravenous contrast	300–350 mgI/mL 3–4 mL/s	300–350 mgI/mL 3–4 mL/s
Reconstruction slice	1.5–3.0 mm	1.5–3.0 mm

suspected appendicitis has a marginal accuracy benefit,[28,38] particularly in patients of low body mass index, but its use may result in some delay in imaging of the patient. MD isometric thin-section imaging with multiplanar reconstructions is essential in bowel wall and vasculature assessment; review of reconstructions in the coronal plane is especially useful for investigating cases of bowel obstruction.

IMAGING FINDINGS/PATHOLOGY
Ischemia

Acute intestinal ischemia is an uncommon condition, accounting for approximately 0.1% of hospital admissions.[39] However, all-cause mortality remains approximately 70%,[4,39] a figure that increases to closer to 90% when infarction has become established.

The causes of acute mesenteric ischemia are as follows:

- Arterial occlusion (50%–60% of cases[5,32])
- Venous thrombosis (5%–10% of cases[5])
- Small vessel disease: vasculitides, radiation, chemotherapy induced
- Mechanical bowel obstruction
- Nonocclusive mesenteric ischemia (shock bowel)

Key imaging findings include:

- Abnormal bowel wall thickness
- Increased bowel wall attenuation from submucosal hemorrhage on the unenhanced CT phase
- Abnormal wall enhancement
- Increased luminal diameter
- Mesenteric arterial or venous occlusion
- Ascites and mesenteric fluid or stranding
- Pneumatosis intestinalis (gas in the bowel wall)
- Pneumatosis portalis (gas in the portovenous system)
- Pneumoperitoneum

Bowel wall thickening

Normal bowel wall thickness ranges from 3 to 5 mm.[40,41] The degree of bowel wall distention is a factor in determining whether the bowel wall is truly thickened and caution is needed when the bowel is collapsed or overdistended. Wall thickening from mucosal/submucosal edema or hemorrhage is the commonest finding in intestinal ischemia, and it is present in most cases that are not caused by acute arterial occlusion; however, bowel wall thickening is not specific for intestinal ischemia (**Fig. 1**).[16,19,21,22,42,43] The degree of

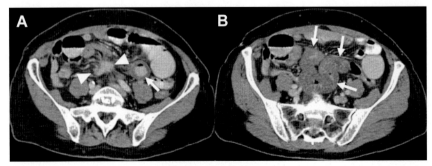

Fig. 1. Axial contrast-enhanced CT scan in a 47-year-old female patient with acute abdominal pain. A hypervascular mesenteric carcinoid mass (*A, arrowheads*) is seen in the mesentery with a marked surrounding desmoplastic reaction. The adjacent small bowel shows signs of venous ischemia (*A and B, arrows*) with wall thickening, submucosal edema, and mucosal hyperenhancement.

wall thickening does not correlate with the severity of ischemic wall damage. However, in the setting of acute arterial occlusion, the wall is frequently thinned (paper-thin wall) (**Fig. 2**) and this seems to be explained by the absence of vascular flow required to produce edema or hemorrhage.

Bowel wall attenuation on control images

Increased bowel wall attenuation from submucosal hemorrhage on unenhanced CT images is a specific sign for bowel ischemia.[37,44] The sign is rarely seen in isolation.[37,45] Like bowel wall thickening, submucosal hemorrhage is rarely present in the setting of arterial occlusion.

Abnormal wall enhancement

Reduced or absent bowel wall enhancement, which is an insensitive but specific sign, may be seen in arterial occlusion without reperfusion (see **Fig. 1**).[5,16,43] Reduced enhancement is also associated with infarction.[46] In cases of incomplete arterial occlusion, arterial occlusion with reperfusion, and other causes of intestinal ischemia, increased bowel wall enhancement is more commonly evident.

Increased luminal diameter

Bowel distention is seen in up to 90% of bowel infarction cases but its presence is variable in cases of reversible ischemia.[5,16,43] The distention is predominantly caused by increased intraluminal fluid and ileus from neuroenteric plexus dysfunction.

Mesenteric arterial or venous occlusion

The finding of arterial (see **Fig. 2**; **Fig. 3**) or venous occlusion (**Fig. 4**) in the mesenteric vessels indicates the cause rather than an effect of mesenteric ischemia. Embolus rather than thrombosis is more common in the SMA in the acute setting. Infarcts may also be seen in the other viscera, such as the kidneys or spleen, as a result of emboli. In the chronic setting, atherosclerosis dominates in terms of cause but incidental mesenteric atherosclerotic disease is common in asymptomatic elderly patients.[47] On the venous side, thrombosis may be caused by a local trigger such as intra-abdominal infection; neoplasm or inflammation; portal hypertension; or a systemic tendency for clot formation, such as antiphospholipid syndrome or oral contraceptive pill use.[5,16,48,49]

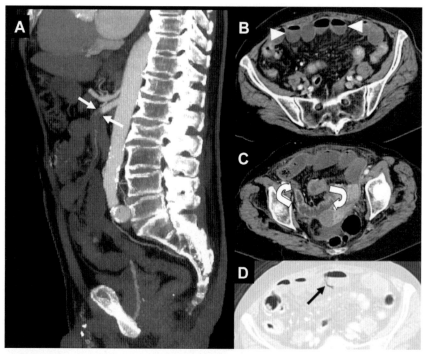

Fig. 2. Axial and sagittal CT images, from an 81-year-old man with a history of atrial fibrillation, who attended the emergency department with acute severe constant abdominal pain. Acute complete occlusion of the SMA (*A, white arrows*) is identified along with poorly enhancing small bowel walls (*B, arrowheads*). Distal small bowel loops show hyperenhancement (*C, curved arrows*) suggesting some reperfusion but ongoing ischemia. Pneumatosis portalis (portovenous gas) is seen in the perienteric veins anteriorly (*D, black arrow*).

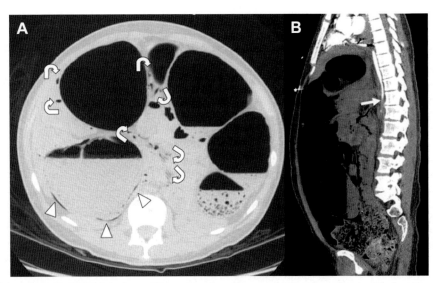

Fig. 3. Axial and sagittal arterial phase CT images of a 48-year-old female patient with long-term cognitive impairment who attended with abdominal pain and distention. Multiple dilated bowel loops from stercoral large bowel obstruction are seen along with pneumatosis intestinalis (*A, arrowheads*) and pneumatosis portalis (portovenous gas) (*A, curved arrows*). The stercoral obstruction led to severe abdominal compartment syndrome resulting in obstruction of the abdominal aorta (*B, arrow*) with resultant ischemia.

Ascites and mesenteric fluid or stranding

As with many other intra-abdominal disorders, the presence of free fluid is a nonspecific sign in the setting of suspected intestinal ischemia. The presence of free fluid in the mesentery (see **Fig. 4**) is reportedly more sensitive (88% vs 75%) and specific (90% vs 76%) than the finding of free ascites in the setting of ischemia from small bowel obstruction.[50,51] The presence of ascites and/or mesenteric stranding may increase the likelihood of infarction in the setting of arterial occlusion.[5] There should be increased suspicion for ischemia

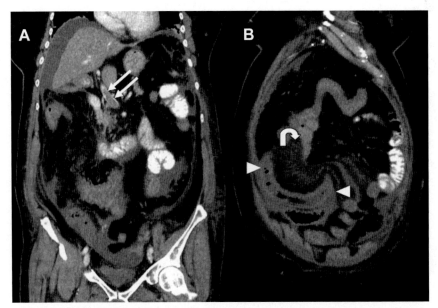

Fig. 4. Coronal reformatted portovenous phase CT images of a 46-year-old female patient with acute abdominal pain and vomiting. Thrombus is identified in the superior mesenteric vein (*A, arrows*). There is resultant ischemia of the small bowel with stranding and fluid in the mesentery (*B, curved arrow*) and mural thickening and hyperenhancement in the mildly dilated small bowel loops (*B, arrowheads*).

in the presence of high-density ascites related to bowel wall compromise and subsequent hemorrhage.

Pneumatosis intestinalis, pneumatosis portalis, and pneumoperitoneum

Detection of pneumatosis intestinalis (gas in the bowel wall) at CT is best performed by using lung-window settings (see Fig. 3). The dependent part of the wall is the best location to detect this finding because the dependent luminal contents can be used to improve conspicuity and localization. Gas may appear as bubbles or rims of gas separating the wall layers. In addition, images have to be scrutinized closely to assess for pneumatosis portalis (gas in the mesenteric or portal veins) (Fig. 5). Distinguishing intrahepatic portovenous gas (Fig. 6) from pneumobilia can be achieved by following the course of the vessel or channel involved. In addition, pneumobilia is more frequently central and does not involve the subcapsular ~2 cm of parenchyma, unlike portovenous gas, which is frequently peripheral and extends much closer to the capsule. In the correct clinical context, the presence of pneumatosis intestinalis or pneumatosis portalis has specificities approaching 100% for ischemia detection, particularly when seen with other findings such as abnormal bowel wall enhancement.[5,16] The presence of both entities has a reported specificity of 83% for infarction, although the sensitivity is only 17%.[52] However, there are multiple other causes of these entities. Alternate, more benign causes of pneumatosis intestinalis or portalis include systemic lupus erythematosus, scleroderma, barotrauma, asthma, chronic obstructive pulmonary disease, intra-abdominal infection, bowel

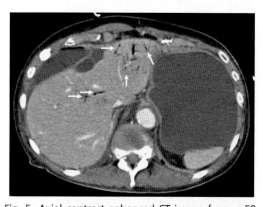

Fig. 5. Axial contrast-enhanced CT image from a 58-year-old man with mesenteric ischemia and perforation related to mechanical obstruction. Intrahepatic pneumatosis portalis (portovenous gas) is seen within the liver (*arrows*), extending almost to the capsule of the liver.

obstruction, iatrogenic bowel distention, and inflammatory bowel disease.[53,54] The presence of free air in the setting of intestinal ischemia strongly suggests transmural infarction.

Obstruction

Obstruction of the small intestine accounts for 80% of mechanical small bowel obstructions, with the remaining 20% being caused by colonic obstruction. The typical presentation is with abdominal pain, distention, vomiting, and absolute constipation.

Small bowel obstruction

Adhesions from prior abdominal surgery represent the commonest cause of small bowel obstruction (SBO), accounting for up to 75% of cases,[1,24,25] with hernias being the next commonest cause. Further causes can be broadly categorized by cause: congenital (eg, ileal atresia, midgut volvulus), extrinsic (eg, volvulus, compression from mass), bowel wall disorders (eg, stricture, intussusception, tumor), and intraluminal disorders (eg, meconium ileus, gallstones, foreign body, bezoar).

Large bowel obstruction

Mechanical obstruction of the colon is most commonly caused by colon cancer, which accounts for 50% to 60%.[10,27,55] Other causes include volvulus, diverticulitis, inflammatory bowel disease, radiation, ischemia, fecal impaction, or hernia.

Imaging findings

Considerations include:

- Proximal bowel distention
- Distal collapsed bowel
- String-of-pearls sign
- Transition point beak sign
- Grading
- Small bowel feces
- Potential closed loop
- Visible-cause SBO
- Visible-cause large bowel obstruction
- Possible mesenteric ischemia

Bowel distention with distal collapse

The key finding in SBO (Fig. 7) or large bowel obstruction (Fig. 8) is dilatation of the loops proximal to, and collapse of loops distal to, a point of obstruction. Small bowel diameter in excess of 2.5 cm and large bowel diameter in excess of 6 cm (9 cm for cecum) are considered dilated. On plain radiography, small bowel loops are dilated centrally with visible transverse valvulae conniventes, whereas the large bowel is peripheral

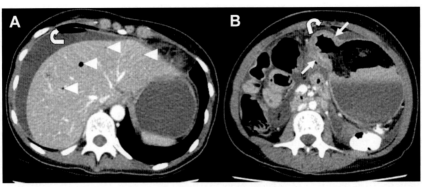

Fig. 6. Axial CT images from a 74-year-old man with an obstructing perforated gastric tumor (*B, arrows*), resulting in mesenteric ischemia with intrahepatic portovenous gas (*A, arrowheads*). Pneumoperitoneum is also evident (*curved arrows*).

in location with haustral folds that are seen to incompletely traverse the wall. The location of distal bowel collapse helps decide whether the obstruction is in the small or large bowel. If the obstruction is in the colon but the ileocecal valve is competent, the small bowel is not dilated. It is important to differentiate mechanical obstruction from paralytic ileus and pseudo-obstruction. Paralytic ileus typically occurs in postoperative patients, is often painless with absent bowel sounds, and shows small and large bowel distention. In contrast, colonic pseudo-obstruction, known as

Ogilvie syndrome in the acute setting, is similar in presentation to large bowel obstruction in that the patients often have pain and distention but frequently have a history of chronic constipation.[56,57] Imaging in pseudo-obstruction shows a dilated proximal colon; distal collapse; and, classically, a caliber change at the splenic flexure, without a lesion at the site of transition.[56] However, the site of transition can be anywhere in the colon.[57] In this syndrome, the small intestine may be dilated if the ileocecal valve is incompetent.

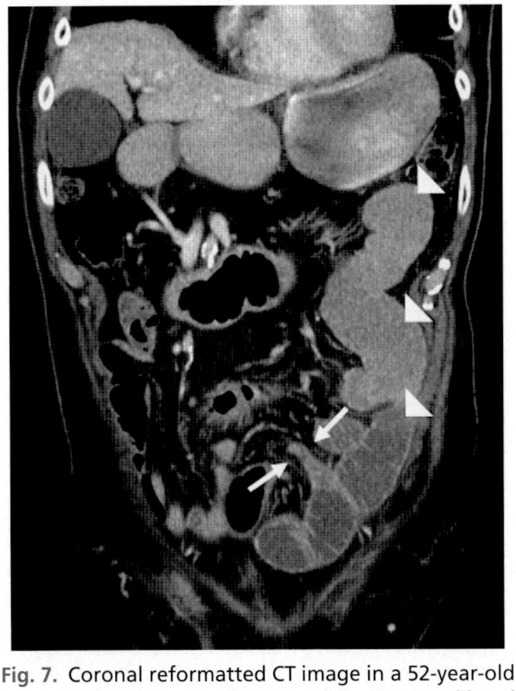

String-of-pearls sign

The string-of-pearls sign is seen on lateral decubitus or erect abdominal radiographs, in addition to CT, when small bubbles of gas are trapped between the valvulae conniventes. It is reported

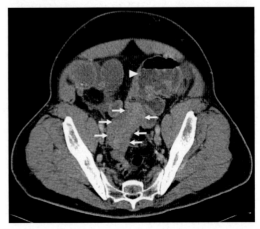

Fig. 8. Axial CT image in a 61-year-old female patient with an obstructing sigmoid tumor (*arrows*) that showed shouldering and asymmetrical bowel wall thickening and proximal colonic dilatation (*arrowhead*).

Fig. 7. Coronal reformatted CT image in a 52-year-old man with high-grade adhesional SBO showing dilated proximal small bowel loops (*arrowheads*) and a beak sign (*arrows*) at the site of obstruction.

to be specific for SBO and absent in the setting of adynamic ileus or gastroenteritis.[58]

Transition point beak sign

Typically, transition from dilated proximal bowel to collapsed distal bowel occurs at the site of obstruction, although this is not always the case. When an abrupt transition occurs, the bowel forms a beak sign whereby the dilated proximal bowel quickly tapers to the transition point, resulting in the shape of a beak (see **Fig. 7**; **Fig. 9**). In a closed-loop obstruction, 2 transition point beak signs may be seen. The absence of a beak sign is associated with successful nonoperative management in the setting of adhesion-related SBO, along with the presence of a small bowel feces sign and an anterior parietal adhesion.[59] In contrast, 2 or more beak signs, a whirl sign, a C-shaped or U-shaped bowel loop, and high-grade obstruction are more likely to require surgical management in the setting of adhesional SBO.[59,60]

Grading

Bowel obstruction is typically graded either into complete or high-grade obstruction, or partial or low-grade obstruction. Incomplete obstruction is suggested when the transition is not abrupt, the distal bowel is not fully collapsed, the proximal bowel is only mildly distended, and ingested contents such as positive oral contrast traverse the

obstruction.[1,10,25] In contrast, complete obstruction is the opposite of these entities. High-grade obstruction is more likely to require operative management in the setting of adhesion-related SBO.[59]

Small bowel feces

The presence of solid heterogeneous feces-like particulate matter mixed with gas in the small bowel proximal to the site of obstruction is a useful sign in the setting of bowel obstruction (**Fig. 10**). The main usefulness seems to be in locating the site and cause of obstruction.[1,61] It is associated with successful nonoperative management in the setting of adhesion-related SBO.[59] However, it is not pathognomonic for obstruction because it is reported to be seen in up to 6% of asymptomatic studies.[62]

Potential closed loop

Closed-loop obstruction occurs when the bowel is obstructed at 2 different points along its length, usually at a single location and from a single cause. It is an important diagnosis to make because it carries a higher risk of bowel ischemia and usually requires prompt surgical

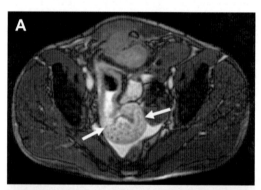

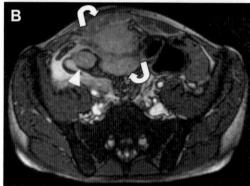

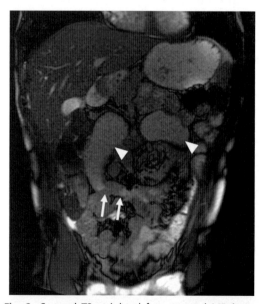

Fig. 9. Coronal T2-weighted fat-saturated MR imaging in a 36-year-old male patient with high-grade SBO from a stricture secondary to underlying Crohn disease (*arrows*). The proximal loops are dilated (*arrowheads*) and there is a benign stricture at the site of transition.

Fig. 10. Axial T2-weighted fat-saturated MR imaging in a 39-year-old male patient showing a small bowel feces sign (*A, arrows*), proximal to a strictured segment of distal ileum (*B, arrowhead*) that has an adjacent phlegmon (*B, curved arrows*).

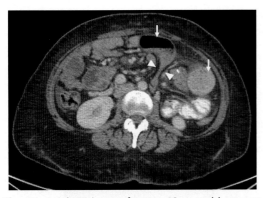

Fig. 11. Axial CT image from a 46-year-old woman with a history of prior bowel surgery who presented with suspected bowel obstruction. An internal hernia through a defect in the transverse mesocolon is shown (*arrowheads*), where there is a visible beak sign. The closed-loop obstruction involves the dilated loops of small bowel (*arrow*).

intervention.[2,10,25,63] Two beak signs may be seen from the 2 points of obstruction, along with a radial or U-shaped configuration of the bowel loops. A whirl (or whirlpool) sign may also be seen, in which the mesenteric vessels have a swirling appearance from torsion of these structures around themselves.[64] Closed-loop obstruction is associated with hernias (particularly internal hernias) (Fig. 11), midgut volvulus, cecal volvulus (Fig. 12), and sigmoid volvulus (Fig. 13). A proximal colonic obstruction with a competent ileocecal valve may also behave like a closed-loop obstruction.

Visible-cause small bowel obstruction
Differentiation of SBO from large bowel obstruction is fundamental in assessing the cause, with the location of the transition point being the key.

Intraluminal causes of SBO, such as bezoar, inspissated contents (distal intestinal obstruction syndrome, seen in cystic fibrosis) (Fig. 14), or gallstone ileus (Fig. 15) appear as intraluminal filling defects. Mural causes have the appearance of focal or segmental wall thickening that may be circumferential (Fig. 16) or eccentric. Extrinsic causes of SBO are the most commonly encountered causes. An adhesional band is rarely evident in the setting of SBO, hence it is a diagnosis of exclusion. Abdominal wall hernias, such as incisional (Fig. 17), epigastric, umbilical, paraumbilical, inguinal (Fig. 18), and femoral (Fig. 19) hernias, may be seen in addition to diaphragmatic, pelvic, and other internal hernias.[63] Internal hernias are increasing in frequency because of the increased volume of surgery, particularly bariatric surgery,[63,65] and their diagnosis can be challenging. Regarding internal herniation, in addition to features of closed-loop obstruction, the herniated bowel loops, most commonly small bowel, have an abnormal location relative to the colon or duodenum.

Visible-cause large bowel obstruction
With regard to large bowel obstruction, the cause of exclusion is a colonic neoplasm, given that it is the cause in 50% to 60% of cases.[10,27,55] A circumferential or eccentric short segment enhancing mass is usually evident in the setting of colon cancer, and is most frequently located in the sigmoid colon (see Fig. 8). Diverticulitis or diverticular stricture involves a longer segment with a greater degree of pericolonic fat stranding and diverticula. If CT findings are equivocal, MR imaging is reported to have a superior sensitivity and specificity for differentiating colonic tumor from diverticulitis.[34] If large bowel obstruction is caused by cecal (see Fig. 12) or sigmoid volvulus

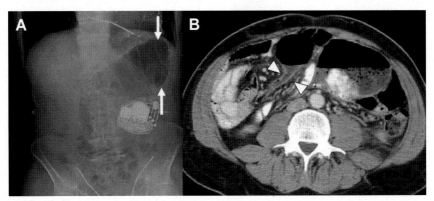

Fig. 12. Abdominal radiograph and axial CT image in a 40-year-old patient with suspected bowel obstruction. The cecal pole has flipped and is now located and pointing to the left upper quadrant (*A, arrows*). A beak sign (*B, arrowheads*) is shown from one of the transition points from the resultant closed-loop obstruction.

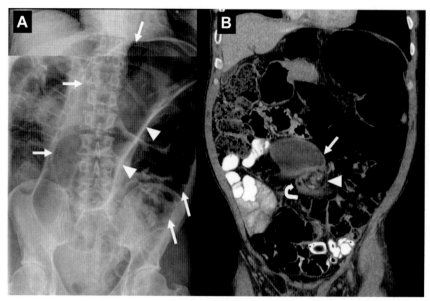

Fig. 13. Abdominal radiograph and coronal reformatted image in an 81-year-old patient with sigmoid volvulus. A dilated loop of colon is seen extending from the pelvis toward the left upper quadrant (*A*, *arrows*) with a resultant coffee bean sign (*A*, *arrows* and *arrowheads*). The subsequent CT image shows a beak sign (*B*, *arrow*), whirl sign (*B*, *arrowhead*), and collapse of the proximal loop (*B*, *curved arrow*).

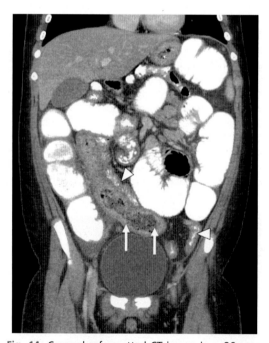

Fig. 14. Coronal reformatted CT image in a 26-year-old patient with cystic fibrosis with distal intestinal obstruction syndrome. Inspissated fecal-type contents are seen in the distal ileum (*arrows*) resulting in proximal bowel obstruction and dilated loops. High-density contents are seen in the nondilated small bowel distal to the obstruction from a prior investigation (*arrowheads*).

(see **Fig. 13**), the diagnosis may be made on abdominal radiography. In cecal volvulus, the cecal pole has an ectopic location, pointing toward or located in the left upper quadrant. Sigmoid volvulus classically has an abnormal loop of large bowel extending out of the pelvis, forming a coffee bean shape.[66] The CT findings are in keeping with those on plain radiographs in addition to closed-loop obstruction.

Possible mesenteric ischemia
Signs of bowel ischemia, as outlined earlier, may be seen in association with bowel obstruction. Ischemia is more likely to occur in the setting of closed-loop and high-grade obstruction.

GASTROINTESTINAL TRACT INFECTION
Small Bowel

Infectious enteritis
Acute infectious enteritis (or gastroenteritis) is usually self-limiting and typically does not require imaging. However, imaging may be performed in atypical presentations, with chronic symptoms and in immunosuppressed patients. Causative organisms include bacteria (*Salmonella, Yersinia, Escherichia coli, Campylobacter, Mycobacterium tuberculosis* [tuberculosis (TB)]), protozoa (*Giardia lamblia, Cryptosporidium*), and viruses (Cytomegalovirus, Norovirus, Rotavirus). Giardia has a

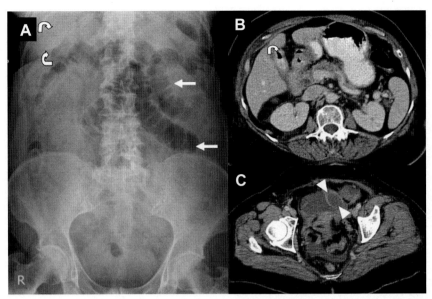

Fig. 15. Abdominal radiograph and axial CT images on a 59-year-old patient with gallstone ileus. Dilated small bowel loops are seen (*A, arrows*) along with pneumobilia (*A and B, curved arrows*) on the radiograph and CT images. The noncalcified gallstone was identified in the lower abdomen (*C, arrowheads*).

preponderance for the proximal small bowel, the CT findings of which are nonspecific, with circumferential wall thickening and lymphadenopathy being the commonest.[67] Most pathogens usually affect the ileum.[22,68] Ninety percent of TB occurs in the ileum or cecum because of the stasis and lymphatic abundance.[69] Ileal TB usually results in asymmetric wall thickening in the ileum and multiple large low-density/necrotic nodes on CT.[68,70] In contrast, Crohn disease is more frequently associated with small nodes, fibrofatty mesenteric proliferation (so-called creeping fat), and potential for fistula formation as a result of the transmural inflammation.[21] Salmonella gives a similar appearance to Crohn disease in terms of segmental circumferential wall thickening.[68,71] Yersinia,

Fig. 16. Coronal T2-weighted fat-saturated MR imaging in a 65-year-old male patient with SBO. Dilated small bowel (*arrows*) is seen superior to a shouldered circumferential lesion (*arrowheads*) with collapsed bowel distally (*curved arrow*). Histology following surgical resection confirmed adenocarcinoma.

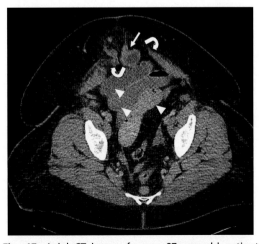

Fig. 17. Axial CT image from a 67-year-old patient with SBO from an incisional hernia. Dilated bowel loops (*arrowheads*) are seen proximal to a transition point beak sign (*arrow*) within the hernia neck (*curved arrows*).

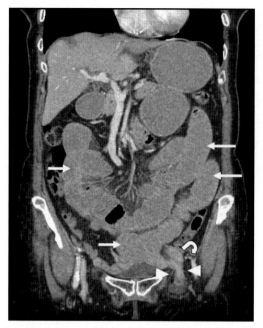

Fig. 18. Coronal reformatted CT image of a 49-year-old female patient with SBO from a left inguinal hernia. Dilated small bowel loops (*arrows*) are seen proximal to the direct left inguinal hernia (*arrowheads*), which lies medial to the inferior epigastric vessels (*curved arrow*).

which often presents with acute pain and tenderness, typically results in mild symmetric bowel wall thickening, aphthous ulceration, and mucosal nodularity.[22] Typhlitis (neutropenic enterocolitis) is discussed later.

Meckel diverticulitis

Approximately 2% of the population has a Meckel diverticulum. Many of these true diverticula are incidental findings but complications or symptoms develop in 4% to 40%.[9,72,73] Diverticular infection/inflammation or diverticulitis (**Fig. 20**) accounts for up to 30% of complications.[9,73] Gastrointestinal bleeding, intussusception, obstruction, perforation, and band strangulation are other common presentations or complications. The right lower quadrant or close to midline are the most likely locations of a Meckel diverticulum at CT examination in the setting of diverticulitis.[74] It appears as a blind-ending pouch of approximately 2.5 cm in (outer wall) diameter and approximately 3.3 cm in length with a mean wall thickness of almost 4 mm. In the setting of Meckel diverticulitis, inflammatory changes in the surrounding fat and some free fluid are evident. Other complications, such as bowel obstruction or perforation, may also be present, making the identification of a Meckel difficult.

Colon

Appendicitis

Acute appendicitis is a common cause of acute abdominal pain, particularly in children and

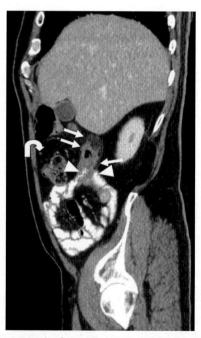

Fig. 20. Sagittal reformatted CT image from a 47-year-old patient with acute abdominal pain from a Meckel diverticulitis. The blind-ending dilated bowel diverticulum is evident (*arrows*) with surrounding fat stranding. The afferent and efferent small bowel loops are seen (*arrowheads*) along with the normal high-lying appendix (*curved arrow*).

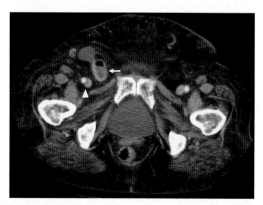

Fig. 19. Axial CT image from a 71-year-old female patient with SBO from a right femoral hernia. The hernia sac (*arrow*) is seen medial to the femoral artery and vein (*arrowhead*).

adolescents, with a lifetime risk of developing acute appendicitis of 6% to 8%.[75] Graded compression ultrasonography[76] is usually the first-line imaging investigation in children, young adults, and pregnancy. The user-dependent nature of the modality likely contributes to variable reported sensitivities of 12% to 90%[77–79] and the commonly encountered lack of confidence in sonographic diagnosis,[80] although high specificities in excess of 85% are routinely reported. MR imaging has reported accuracies, in excess of 90%, that are similar to those of CT in diagnosis of acute appendicitis.[20,33,77,78,81] As a result, the use of MR imaging in this setting continues to increase. Regardless of the imaging modality, typical findings include an appendix diameter of greater than 6 mm, luminal obliteration, noncompressible appendix, appendicolith, periappendiceal inflammatory fat changes, free fluid, inflammatory phlegmon, and abscess (**Figs. 21 and 22**).[75,78,79,81–83]

Colitis and cecitis

Like infectious enteritis, patients with infectious colitis often do not require imaging, unless there is doubt about the diagnosis or complications are suspected. The causes are similar to those of infectious enteritis with the addition of *Clostridium difficile* (pseudomembranous colitis), the protozoon infection amebiasis (*Entamoeba histolytica*), the parasitic infection schistosomiasis, *Chlamydia trachomatis*, *Neisseria gonorrhoeae*, and Herpes species.

In Western countries, bacteria most commonly cause infectious colitis. In particular, the number of cases of pseudomembranous colitis has markedly increased in recent times as a result of

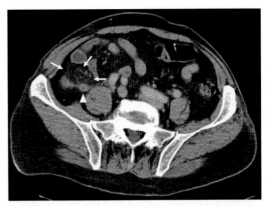

Fig. 22. Axial CT image of a 41-year-old patient with acute appendicitis. The dilated appendix (*arrowhead*), seen in cross section, is enlarged, has luminal obliteration, and shows mural enhancement. Surrounding inflammatory fat stranding is also evident (*arrows*).

increased usage of broad-spectrum and prophylactic antibiotics.[84,85] *C difficile* is not a normal bowel commensal organism but colonizes the colon after antibiotics or chemotherapy have disrupted the normal colonic biology.[85,86] The bacteria produce 2 toxins (A and B) that result in the colonic inflammation. Typical CT findings of pseudomembranous colitis (**Fig. 23**) are wall thickening

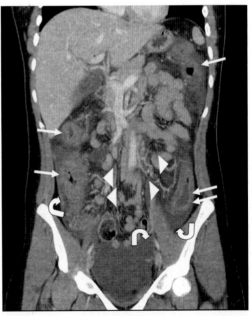

Fig. 23. Coronal reformatted CT image from a 41-year-old oncology patient with pseudomembranous colitis involving the entire colon. Diffuse wall thickening, with submucosal edema (*arrows*), an elongated target sign in the left iliac fossa, mesenteric hypervascularity (*arrowheads*), and ascites (*curved arrows*) are shown.

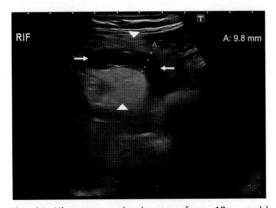

Fig. 21. Ultrasonography image of an 18-year-old male patient with acute appendicitis. The appendix (*arrows*) measures almost 10 mm in diameter and was noncompressible with surrounding echogenic fat (*arrowheads*).

of 11 to 14 mm, submucosal low attenuation from edema, and an irregular mucosal contour.[85,87,88] The so-called accordion sign, in which positive oral contrast interspersed between thickened haustral folds is said to look like an accordion, may also be seen, although it can be seen in any severe colitis (**Fig. 24**).[89] In addition, the target sign, in which postcontrast enhancement of the mucosa and muscularis propria with intervening submucosal edema has the appearance of a target, may also be evident (see **Fig. 23**). The fat-halo sign is similar but occurs when the submucosa shows fat deposition, although it predominantly occurs in ulcerative colitis.[90]

Amebic colitis occurs as a result of colon invasion from the trophozoite form of the organism. The inflammation usually starts in the cecum, often involves the rectum, and may result in diffuse colitis.[87] The most distal part of the ileum may be involved. Amebic colitis results in wall thickening, ulceration, pseudopolyps, and skip lesions that are similar to Crohn colitis. The classic coned cecum, in which the cecum resembles an inverted cone pointing at the appendix base, develops after subacute infection.[87] However, the cone-shaped cecum can be seen in multiple inflammatory, infectious, or neoplastic conditions. Amebomas are focal areas of granulation that can closely mimic colonic neoplasms,[87,91,92] particularly if hepatic amebic disease is present.[93,94] Residual colonic scarring is common after infection.

There is huge overlap in the location and appearances of most bacterial and viral infectious colitides, hence stool culture and history are of key importance in identifying the causative organism. However, certain patterns of involvement are associated with certain organisms. Cytomegalovirus and *E coli* often result in diffuse colitis; shigella and salmonella colitides are frequently confined to the right colon; schistosomiasis is usually confined to the left colon; and *C trachomatis, N gonorrhoeae*, and Herpes species are confined to the rectosigmoid region.

Typhlitis, also known as neutropenic enterocolitis, has an incidence of up to 26% in certain patient groups undergoing chemotherapy,[95] but can occur in any immunosuppressed patient. The mortality remains in excess of 50% despite increased awareness and aggressive management with bowel rest, fluids, broad-spectrum antimicrobial therapy, and blood products if necessary.[95] It is likely multifactorial in cause with neutropenia, bowel wall injury from treatment or neoplasm, and intramural hemorrhage from thrombocytopenia resulting in invasive polymicrobial infection from commensal bowel organisms.[95–97] Clinical symptoms and signs include abdominal pain, localized tenderness, distention, nausea, vomiting, bloody diarrhea, and fever. CT is the imaging modality of choice and shows increased wall thickening (typically ~7 mm) involving the cecum, and often the ileum and remaining colon (**Fig. 25**).[87,96,98] The disease is

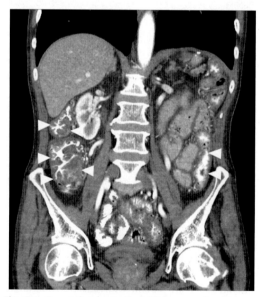

Fig. 24. Coronal reformatted CT image of a 64-year-old patient with acute infectious (coliform) colitis showing the accordion sign (*arrowheads*), in which the positive oral contrast is interspersed between the enlarged haustral folds.

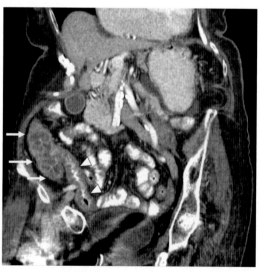

Fig. 25. Coronal reformatted CT image from a 67-year-old oncology patient with typhlitis. Wall thickening involving the terminal ileum (*arrowheads*), cecum, and ascending colon (*arrows*) is shown.

reportedly limited to the cecum in 28% of cases.[96] Pneumatosis, mucosal enhancement, free fluid, and fat stranding may also be seen.[87,96] Neutropenic patients are also at increased risk of other colitides, including cytomegalovirus colitis and pseudomembranous colitis.[96]

For any infectious colitis, the main differential diagnoses include noninfectious causes of colitis, such as inflammatory bowel disease, with radiation colitis and ischemic colitis being less common. Diverticulitis, neoplasm, or graft-versus-host disease are additional alternate diagnoses to consider. Amebic, TB, and pseudomembranous colitis most closely mimic inflammatory bowel disease. Radiation colitis is likely to be suspected from the history and ischemic colitis is found in the older age group, with a vascular distribution and features mentioned earlier. Bowel wall thickness, bowel wall attenuation, degree of wall thickening, symmetry of wall thickening, length of segment involved, and associated findings such as stranding, lymphadenopathy, and abscess are key factors that aid in delineating the cause.[41,90]

Complications of colitis are readily assessed using CT. They include perforation, abscess, ischemia, and toxic megacolon. Toxic megacolon is among the most serious and is most commonly caused by ulcerative colitis or, increasingly, pseudomembranous colitis,[99] but may be associated with any severe form of colitis. Nitric oxide and interleukins seem to be important in the pathogenesis.[99] The key imaging findings are dilatation of the colon, typically the transverse colon, to greater than 6 cm in diameter with loss of the haustral folds and wall thinning,[100,101] findings that help distinguish it from acute severe colitis. Radiographs are useful in assessing bowel diameter in the setting of toxic megacolon,[102] but CT is the superior investigation because it can detect small perforations and abscesses in addition to making a more accurate diagnosis.[99]

Diverticulitis

Colonic diverticula are acquired pseudodiverticula that may result from increased intraluminal pressure and occur at weak points in the circular muscle where mucosal vasculature penetrates on the mesenteric wall.[103] They predominantly occur in the descending and sigmoid colon but can be found anywhere in the colon apart from the rectum. Diverticulosis is common in the Western world, is predominantly a disease of older adults, and is found in greater than 70% of people more than 80 years of age and approximately 5% of people at 40 years of age.[104,105] Traditional thinking about cause was that it occurred in patients lacking in dietary fiber,[106] but studies to

confirm this are conflicting.[107,108] Diverticulitis occurs when one or more of these diverticula become obstructed at the neck, resulting in stasis, inflammation, infection, and perforation. Diverticulitis occurs in between 1% and 25% of patients with diverticular disease, although recent studies suggest that rates of development of acute diverticulitis are at the lower end of that range.[105] It is among the commonest inpatient gastrointestinal diagnoses.[104] Typical presentations include symptoms and signs of left iliac fossa pain and tenderness, altered bowel habit, nausea, pyrexia, possibly a palpable mass, and increased inflammatory markers. CT is the investigation of choice in suspected acute diverticulitis. Findings include mesenteric fat stranding that is disproportionate to the degree of colonic wall thickening, mural hyperemia, segmental involvement, fluid accumulation in the mesenteric root (the comma sign), mesenteric hypervascularity (the centipede sign), and the presence of diverticula (**Fig. 26**).[87,109,110] Associated findings may include an abscess (present in up to 30% of cases) (see **Fig. 26**; **Fig. 27**), localized perforation, generalized perforation, or fistula. Fistulae may be from the involved colon to colon, small bowel, vagina, bladder, or skin. Classification of the severity of acute diverticulitis is advantageous and several scales exist. One such surgical scale is the Hinchey classification[111]: stage Ia, phlegmon; stage Ib, with pericolic or mesenteric abscess; stage II, with walled-off pelvic abscess; stage III, with generalized purulent peritonitis; stage IV, with generalized feculent peritonitis. Although the described classification system has a surgical basis and classification may not be used commonly in practice, the elements should be mentioned in the radiology report to indicate severity.

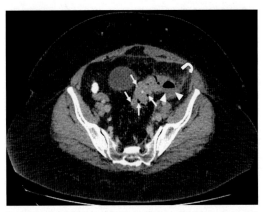

Fig. 26. Axial CT image in a 49-year-old woman with acute diverticulitis. Multiple diverticula are visible (*arrows*) along with surrounding fat stranding (*curved arrow*) and a pericolic abscess (*arrowheads*).

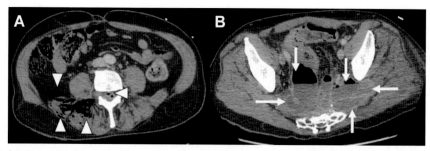

Fig. 27. Axial CT images of 75-year-old male patient with severe complex pelvic sepsis from acute diverticulitis. Large abscesses are seen in the pelvis (*B, arrows*), extending into the buttock via the sciatic notch. In addition, gas is seen in the spinal canal and right paraspinal muscles (*A, arrowheads*) as a result of local spreading of infection.

Differentiating diverticulitis from colonic neoplasm is challenging. The presence of diverticula, disproportionate fat stranding, comma or centipede signs, mesenteric root fluid, mild smooth concentric wall thickening, gradual transition from normal to abnormal bowel thickness, long (5–10 cm) affected segment, and minimal or no lymphadenopathy are associated with acute diverticulitis. In contrast, the absence of diverticula, fat stranding, comma or centipede signs, and mesenteric fluid along with the presence of lymphadenopathy, bowel wall shouldering, increased density of the focal bowel wall thickening or mass after contrast administration, and irregular eccentric short segment (<5 cm) wall thickening is associated with colonic neoplasm.[110,112–114] MR imaging may have an advantage compared with CT in differentiating tumor from diverticulitis.[34] Epiploic appendagitis is another important differential diagnosis in patients with suspected diverticulitis. The key finding is an ovoid fat-density lesion with surrounding inflammation adjacent to the colon with little if any wall thickening (**Fig. 28**).[115]

All patients should undergo endoscopy after an episode of diverticulitis, predominantly to ensure that there is no underlying neoplasm.[105]

Sepsis from gastrointestinal perforation

Hollow viscus perforation and associated abdominal sepsis remains a common problem but the radiological diagnosis of pneumoperitoneum can readily be made on chest and/or abdominal radiographs.[116,117] Subdiaphragmatic free air on erect chest radiography, or the double wall (Rigler sign), lucent liver sign, or football sign on abdominal radiography indicates pneumoperitoneum (**Fig. 29**). The lateral decubitus abdominal radiograph is rarely required but useful if the erect chest radiograph is inclusive, CT is unavailable, or the patient is too unstable for transfer (**Fig. 30**). Perforated peptic ulcer disease (PUD) is less common

than in the era before proton pump inhibitor therapy but it is still a leading cause of pneumoperitoneum. In one recent US series, PUD (16%), diverticulitis (16%), trauma (14%), malignancy (14%), bowel ischemia (10%), appendicitis (6%), and endoscopy (4%) were the leading causes of pneumoperitoneum when postoperative pneumoperitoneum was excluded.[118] Further imaging is often not required if the clinical picture clarifies the likely cause and if further imaging would delay surgical management. CT imaging has a role in planning the type of operative treatment, the prognosis, and in assessing those patients who have clinical symptoms of peritonitis but no radiographic signs of perforation. One scenario in which there may be symptoms of peritonitis but no radiographic signs of perforation, is in the setting of PUD perforation into the lesser sac (**Fig. 31**). In this scenario, a collection of gas and fluid is often seen in the lesser sac, posterior to the stomach. When CT imaging is performed in the setting of known pneumoperitoneum, a careful search for the likely causes should be completed. The

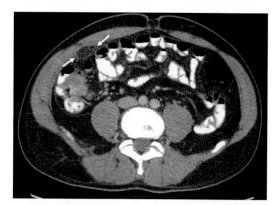

Fig. 28. Axial CT image of a 29-year-old man with right-sided epiploic appendagitis. The typical central ovoid fat density is seen with a surrounding halo of inflammation (*arrows*).

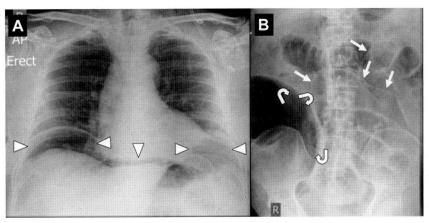

Fig. 29. Erect frontal chest radiograph and frontal abdominal radiograph in a 61-year-old man with pneumoperitoneum from colonic perforation. A large volume of subdiaphragmatic free air is seen (*A, arrowheads*). Multiple double wall (Rigler) signs are seen (*B, arrows*) along with pneumatosis intestinalis and portalis (*B, curved arrows*).

presence of fat stranding, abscess, wall thickening, and potential mural defect helps to localize the site of perforation (**Fig. 32**).

DIAGNOSTIC CRITERIA

Intestinal ischemia
1. Abnormal bowel wall thickness
   a. Paper-thin in acute complete arterial occlusion without reperfusion
   b. Diffusely thickened, possibly with submucosal hemorrhage in other causes of ischemia
2. Abnormal wall enhancement
   a. Absent or hypoenhancement in acute complete arterial occlusion without reperfusion
   b. Hyperenhancement in other causes of ischemia
3. Increased luminal diameter

4. Arterial or venous occlusion
5. Mesenteric fluid or stranding
6. Pneumatosis intestinalis
7. Pneumatosis portalis

Obstruction
1. Dilated proximal bowel (>2.5 cm for small bowel, >9 cm for cecum, >6 cm for remaining colon)
2. Collapsed or nondistended bowel distally
3. Transition point with or without beak sign
4. Possible visible cause at transition point

Infection
1. Enteritis
   a. Circumferential wall thickening

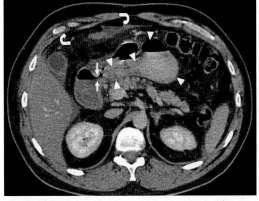

Fig. 30. Lateral decubitus abdominal radiograph in an 87-year-old patient with pneumoperitoneum from perforated peptic ulcer disease. A large volume of free air (*arrowheads*) is seen adjacent to the liver (*arrows*) in the right upper quadrant.

Fig. 31. Axial CT image from a 41-year-old patient with a perforated ulcer in the first part of the duodenum. A defect is seen in the medial duodenum (*arrows*), a large collection is seen in the lesser sac posterior to the stomach (*arrowheads*), and further pneumoperitoneum is also seen anteriorly (*curved arrows*).

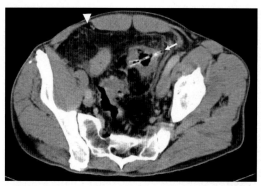

Fig. 32. Axial CT image from a 51-year-old man with a sigmoid perforation secondary to an ingested chicken bone (*arrow*). Considerable stranding is seen adjacent to the foreign body as well as an anterior pneumoperitoneum (*arrowhead*).

b. Asymmetric nodular wall thickening in TB ileitis
c. Mural hyperenhancement
d. Fat stranding
e. Lymphadenopathy (particularly in TB ileitis)
2. Meckel diverticulitis
a. Blind-ending tubular structure approximately 60 cm (2 feet) from the ileocecal valve
b. Wall thickening
c. Surrounding fat stranding
3. Appendicitis
a. Appendix diameter of greater than 6 mm
b. Luminal obliteration
c. Noncompressible appendix at ultrasonography
d. Appendicolith
e. Periappendiceal inflammatory fat changes
4. Colitis
a. Circumferential segmental wall thickening
b. Mucosal hyperenhancement
c. Accordion sign
d. Halo sign
e. Pericolonic fat stranding
f. Submucosal edema
5. Typhlitis
a. As for colitis but may be confined to cecum or involve the ileum
6. Diverticulitis
a. Diverticula
b. Fat stranding that is disproportionate to the mild, smooth, concentric wall thickening
c. Comma or centipede signs
d. Mesenteric root fluid
e. Gradual transition from normal to abnormal bowel thickness

f. Long (5–10 cm) affected segment
g. Minimal or no lymphadenopathy

PEARLS, PITFALLS, VARIANTS

Ischemia
- Bowel wall thickness is difficult to assess in underdistended or overdistended bowel, hence the level of distention should be taken into account. Oral intake of water or perrectal administration of water or air facilitates adequate distention.
- Ischemic bowel, particularly ischemic colon, may contract as a result of ischemia. Again, adequate distention with oral water or perrectal water or air is important.
- Bowel distention with intraluminal fluid and mural thickening as a result of ischemia may be mistaken for mechanical obstruction. Clinical findings, transition point appearance, and ancillary findings are key in this regard.

Obstruction
- As mentioned in the final point regarding ischemia, it is important to differentiate bowel that is dilated as a result of ischemia, from obstructed bowel.
- Paralytic ileus and colonic pseudo-obstruction can be mistaken for adhesional obstruction. The presence of collapsed distal bowel, a transition point beak sign, and visible cause are important differentiating factors.

Infection
- As with mesenteric ischemia, bowel wall thickness in the context of underdistention or overdistention needs careful assessment in patients with colitis or enteritis. Adequate distention with oral or rectal contrast or air is important in optimizing bowel distention.
- Regarding diverticulitis, the findings described earlier are useful in differentiating diverticulitis from colon adenocarcinoma.
- The retrogastric lesser sac needs to be scrutinized in patients with upper abdominal peritonitis to assess for a PUD perforation into the lesser sac.

What the Referring Physician Needs to Know

Ischemia
- Location and length of involved segment
- Cause

- Features raising concern for bowel infarction: pneumatosis intestinalis, pneumatosis portalis, pneumoperitoneum

Obstruction
- Small or large bowel obstruction
- Closed loop or not
- High-grade (complete) or low-grade (incomplete) obstruction
- Cause
- Presence of ischemia
- Presence of perforation

Infection
1. Enteritis
   a. Extent of involvement
   b. Possible cause
   c. Complications
2. Appendicitis
   a. Simple or complicated (phlegmon, abscess)
3. Meckel diverticulitis
   a. Suspected diagnosis
   b. Presence of complications (abscess, bowel obstruction)
4. Colitis, cecitis, and typhlitis
   a. Segment and extent of bowel involved
   b. Likely causes
   c. Presence of complications (toxic megacolon, ischemia, abscess, perforation)
5. Diverticulitis
   a. Location and length of involved segment
   b. Presence of pericolic phlegmon or abscess
   c. Presence of pelvic abscess
   d. Presence of localized walled-off perforation
   e. Presence of generalized pneumoperitoneum
   f. Presence of feculent peritoneal contamination

SUMMARY

Ischemia, obstruction, and gastrointestinal infection are serious conditions frequently associated with significant morbidity and mortality in addition to being entities frequently encountered by emergency radiologists. CT remains the investigation of choice, although other modalities, MR imaging in particular, are going to play a greater role in the future. It is of key importance to ensure that the CT protocol is set up correctly in suspected intestinal ischemia, because multiphase imaging is required for optimal assessment. Measures should also be taken to ensure adequate bowel distention.

DIFFERENTIAL DIAGNOSIS

Intestinal ischemia differentials

1. Bowel obstruction
2. Dilated bowel after endoscopy or contrast enema with pneumatosis
3. Infectious or inflammatory enteritis or colitis
4. Scleroderma, vasculitis with pneumatosis
5. Bowel wall hematoma
6. Gastrointestinal lymphoma
7. Graft-versus-host disease
8. Angioedema

Bowel obstruction differentials

1. Paralytic ileus or pseudo-obstruction
   a. Recent surgery or trauma
   b. Shock
   c. Medications
   d. Electrolyte abnormalities
2. Celiac disease
3. Scleroderma
4. Mesenteric ischemia

Bowel infection differentials

1. Appendicitis or Meckel diverticulitis
   a. Omental infarct
   b. Epiploic appendagitis
   c. Ileitis
   d. Right-sided colonic diverticulitis
   e. Pelvic inflammatory disease
2. Enteritis/ileitis
   a. Crohn disease
   b. Intestinal ischemia
   c. Spondyloarthropathy associated ileitis
   d. Vasculitis
   e. Neoplasm (eg, lymphoma)
   f. Radiation
3. Infectious colitis
   a. Inflammatory bowel disease
   b. Typhlitis
   c. Radiation colitis

d. Diverticulitis

e. Neoplasm

f. Graft-versus-host disease

4. Diverticulitis

a. Colonic neoplasm

b. Colitis

c. Epiploic appendagitis

d. Omental infarct

5. Perforation/pneumoperitoneum

a. Residual postoperative air

b. PUD

c. Diverticulitis

d. Trauma

e. Bowel malignancy

f. Bowel ischemia

g. Appendicitis

h. Endoscopy

REFERENCES

1. Nicolaou S, Kai B, Ho S, et al. Imaging of acute small-bowel obstruction. AJR Am J Roentgenol 2005;185(4):1036–44.

2. Silva AC, Pimenta M, Guimarães LS. Small bowel obstruction: what to look for. Radiographics 2009; 29(2):423–39.

3. Foster NM, McGory ML, Zingmond DS, et al. Small bowel obstruction: a population-based appraisal. J Am Coll Surg 2006;203(2):170–6.

4. Chang RW, Chang JB, Longo WE. Update in management of mesenteric ischemia. World J Gastroenterol 2006;12(20):3243–7.

5. Wiesner W, Khurana B, Ji H, et al. CT of acute bowel ischemia. Radiology 2003;226(3):635–50.

6. Qamar MI, Read AE. Intestinal blood flow. Q J Med 1985;56(220):417–9.

7. Pickhardt PJ, Bhalla S. Intestinal malrotation in adolescents and adults: spectrum of clinical and imaging features. AJR Am J Roentgenol 2002; 179(6):1429–35.

8. Smith HF, Fisher RE, Everett ML, et al. Comparative anatomy and phylogenetic distribution of the mammalian cecal appendix. J Evol Biol 2009; 22(10):1984–99.

9. Elsayes KM, Menias CO, Harvin HJ, et al. Imaging manifestations of Meckel's diverticulum. AJR Am J Roentgenol 2007;189(1):81–8.

10. Khurana B, Ledbetter S, McTavish J, et al. Bowel obstruction revealed by multidetector CT. AJR Am J Roentgenol 2002;178(5):1139–44.

11. Fukuya T, Hawes DR, Lu CC, et al. CT diagnosis of small-bowel obstruction: efficacy in 60 patients. AJR Am J Roentgenol 1992;158(4):765–9 [discussion: 771–2].

12. Thompson WM, Kilani RK, Smith BB, et al. Accuracy of abdominal radiography in acute small-bowel obstruction: does reviewer experience matter? AJR Am J Roentgenol 2007;188(3):W233–8.

13. Gans SL, Stoker J, Boermeester MA. Plain abdominal radiography in acute abdominal pain; past, present, and future. Int J Gen Med 2012;5:525–33.

14. Mendez D, Caviness AC, Ma L, et al. The diagnostic accuracy of an abdominal radiograph with signs and symptoms of intussusception. Am J Emerg Med 2012;30(3):426–31.

15. Maglinte DD, Reyes BL, Harmon BH, et al. Reliability and role of plain film radiography and CT in the diagnosis of small-bowel obstruction. AJR Am J Roentgenol 1996;167(6):1451–5.

16. Furukawa A, Kanasaki S, Kono N, et al. CT diagnosis of acute mesenteric ischemia from various causes. AJR Am J Roentgenol 2009;192(2):408–16.

17. Lee SS, Park SH. Computed tomography evaluation of gastrointestinal bleeding and acute mesenteric ischemia. Radiol Clin North Am 2013;51(1): 29–43.

18. Kwok HC, Dirkzwager I, Duncan DS, et al. The accuracy of multidetector computed tomography in the diagnosis of non-occlusive mesenteric ischaemia in patients after cardiovascular surgery. Crit Care Resusc 2014;16(2):90–5.

19. Murphy KP, McLaughlin PD, O'Connor OJ, et al. Imaging the small bowel. Curr Opin Gastroenterol 2014;30(2):134–40.

20. Karul M, Berliner C, Keller S, et al. Imaging of appendicitis in adults. Rofo 2014;186(6):551–8.

21. McLaughlin PD, Maher MM. Nonneoplastic diseases of the small intestine: differential diagnosis and Crohn disease. AJR Am J Roentgenol 2013; 201(2):W174–82.

22. McLaughlin PD, Maher MM. Nonneoplastic diseases of the small intestine: clinical, pathophysiologic, and imaging characteristics. AJR Am J Roentgenol 2013;201(3):W382–90.

23. Barnett RE, Younga J, Harris B, et al. Accuracy of computed tomography in small bowel obstruction. Am Surg 2013;79(6):641–3.

24. Santillan CS. Computed tomography of small bowel obstruction. Radiol Clin North Am 2013; 51(1):17–27.

25. Mullan CP, Siewert B, Eisenberg RL. Small bowel obstruction. AJR Am J Roentgenol 2012;198(2): W105–17.

26. Suri S, Gupta S, Sudhakar PJ, et al. Comparative evaluation of plain films, ultrasound and CT in the diagnosis of intestinal obstruction. Acta Radiol 1999;40(4):422–8.

27. Hayakawa K, Tanikake M, Yoshida S, et al. Radiological diagnosis of large-bowel obstruction: neoplastic etiology. Emerg Radiol 2013;20(1):69–76.

28. Mun S, Ernst RD, Chen K, et al. Rapid CT diagnosis of acute appendicitis with IV contrast material. Emerg Radiol 2006;12(3):99–102.

29. Beall DP, Fortman BJ, Lawler BC, et al. Imaging bowel obstruction: a comparison between fast magnetic resonance imaging and helical computed tomography. Clin Radiol 2002;57(8):719–24.

30. Taylor MR, Lalani N. Adult small bowel obstruction. Acad Emerg Med 2013;20(6):528–44.

31. Shih MC, Hagspiel KD. CTA and MRA in mesenteric ischemia: part 1, role in diagnosis and differential diagnosis. AJR Am J Roentgenol 2007; 188(2):452–61.

32. Rha SE, Ha HK, Lee SH, et al. CT and MR imaging findings of bowel ischemia from various primary causes. Radiographics 2000;20(1):29–42.

33. Aspelund G, Fingeret A, Gross E, et al. Ultrasonography/MRI versus CT for diagnosing appendicitis. Pediatrics 2014;133(4):586–93.

34. Öistämö E, Hjern F, Blomqvist L, et al. Cancer and diverticulitis of the sigmoid colon. Differentiation with computed tomography versus magnetic resonance imaging: preliminary experiences. Acta Radiol 2013;54(3):237–41.

35. Hefny AF, Corr P, Abu-Zidan FM. The role of ultrasound in the management of intestinal obstruction. J Emerg Trauma Shock 2012;5(1):84–6.

36. Reginelli A, Genovese E, Cappabianca S, et al. Intestinal ischemia: US-CT findings correlations. Crit Ultrasound J 2013;5(Suppl 1):S7.

37. Schieda N, Fasih N, Shabana W. Triphasic CT in the diagnosis of acute mesenteric ischaemia. Eur Radiol 2013;23(7):1891–900.

38. Lee SY, Coughlin B, Wolfe JM, et al. Prospective comparison of helical CT of the abdomen and pelvis without and with oral contrast in assessing acute abdominal pain in adult emergency department patients. Emerg Radiol 2006;12(4):150–7.

39. Vokurka J, Olejnik J, Jedlicka V, et al. Acute mesenteric ischemia. Hepatogastroenterology 2008; 55(85):1349–52.

40. Desai RK, Tagliabue JR, Wegryn SA, et al. CT evaluation of wall thickening in the alimentary tract. Radiographics 1991;11(5):771–83 [discussion: 784].

41. Macari M, Balthazar EJ. CT of bowel wall thickening: significance and pitfalls of interpretation. AJR Am J Roentgenol 2001;176(5):1105–16.

42. Lee R, Tung HK, Tung PH, et al. CT in acute mesenteric ischaemia. Clin Radiol 2003;58(4):279–87.

43. Horton KM, Fishman EK. Multidetector CT angiography in the diagnosis of mesenteric ischemia. Radiol Clin North Am 2007;45(2):275–88.

44. Geffroy Y, Boulay-Coletta I, Jullès MC, et al. Increased unenhanced bowel-wall attenuation at multidetector CT is highly specific of ischemia complicating small-bowel obstruction. Radiology 2014;270(1):159–67.

45. Tseng CY, Chiu YH, Chuang JL, et al. How to differentiate spontaneous intramural intestinal hemorrhage from acute mesenteric ischemia. Am J Emerg Med 2013;31(11):1586–90.

46. Chou CK, Mak CW, Tzeng WS, et al. CT of small bowel ischemia. Abdom Imaging 2004;29(1): 18–22.

47. Cardin F, Fratta S, Perissinotto E, et al. Clinical correlation of mesenteric vascular disease in older patients. Aging Clin Exp Res 2012;24(Suppl 3):43–6.

48. Grendell JH, Ockner RK. Mesenteric venous thrombosis. Gastroenterology 1982;82(2):358–72.

49. Oldenburg WA, Lau LL, Rodenberg TJ, et al. Acute mesenteric ischemia: a clinical review. Arch Intern Med 2004;164(10):1054–62.

50. Hayakawa K, Tanikake M, Yoshida S, et al. CT findings of small bowel strangulation: the importance of contrast enhancement. Emerg Radiol 2013;20(1):3–9.

51. Zalcman M, Sy M, Donckier V, et al. Helical CT signs in the diagnosis of intestinal ischemia in small-bowel obstruction. AJR Am J Roentgenol 2000;175(6):1601–7.

52. Milone M, Di Minno MN, Musella M, et al. Computed tomography findings of pneumatosis and portomesenteric venous gas in acute bowel ischemia. World J Gastroenterol 2013;19(39): 6579–84.

53. Feczko PJ, Mezwa DG, Farah MC, et al. Clinical significance of pneumatosis of the bowel wall. Radiographics 1992;12(6):1069–78.

54. Sebastià C, Quiroga S, Espin E, et al. Portomesenteric vein gas: pathologic mechanisms, CT findings, and prognosis. Radiographics 2000;20(5): 1213–24 [discussion: 1224–6].

55. Hayakawa K, Tanikake M, Yoshida S, et al. Radiological diagnosis of large-bowel obstruction: nonneoplastic etiology. Jpn J Radiol 2012;30(7): 541–52.

56. Choi JS, Lim JS, Kim H, et al. Colonic pseudoobstruction: CT findings. AJR Am J Roentgenol 2008;190(6):1521–6.

57. Lee KJ, Jung KW, Myung SJ, et al. The clinical characteristics of colonic pseudo-obstruction and the factors associated with medical treatment response: a study based on a multicenter database in Korea. J Korean Med Sci 2014;29(5):699–703.

58. Nevitt PC. The string of pearls sign. Radiology 2000;214(1):157–8.

59. Millet I, Ruyer A, Alili C, et al. Adhesive small-bowel obstruction: value of CT in identifying findings associated with the effectiveness of nonsurgical treatment. Radiology 2014;273(2):425–32.

60. Suri RR, Vora P, Kirby JM, et al. Computed tomography features associated with operative

management for nonstrangulating small bowel obstruction. Can J Surg 2014;57(4):254–9.

61. Lazarus DE, Slywotsky C, Bennett GL, et al. Frequency and relevance of the "small-bowel feces" sign on CT in patients with small-bowel obstruction. AJR Am J Roentgenol 2004;183(5):1361–6.

62. Jacobs SL, Rozenblit A, Ricci Z, et al. Small bowel faeces sign in patients without small bowel obstruction. Clin Radiol 2007;62(4):353–7.

63. Murphy KP, O'Connor OJ, Maher MM. Adult abdominal hernias. AJR Am J Roentgenol 2014; 202(6):W506–11.

64. Epelman M. The whirlpool sign. Radiology 2006; 240(3):910–1.

65. Levine MS, Carucci LR. Imaging of bariatric surgery: normal anatomy and postoperative complications. Radiology 2014;270(2):327–41.

66. Ladizinski B, Amjad H, Rukhman E, et al. The coffee bean sign and sigmoid volvulus in an elderly adult. J Am Geriatr Soc 2013;61(10):1843–4.

67. Orchard JL, Petorak V. Abnormal abdominal CT findings in a patient with giardiasis. Resolution after treatment. Dig Dis Sci 1995;40(2):346–8.

68. Dilauro S, Crum-Cianflone NF. Ileitis: when it is not Crohn's disease. Curr Gastroenterol Rep 2010; 12(4):249–58.

69. Paustian FF, Bockus HL. So-called primary ulcerohypertrophic ileocecal tuberculosis. Am J Med 1959;27:509–18.

70. Boudiaf M, Zidi SH, Soyer P, et al. Tuberculous colitis mimicking Crohn's disease: utility of computed tomography in the differentiation. Eur Radiol 1998; 8(7):1221–3.

71. Balthazar EJ, Charles HW, Megibow AJ. *Salmonella*- and *Shigella*-induced ileitis: CT findings in four patients. J Comput Assist Tomogr 1996; 20(3):375–8.

72. Thurley PD, Halliday KE, Somers JM, et al. Radiological features of Meckel's diverticulum and its complications. Clin Radiol 2009;64(2):109–18.

73. Kusumoto H, Yoshida M, Takahashi I, et al. Complications and diagnosis of Meckel's diverticulum in 776 patients. Am J Surg 1992;164(4):382–3.

74. Bennett GL, Birnbaum BA, Balthazar EJ. CT of Meckel's diverticulitis in 11 patients. AJR Am J Roentgenol 2004;182(3):625–9.

75. Callahan MJ, Rodriguez DP, Taylor GA. CT of appendicitis in children. Radiology 2002;224(2): 325–32.

76. Puylaert JB. Acute appendicitis: US evaluation using graded compression. Radiology 1986;158(2): 355–60.

77. Orth RC, Guillerman RP, Zhang W, et al. Prospective comparison of MR imaging and US for the diagnosis of pediatric appendicitis. Radiology 2014;272(1):233–40.

78. Ramalingam V, LeBedis C, Kelly JR, et al. Evaluation of a sequential multi-modality imaging algorithm for the diagnosis of acute appendicitis in the pregnant female. Emerg Radiol 2014. [Epub ahead of print].

79. Sivit CJ, Applegate KE, Stallion A, et al. Imaging evaluation of suspected appendicitis in a pediatric population: effectiveness of sonography versus CT. AJR Am J Roentgenol 2000;175(4):977–80.

80. Peña BM, Taylor GA. Radiologists' confidence in interpretation of sonography and CT in suspected pediatric appendicitis. AJR Am J Roentgenol 2000;175(1):71–4.

81. Koning JL, Naheedy JH, Kruk PG. Diagnostic performance of contrast-enhanced MR for acute appendicitis and alternative causes of abdominal pain in children. Pediatr Radiol 2014;44(8):948–55.

82. Pinto Leite N, Pereira JM, Cunha R, et al. CT evaluation of appendicitis and its complications: imaging techniques and key diagnostic findings. AJR Am J Roentgenol 2005;185(2):406–17.

83. Rodgers PM, Verma R. Transabdominal ultrasound for bowel evaluation. Radiol Clin North Am 2013; 51(1):133–48.

84. Issa M, Ananthakrishnan AN, Binion DG. *Clostridium difficile* and inflammatory bowel disease. Inflamm Bowel Dis 2008;14(10):1432–42.

85. Ramachandran I, Sinha R, Rodgers P. Pseudomembranous colitis revisited: spectrum of imaging findings. Clin Radiol 2006;61(7):535–44.

86. Kirkpatrick ID, Greenberg HM. Evaluating the CT diagnosis of *Clostridium difficile* colitis: should CT guide therapy? AJR Am J Roentgenol 2001; 176(3):635–9.

87. Thoeni RF, Cello JP. CT imaging of colitis. Radiology 2006;240(3):623–38.

88. Fishman EK, Kavuru M, Jones B, et al. Pseudomembranous colitis: CT evaluation of 26 cases. Radiology 1991;180(1):57–60.

89. Macari M, Balthazar EJ, Megibow AJ. The accordion sign at CT: a nonspecific finding in patients with colonic edema. Radiology 1999;211(3):743–6.

90. Wittenberg J, Harisinghani MG, Jhaveri K, et al. Algorithmic approach to CT diagnosis of the abnormal bowel wall. Radiographics 2002;22(5): 1093–107 [discussion: 1107–9].

91. Sinharay R, Atkin G, Mohamid W, et al. Caecal amoebic colitis mimicking a colorectal cancer. J Surg Case Rep 2011;2011(11):1.

92. Saha K, Sengupta M, Mitra S, et al. Amoeboma of colon mimicking colonic carcinoma. Trop Parasitol 2014;4(2):122–4.

93. Mourra N, Colignon N, Broudin C, et al. Amoebic hepatic and renal abscesses complicating amoebic colitis. Clin Res Hepatol Gastroenterol 2014;38(5):541–2.

94. Moorchung N, Singh V, Srinivas V, et al. Caecal amebic colitis mimicking obstructing right sided colonic carcinoma with liver metastases: a rare case. J Cancer Res Ther 2010;10(2):440–2.

95. Nesher L, Rolston KV. Neutropenic enterocolitis, a growing concern in the era of widespread use of aggressive chemotherapy. Clin Infect Dis 2013; 56(5):711–7.

96. Kirkpatrick ID, Greenberg HM. Gastrointestinal complications in the neutropenic patient: characterization and differentiation with abdominal CT. Radiology 2003;226(3):668–74.

97. Gomez L, Martino R, Rolston KV. Neutropenic enterocolitis: spectrum of the disease and comparison of definite and possible cases. Clin Infect Dis 1998;27(4):695–9.

98. Hoeffel C, Crema MD, Belkacem A, et al. Multi-detector row CT: spectrum of diseases involving the ileocecal area. Radiographics 2006;26(5):1373–90.

99. Gan SI, Beck PL. A new look at toxic megacolon: an update and review of incidence, etiology, pathogenesis, and management. Am J Gastroenterol 2003;98(11):2363–71.

100. Moulin V, Dellon P, Laurent O, et al. Toxic megacolon in patients with severe acute colitis: computed tomographic features. Clin Imaging 2011;35(6):431–6.

101. Imbriaco M, Balthazar EJ. Toxic megacolon: role of CT in evaluation and detection of complications. Clin Imaging 2001;25(5):349–54.

102. Benchimol EI, Turner D, Mann EH, et al. Toxic megacolon in children with inflammatory bowel disease: clinical and radiographic characteristics. Am J Gastroenterol 2008;103(6):1524–31.

103. Slack WW. The anatomy, pathology, and some clinical features of diverticulitis of the colon. Br J Surg 1962;50:185–90.

104. Peery AF, Dellon ES, Lund J, et al. Burden of gastrointestinal disease in the United States: 2012 update. Gastroenterology 2012;143(5):1179–87.e1–3.

105. Peery AF, Sandler RS. Diverticular disease: reconsidering conventional wisdom. Clin Gastroenterol Hepatol 2013;11(12):1532–7.

106. Painter NS, Truelove SC, Ardran GM, et al. Segmentation and the localization of intraluminal pressures in the human colon, with special reference to the pathogenesis of colonic diverticula. Gastroenterology 1965;49:169–77.

107. Peery AF, Barrett PR, Park D, et al. A high-fiber diet does not protect against asymptomatic diverticulosis. Gastroenterology 2012;142(2):266–72.e1.

108. Crowe FL, Balkwill A, Cairns BJ, et al. Source of dietary fibre and diverticular disease incidence: a prospective study of UK women. Gut 2014;63(9): 1450–6.

109. Horton KM, Corl FM, Fishman EK. CT evaluation of the colon: inflammatory disease. Radiographics 2000;20(2):399–418.

110. Pereira JM, Sirlin CB, Pinto PS, et al. Disproportionate fat stranding: a helpful CT sign in patients with acute abdominal pain. Radiographics 2004; 24(3):703–15.

111. Hinchey EJ, Schaal PG, Richards GK. Treatment of perforated diverticular disease of the colon. Adv Surg 1978;12:85–109.

112. Chintapalli KN, Chopra S, Ghiatas AA, et al. Diverticulitis versus colon cancer: differentiation with helical CT findings. Radiology 1999;210(2): 429–35.

113. Jang HJ, Lim HK, Lee SJ, et al. Acute diverticulitis of the cecum and ascending colon: the value of thin-section helical CT findings in excluding colonic carcinoma. AJR Am J Roentgenol 2000;174(5): 1397–402.

114. Padidar AM, Jeffrey RB, Mindelzun RE, et al. Differentiating sigmoid diverticulitis from carcinoma on CT scans: mesenteric inflammation suggests diverticulitis. AJR Am J Roentgenol 1994; 163(1):81–3.

115. Singh AK, Gervais DA, Hahn PF, et al. CT appearance of acute appendagitis. AJR Am J Roentgenol 2004;183(5):1303–7.

116. Baker SR. Pneumoperitoneum—the radiographic and clinical virtues of the supine abdominal film. Emerg Radiol 2012;19(6):547–8.

117. Kasznia-Brown J, Cook C. Radiological signs of pneumoperitoneum: a pictorial review. Br J Hosp Med (Lond) 2006;67(12):634–9.

118. Kumar A, Muir MT, Cohn SM, et al. The etiology of pneumoperitoneum in the 21st century. J Trauma Acute Care Surg 2012;73(3):542–8.

Imaging of Nontraumatic Neuroradiology Emergencies

Kathleen R. Fink, MD[a],*, Jayson L. Benjert, DO[b]

KEYWORDS

- Subarachnoid hemorrhage • Vasogenic edema • Hydrocephalus • Neurologic abnormalities

KEY POINTS

- Emergency neuroradiology can be challenging because of the wide range of conditions that present with acute neurologic symptoms or signs.
- Nonenhanced computed tomography (NECT) of the head is almost always the most appropriate first imaging test and is extremely useful for excluding life-threatening conditions.
- The imaging findings of a variety of neurologic abnormalities overlap on NECT, however, and the differential diagnosis may be extremely broad.
- The first step to narrowing the differential diagnosis and providing imaging workup includes classifying the NECT findings into a broad category, as the authors have tried to do in this article.
- Based on the type of imaging abnormality, further imaging workup may include computed tomographic angiography (CTA), digital subtraction angiography (DSA), and/or MR imaging.
- Familiarity with specific imaging finding that suggests a specific diagnosis may help further facilitate appropriate clinical workup and treatment.

INTRODUCTION

NECT is the imaging study of choice for the evaluation of acute neurologic conditions referable to the brain. NECT is fast, widely available, and well tolerated by critically ill patients. NECT is excellent at excluding most life-threatening conditions including intracranial hemorrhage, brain herniation, acute hydrocephalus, and large mass. The emergency radiologist must be able to not only identify these conditions but also come up with a succinct, relevant differential diagnosis in order to facilitate patient triage, direct further evaluation and management, and alert the referring provider to diagnoses, which may not have been considered.

This article approaches the broad spectrum of nontraumatic neurologic emergencies by discussing patterns of findings on NECT and differential diagnoses, suggesting algorithms for further workup, and highlighting key difficult or important diagnoses. Specific angiographic or MR imaging features that might lead to a particular diagnosis are also discussed.

SCENARIO 1: SUBARACHNOID HEMORRHAGE
Imaging Protocol

Thunderclap headache is the classic presenting symptom of patients with spontaneous

---

K.R. Fink has the following disclosures: spouse is site coinvestigator for contrast agent clinical trials involving Bayer Pharmaceuticals, Guerbet, and Bracco. J.L. Benjert has no conflicts of interest to disclose.
[a] Department of Radiology, University of Washington, Box 359728, 325 9th Avenue, Seattle, WA 98104, USA;
[b] Department of Radiology, VA Puget Sound Health Care System, 1660 South Columbian Way, Seattle, WA 98108, USA
* Corresponding author.
E-mail address: ktozer@u.washington.edu

subarachnoid hemorrhage (SAH), and NECT is the preferred imaging study for suspected SAH.[1] If the result is negative, lumbar puncture should be performed.[2]

Because ruptured aneurysms account for approximately 85% of spontaneous SAHs,[3] excluding aneurysm is crucial. DSA is the gold standard, although CTA is sensitive for aneurysms greater than 3 mm.[4,5] Magnetic resonance (MR) angiography is not sensitive enough to conclusively exclude small aneurysm. If the result of CTA is negative, DSA is the next step, unless the pattern of blood meets criteria for perimesencephalic hemorrhage (PMH, see below). Some investigators suggest that negative result of CTA is sufficient to exclude aneurysm in this setting,[6] although practice varies, with most centers obtaining at least 1 and possibly 2 subsequent DSAs. If the criteria for PMH are not met, DSA is indicated, and if the result is negative, the examination is often repeated at 1 week.[4]

Findings

SAH manifests as hyperdense blood in the cerebrospinal fluid (CSF) spaces, including the basilar cisterns and sulci, with possible redistribution into the ventricles. The pattern of SAH may suggest the underlying cause.[7]

Differential Diagnosis

Diffuse or basilar predominant subarachnoid hemorrhage

Aneurysmal subarachnoid hemorrhage About 85% of spontaneous SAH is caused by rupture of aneurysm.[3] Aneurysms appear as saccular outpouchings at vascular branch points, and SAH patterns may suggest a particular aneurysm. For example, SAH centered on the sylvian fissure suggests middle cerebral artery aneurysm, whereas SAH in the anterior interhemispheric fissure suggests anterior cerebral artery aneurysm. Asymmetric SAH around the medulla or inferiorly in the posterior fossa should suggest anterior or posterior inferior cerebellar artery aneurysm.

Focal contour abnormality of the aneurysm sac on vascular imaging suggests a rupture point. Aneurysms occur most commonly in the anterior circulation, but specific areas to inspect when evaluating CTA for aneurysm include terminal internal carotid artery, anterior communicating artery, middle cerebral artery bifurcation/trifurcation, posterior communicating artery, basilar tip, and posterior inferior cerebral artery origin.

Benign perimesencephalic subarachnoid hemorrhage Spontaneous SAH can be classified as non-aneurysmal or benign PMH approximately 10% of the time.[8] Specific imaging criteria are required to make this diagnosis: NECT obtained within 3 days of ictus showing hemorrhage centered anterior to the midbrain or within the quadrigeminal plate cistern. The hemorrhage cannot extend to the lateral portions of the sylvian fissures or anterior part of the interhemispheric fissure. Some layering of blood in the lateral ventricles is permitted, but frank intraventricular hemorrhage is not and no parenchymal hematoma is allowed (**Fig. 1**).[9]

Patients with PMH tend to have a less severe clinical course than those with aneurysmal SAH, and rebleeding does not occur. Venous bleeding from a cisternal vein is believed to be the cause.[3]

Other As listed in **Table 1**, a variety of other vascular lesions may also cause diffuse or perimesencephalic SAH, most of which can be excluded

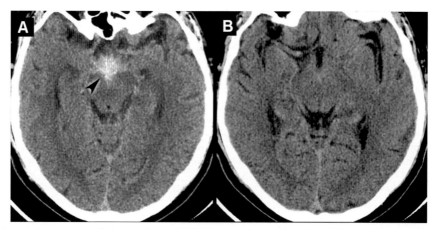

Fig. 1. Benign perimesencephalic hemorrhage. NECT demonstrates subarachnoid hemorrhage centered anterior to the midbrain (*arrowhead, A*). There is no extension to the sylvian fissures or anterior interhemispheric fissure (*B*).

Table 1 Differential diagnosis of spontaneous SAH by location	
Diffuse or Perimesencephalic	**Convexity**

• Saccular aneurysm
• PMH (specific criteria, see text)
• Nonsaccular aneurysm
  ○ Fusiform
  ○ Dissecting
• Arterial dissection
• Vascular malformation
  ○ AVM
  ○ Dural AVF
• Tumor
• Vasculitis
	• RCVS
	• Cerebral amyloid angiopathy
	• PRES
	• Cerebral venous thrombosis
	• Septic emboli, septic aneurysm
	• Coagulopathy
	• Moyamoya disease
	• Superficial vascular malformation
	• Tumor
	• Vasculitis

Abbreviations: AVF, arteriovenous fistulas; AVM, arteriovenous malformation; PRES, posterior reversible encephalopathy syndrome; RCVS, reversible cerebral vasoconstriction syndrome.
Adapted from Marder CP, Narla V, Fink JR, et al. Subarachnoid hemorrhage: beyond aneurysms. AJR Am J Roentgenol 2014;202(1):27.

by CTA and/or DSA. In rare cases, posterior fossa or spinal tumors or vascular malformations may cause low SAH, in which case MR imaging may be helpful to make the diagnosis.[7]

Convexity subarachnoid hemorrhage

Convexity SAH has a different differential diagnosis than basilar or diffuse SAH[7] and includes reversible cerebral vasoconstriction syndrome (RCVS) in patients younger than 60 years, and cerebral amyloid angiopathy (CAA) in those older than 60 years. **Table 1** lists additional causes.

Reversible cerebral vasoconstriction syndrome RCVS is a clinical syndrome of headache and variable neurologic deficits with hemorrhage or ischemia evident on imaging. A variety of possible triggers are reported, including vasoactive medications, stimulants, serotonergic medications, and strenuous activity. RCVS may cause isolated convexity SAH, intraparenchymal hemorrhage (IPH), or subdural hematoma (SDH) as well as ischemic infarcts. Vascular imaging demonstrates segmental areas of vasoconstriction that may not be initially evident (**Fig. 2**), which resolve with time and removal of the inciting factor.[10,11]

Other CAA is associated with cortical SAH, and is described further below in the section on IPH. Posterior reversible encephalopathy syndrome (PRES) may also manifest as SAH and is described further below in the section on vasogenic edema. Cortical or dural venous thrombosis is an uncommon cause of convexity SAH but an important diagnosis because it is difficult to make both clinically and by imaging (**Fig. 3**).[12]

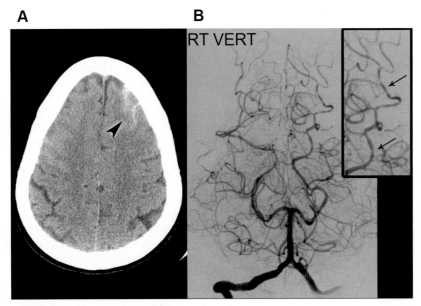

Fig. 2. Reversible cerebral vasoconstriction syndrome. NECT demonstrates convexity SAH (*arrowhead, A*). Right vertebral artery injection from digital subtraction angiography (*B*) demonstrates irregular segmental narrowing in the posterior cerebral arteries (*arrows, inset*).

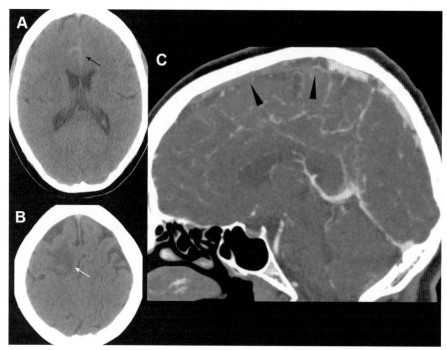

Fig. 3. Superior sagittal sinus thrombosis. NECT (*A, B*) demonstrates SAH in the anterior interhemispheric fissure (*black arrow*) as well as right frontal vasogenic edema (*white arrow*). Venous phase CT (*C*) demonstrates nonfilling of the anterior portion of the superior sagittal sinus (*arrowheads*), consistent with thrombosis.

Key Points

- Spontaneous basilar SAH is commonly caused by a saccular aneurysm, and exclusion of aneurysm by angiography is critical.
- PMH meeting specific imaging criteria is usually not caused by an underlying aneurysm and confers a more benign clinical course.
- The differential diagnosis of convexity SAH is different from that of basilar or diffuse SAH, and includes RCVS in younger adults.

SCENARIO 2: INTRAPARENCHYMAL HEMORRHAGE
Imaging Protocol

NECT is the first test of choice in the setting of suspected IPH. If present, further evaluation with CTA, DSA, or MR imaging with contrast may all be appropriate depending on the clinical scenario, although practice patterns are variable and differ based on patient age and IPH location.[13] T2*-weighted MR imaging is helpful to detect additional hemorrhages, the pattern of which may suggest a specific diagnosis.

One recently proposed imaging algorithm by Ciura and Romero[14] is similar to that followed at the authors' institution, whereby most patients with IPH diagnosed by computed tomography (CT) undergo immediate CTA. DSA is reserved for those patients with suspicious findings at CTA or patients with a negative result of CTA in whom clinical suspicion is high, such as younger or nonhypertensive patients. Contrast-enhanced MR imaging is a useful adjunct to evaluate underlying enhancing mass or the presence of additional microhemorrhages.

Findings

IPH appears as hyperdense acute hemorrhage in the brain parenchyma and may be classified by location: lobar, deep, or posterior fossa. On MR imaging, parenchymal blood products have characteristic T1 and T2 appearance as the blood products break down, which may help to date the IPH.

Angiography may reveal an underlying vascular malformation. Contrast-enhanced MR imaging may identify surrounding enhancement, although care must be taken to differentiate inherent T1 hyperintensity from true enhancement. Variable surrounding vasogenic edema is present. T2*-weighted MR imaging shows blooming of the hemorrhage, as well as microhemorrhages, which appear as punctate areas of blooming artifact.

Differential Diagnosis

The differential diagnosis of IPH is broad, with many possible causes (**Table 2**).[15] Hypertension and amyloid angiopathy are the most common

Table 2
Classification for nontraumatic IPH based on the cause

Primary	
Hypertension	Most common cause of deep hemorrhage.
Amyloid angiopathy	Favors lobar/cortical location Older patients, >55 y
Secondary	
Coagulopathy	• Medication ○ Warfarin, heparin, enoxaparin • Congenital bleeding disorder
Structural vascular lesion	• Cavernous malformation • Arteriovenous malformation • Aneurysm

Tumor	• Metastasis
	• Primary
	  ○ Glioblastoma
	  ○ Oligodendrogial tumors

Systemic disease	• Liver disease • Thrombocytopenia
Rare others	• Cerebral venous thrombosis • Amphetamine use • Vasculitis • RCVS • Moyamoya disease

nontraumatic causes reported,[15,16] with hemorrhagic tumors, structural vascular lesions, and anticoagulation being other frequent causes. Localizing the hemorrhage as lobar or cortical versus deep helps refine the differential diagnosis. The patient's age and clinical history, including the use of anticoagulants, also informs the differential.

Deep intraparenchymal hemorrhage

Deep IPH includes hemorrhage into the basal ganglia, thalamus, brain stem, and posterior fossa. In most cases of older patients with hypertension and basal ganglia IPH, hypertensive hemorrhage is the diagnosis, although reports find that 13% or more patients may have an underlying structural vascular lesion such as aneurysm, cavernous malformation (CM), arteriovenous malformation (AVM), or moyamoya disease,[17] regardless of the age or coincident hypertension. Diagnostic yield of angiography seems to be higher in younger adults (age <45 years) and in those without hypertension[18] and should be strongly considered in the

evaluation of these patients. Uniform imaging guidelines, however, do not exist.[13]

Lobar intraparenchymal hemorrhage

Lobar hemorrhage refers to bleeding involving the cortex and adjacent white matter of a hemisphere and is also called cortical-subcortical hemorrhage. Lobar hemorrhage is often associated with CAA in older patients,[19] but may be due to a variety of causes.

Hypertensive hemorrhage Hypertensive hemorrhage commonly involves deep structures, particularly the basal ganglia/external capsule (60%–65%), thalamus (15%–20%), as well as cerebellum and pons (10% combined)[14] and may extend to the ventricles. Hemorrhage in these locations, particularly in a patient with a history of hypertension, should favor this diagnosis.[19] The presence of microbleeds isolated to the deep structures is a helpful confirmatory finding (**Fig. 4**).[20]

As mentioned above, there may be other causes of deep hemorrhages, including anticoagulation or underlying tumor or vascular lesion. Conversely, hypertensive hemorrhages occur in a cortical location 5% to 10% of the time.[14,15]

Cerebral amyloid angiopathy The diagnosis of CAA is definitively made by tissue analysis, which is often not available. Thus, a set of imaging criteria supporting this diagnosis have been reported (**Table 3**) and include primary lobar hemorrhage in a patient aged 55 years or older.[21] SAH is also associated with CAA. T2*-weighted MR imaging may show additional microhemorrhages at the gray-white junction[20] or convexity hemosiderosis (**Fig. 5**). Recent early work suggests that dilated perivascular spaces (specifically >20) in the centrum semiovale may improve the sensitivity of the Boston criteria without altering the specificity.[22]

Coagulopathy Coagulopathy, usually related to medication but rarely caused by a congenital or acquired condition, can cause IPH, and accounts for 10% to 20% of cases of nontraumatic IPH.[14] Clinical history and laboratory evaluation are the key to making this diagnosis. Medications associated with IPH include warfarin, heparin, and enoxaparin. Antiplatelet agents such as aspirin are associated with a slightly increased risk of ICH. Most IPHs associated with anticoagulant medications are lobar.[14] SDHs are also seen.

Structural vascular lesion Although more commonly reported with lobar hemorrhages, vascular lesions may also cause deep IPH and account for approximately 15% of spontaneous

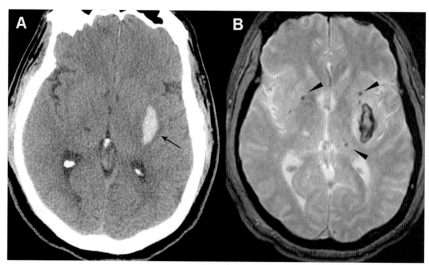

Fig. 4. Hypertensive hemorrhage. NECT (*A*) demonstrates deep intraparenchymal hemorrhage (*arrow*) centered in the left putamen/external capsule. T2*-weighted MR imaging (*B*) redemonstrates the hemorrhage, as well as multiple deep microhemorrhages, consistent with hypertensive hemorrhages.

ICH.[14] Causes include CMs, AVMs, and aneurysms, and most can be identified with CTA.[23]

Most AVMs appear on CTA as a tangle of abnormal vessels with a large draining vein. DSA is usually the next step to better characterize feeding arteries and venous drainage and for treatment planning. Dural arteriovenous fistulas rarely present with IPH and may be difficult to identify on CTA. DSA is diagnostic. Aneurysms may cause IPH, although usually there is associated SAH or SDH. Infectious (mycotic) aneurysms are located in atypical locations often over the cortical surface, and a careful search is required for diagnosis.

CMs may acutely hemorrhage and are in the differential for IPH. CMs have a characteristic appearance on MR imaging, including locules of

Table 3
Boston criteria for CAA-related hemorrhage

Category	Description
Definite CAA	Postmortem examination: Lobar, cortical, or corticosubcortical hemorrhage Severe CAA with vasculopathy No other cause
Probable CAA with supporting pathology	Clinical data with pathologic tissue (biopsy or evacuated hematoma) showing: Lobar, cortical, or corticosubcortical hemorrhage Some CAA in specimen No other cause
Probable CAA	Clinical data and MR imaging or CT showing: Multiple lobar, cortical, or corticosubcortical hemorrhages Age $\geq$55 y No other cause
Possible CAA	Clinical data and MR imaging or CT showing: Single lobar, cortical, or corticosubcortical hemorrhage Age $\geq$55 y No other cause

Abbreviation: CT, computed tomography.
Adapted from Knudsen KA, Rosand J, Karluk D, et al. Clinical diagnosis of cerebral amyloid angiopathy: validation of the Boston criteria. Neurology 2001;56(4):539.

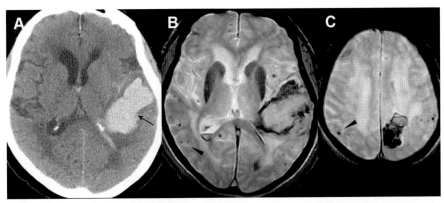

Fig. 5. Cerebral amyloid angiopathy. NECT (*A*) demonstrates a left temporal lobar hemorrhage (*arrow*). T2*-weighted MR imaging redemonstrates the hemorrhage (*B*), as well as multiple microhemorrhages (*arrowheads B, C*) at the gray-white junction. There is an additional nonacute left frontoparietal lobar hemorrhage (*C*). These imaging findings meet Boston criteria for probable CAA.

T1 and T2 signal hyperintensity and a complete hemosiderin ring (**Fig. 6**). Enhancement, if present, is minimal. On CT, CMs that have not recently hemorrhaged may appear hyperdense and can mimic acute IPH (see **Fig. 6**). The presence of an associated developmental venous anomaly, appearing as a confluence of veins into a central trunk ("medusa head"), is a confirmatory finding.[24] CMs may be multiple.

Other vascular abnormalities such as vasculitis (infectious or drug induced), RCVS, and moyamoya disease may also cause IPH. Angiography, either CTA or DSA, is helpful to make these diagnoses.

Underlying mass lesion Hemorrhagic neoplasms cause up to 5% of spontaneous IPH.[14] Certain mass lesions have a propensity to hemorrhage, including metastases. While hypervascular metastases such as those from renal cell carcinoma, melanoma, choriocarcinoma, and thyroid cancer have a particular propensity to hemorrhage, lung and breast cancers are common hemorrhagic metastases because of their overall prevalence.[25]

Brain metastases tend to occur in the cerebral hemispheres (up to 80%), although cerebellar and basal ganglia metastases also occur.[25] Thus hemorrhagic metastases tend to cause lobar IPH, although IPH can occur anywhere a metastasis occurs.

Primary brain tumors may also hemorrhage, particularly oligodendroglial tumors and glioblastoma.[26] These tumors tend to occur in the cerebral hemispheres, thus causing a lobar distribution of hemorrhage.

While bland hemorrhages may exhibit a smooth rim of enhancement acutely, the persistence of enhancement or the presence of nodular enhancement should raise the possibility of underlying mass. Follow-up MR imaging may help differentiate bland from tumor hemorrhage.[14]

Hemorrhagic venous infarct Cerebral venous infarction is an uncommon but clinically important cause of IPH. Venous sinus thrombosis may occur without parenchymal sequela, or may cause venous congestion, bland infarction, or hemorrhagic infarction.

Certain patterns of hemorrhage should suggest venous thrombosis. Unusual-appearing bilateral frontoparietal lobar hemorrhages should prompt evaluation for superior sagittal sinus thrombosis. Unilateral temporal hemorrhage with edema may indicate vein of Labbe or transverse/sigmoid sinus thrombosis. Bilateral thalamic hemorrhages suggest vein of Galen or straight sinus thrombosis.[27]

Key Points

- In an older patient (>60 years) with known hypertension, basal ganglia hemorrhage is likely hypertensive. However, underlying structural vascular lesions do occur in older adults and vascular evaluation should be considered.
- CAA is a common cause of lobar hemorrhage in patients older than 55 years, but the differential diagnosis is broad and this is a diagnosis of exclusion. Contrast-enhanced MR imaging and vascular evaluation can exclude most other causes.
- Bland IPH can enhance peripherally acutely. Persistent or nodular enhancement should suggest underlying neoplasm.
- Hemorrhagic venous infarct is an important diagnosis to consider with unusual-appearing or bilateral IPH, particularly in a younger person.

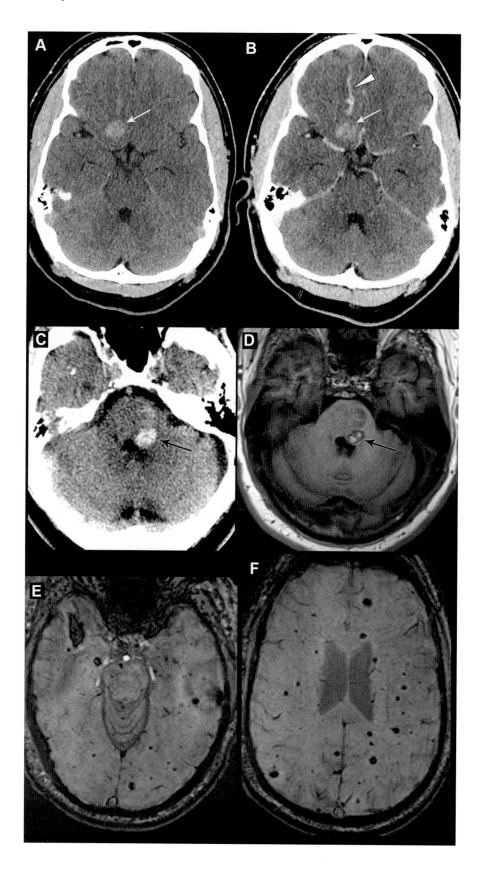

SCENARIO 3: VASOGENIC EDEMA WITH MASS LESION

Imaging Protocol

If vasogenic edema is evident on NECT, a contrast-enhanced study is next indicated. Contrast-enhanced CT could be considered, particularly if contrast-enhanced MR imaging is not available within a reasonable time frame. MR imaging is more sensitive than CT for detecting additional lesions as in the case of metastasis[28–31] and often reveals additional clues to direct the differential diagnosis.

Findings

Vasogenic edema appears as an area of gyral expansion and exaggeration of gray-white differentiation on NECT; it may suggest an underlying mass within the area of edema.

Contrast-enhanced imaging often shows solid, ring, or discontinuous ring enhancement. Diffusion-weighted imaging (DWI) may show restricted diffusion (ie, bright DWI signal with decreased apparent diffusion coefficient [ADC] values) or facilitated diffusion (bright DWI and increased ADC values). T2*-weighted MR imaging may show the presence of blood products or calcium.

Differential Diagnosis

The differential diagnosis for a solitary mass lesion includes metastasis, primary brain tumor, pyogenic abscess, lymphoma, tumefactive demyelination, and subacute ischemic infarct or hemorrhage. Multiple enhancing mass lesions usually are metastases, although abscesses and demyelinating lesions may also be multiple. Primary brain tumors such as glioblastoma may be multiple or have multifocal areas of enhancement within an encompassing area of T2 signal abnormality. MR imaging features may help differentiate these various causes (**Table 4**).

Metastasis and primary high-grade glioma

Metastases are solitary up to half the time, but when multiple, they tend to have 3 or more lesions.[25] Metastases are usually ring enhancing, supratentorial, and located at the gray-white junction. Solitary brain metastases often cannot be distinguished from high-grade gliomas on standard MR imaging, although advanced techniques including MR spectroscopy and perfusion may help differentiate the two.[25,32]

DWI is variable, with either facilitated diffusion or mildly restricted diffusion of the enhancing portion of the tumor. Either tumor types can hemorrhage. Glioblastomas typically exhibit thick irregular enhancement, which may slightly favor this diagnosis, but imaging features overlap.

Abscess

Pyogenic abscesses are in the differential for ring-enhancing mass lesions, but several MR imaging characteristics suggest this diagnosis (**Fig. 7**). The central necrotic core of pyogenic abscesses typically shows intensely restricted diffusion.[33] Rim enhancement is often thick and smooth, although there may be thinning toward the ventricle. The fibrous capsule appears on T2 as a hypointense rim, but may also be evident on noncontrast CT as a hyperdense rim.[34] Daughter nodules may occur if the capsule ruptures focally.[35]

Cerebral abscesses may result from direct extension of local infection or from hematogenous spread. Local infections implicated in cerebral abscess formation include sinusitis, odontogenic infections, and otomastoiditis,[36] and imaging evidence of these infections in conjunction with a brain mass should raise suspicion of a cerebral abscess.

In immunocompromised patients, abscesses may show little enhancement and only mild surrounding vasogenic edema, so a high index of suspicion is required in these patients to make the diagnosis.

Abscesses have a propensity to rupture into the ventricles, causing ventriculitis. Imaging findings include layering debris in the lateral ventricles and ependymal enhancement (see **Fig. 7**). Debris appears hyperdense on CT, hyperintense on fluid-attenuated inversion recovery (FLAIR) to CSF, and may show restricted diffusion. Ventricular rupture confers a more serious clinical course[37] requiring aggressive treatment.

Lymphoma

Lymphoma has unique imaging features on CT and MR imaging (**Fig. 8**). In immunocompetent patients, lymphoma is typically uniformly hyperdense. MR imaging reveals uniform

Fig. 6. Cavernomas in 2 patients. CT without (*A*) and with (*B*) contrast demonstrates a right inferior frontal hyperdense masses (*white arrows*), with developmental venous anomaly evident on postcontrast image (*arrowhead*). NECT (*C*) and MR imaging (*D–F*) in a second patient shows a hyperdense left pontine mass (*black arrow, C*) with internal locules of T1 signal hyperintensity (*black arrow, D*). Susceptibility-weighted T2* MR imaging (*E, F*) demonstrates a randomly distributed pattern of hemorrhages of variable sizes scattered throughout the superficial and deep areas of the brain. Findings are consistent with multiple cavernous malformations.

Table 4
Characteristics helping differentiate solitary enhancing masses on MR imaging

Lesion	Clues	Pitfalls	Pearls
Metastasis	Multiple 50% of time Rim enhancing, at gray-white junction	Often indistinguishable from high-grade glioma	If solitary, primary brain tumor should be on differential
High-grade glioma	Usually solitary Thick irregular enhancement	Often indistinguishable from solitary metastasis	Metastasis should be on differential
Pyogenic abscess	Markedly restricted diffusion of central necrotic core Thick smooth rim enhancement Daughter nodules	Fungal abscesses generally do not show restricted central core	Check for ventricular rupture
Lymphoma	Hyperdense on CT Solid enhancement if immunocompetent Restricted diffusion	Restricted diffusion is less intense than abscess	May be ring enhancing if patients is immunocompromized
Tumefactive demyelinating lesion	Open ring of enhancement Discontinuous enhancement toward cortex	Uncommon and often mistaken for neoplasm	Mass effect and edema may be less than expected for size
Subacute infarct	Infarcts may enhance from 1 wk to several months	May be multiple if embolic origin	FLAIR abnormality matches enhancing mass; ie, no surrounding vasogenic edema
Subacute IPH	Complex heterogeneous appearance, may rim enhance	Subacute IPH may have vasogenic edema	Compare precontrast and postcontrast images to differentiate enhancement from blood products

Abbreviation: FLAIR, fluid-attenuated inversion recovery.

toothpaste-like enhancement with restricted diffusion indicating the densely cellular nature of the tumor. Unlike pyogenic abscess, the restricted diffusion corresponds to the enhancing tumor and not the central necrotic core. In addition, the intensity of diffusion restriction is less. Often but not always solitary, lymphoma can also manifest as a butterfly lesion crossing the corpus callosum.[38] In immunocompromised patients, lymphoma often appears as a ring-enhancing mass.

Tumefactive demyelinating lesion
Tumefactive demyelinating lesions (TDLs) are a great mimic in neuroradiology and may come to biopsy or resection if not recognized as such. TDLs appear as irregular rim-enhancing masses with relatively little mass effect or surrounding vasogenic edema. The key to recognizing this entity is to look for an incomplete rim of enhancement, with the nonenhancing portion facing the cortex.[39]

Subacute ischemic infarct and hemorrhage
Subacute ischemic infarcts may enhance, typically beginning at 1 week and lasting 2 to 3 months.[40] Comparison imaging showing the original infarct or rapidly developing enhancement may be helpful. Subacute IPH often has a complex appearance and may induce a rim of enhancement as the hematoma breaks down.[14] Differentiating this from a hemorrhagic mass may be difficult and may require follow-up imaging to be sure.

Multiple lesions
Multiple enhancing lesions should suggest a diagnosis of metastasis, although as mentioned primary high-grade brain tumors are occasionally multiple. Important considerations on the

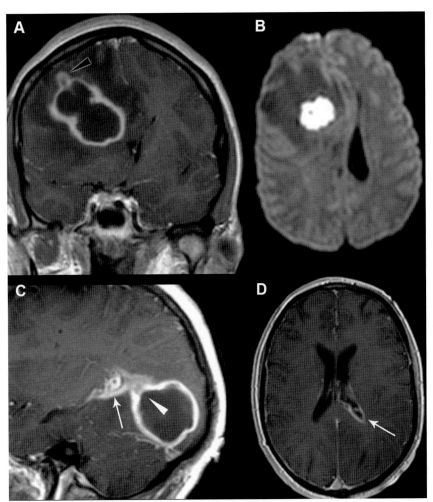

Fig. 7. Pyogenic abscesses in 2 patients. T1-weighted enhanced MR imaging (*A*) demonstrates a ring-enhancing right frontal mass with daughter lesions (*arrowhead*). DWI (*B*) demonstrates markedly restricted diffusion. T1-weighted enhanced MR imaging in a second patient (*C, D*) demonstrates a rim enhancing mass with thinning of the wall toward the ventricle (*arrowhead, C*) and ventricular extension (*white arrows*).

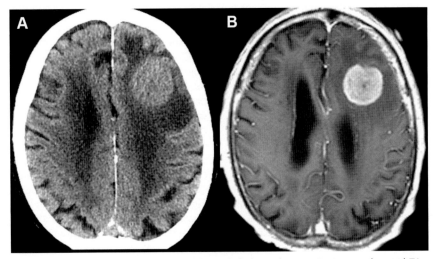

Fig. 8. Lymphoma. NECT (*A*) demonstrates a hyperdense left frontal mass. Contrast-enhanced T1-weighted MR imaging (*B*) demonstrates uniform enhancement.

differential include demyelinating lesions such as with active multiple sclerosis or acute disseminated encephalomyelitis, multiple subacute ischemic infarcts, and multiple abscesses. In immunocompromised patients in particular, toxoplasmosis should be considered. Other infectious causes of multiple enhancing masses include central nervous system tuberculosis, which is often associated with basilar meningitis.

Key Points

- Metastasis and high-grade gliomas often cannot be distinguished on standard MR imaging. Multiplicity should favor the diagnosis of metastasis.
- Light-bulb bright restricted diffusion of the central necrotic core of a lesion should favor the diagnosis of pyogenic abscess. Ventricular rupture and ventriculitis should be evaluated for.
- Tumefactive demyelination should be kept in mind—although uncommon, this entity should be recognized prior to biopsy.

SCENARIO 4: VASOGENIC EDEMA WITHOUT MASS LESION
Imaging Protocol

NECT is the typical first-line imaging study for evaluation of the symptoms most commonly associated with this abnormality, including headache, mental status changes, seizure, and visual changes. Once evidence of vasogenic edema is established, contrast-enhanced study is required for further evaluation. Gadolinium-enhanced MR imaging provides the most information for differentiating between the myriad of conditions present in the differential diagnosis.

Findings

The appearance on NECT is similar to that of vasogenic edema caused by mass lesions. There is low attenuation within the white matter, which spares the gray matter and causes exaggeration of the gray-white interface. There may be gyral enlargement with effacement of the sulci.

Depending on the cause of the vasogenic edema, enhancement may be seen within the area of edema. The enhancement may be variable and can be visualized as solid, rim, or patchy enhancement. Diffuse restriction also variably occurs in the bulk of these conditions. T2*-weighted sequences are useful for determining the presence of hemorrhage or calcification.

Differential Diagnosis

The differential diagnosis is broad and varied because many different conditions can cause vasogenic edema. This article focuses on conditions in which rapid identification and treatment can have great positive impact on the prognosis of the patient. These include PRES, herpes encephalitis, progressive multifocal leukoencephalopathy (PML), and venous infarct.

Posterior reversible encephalopathy syndrome
PRES is also known as acute hypertensive encephalopathy. This condition may occur in patients presenting with hypertensive urgency or emergency. This syndrome should also be suspected in pregnant woman presenting with symptoms of preeclampsia or eclampsia.[41] It should, however, be remembered that in some patients, especially children, blood pressure may be normal or only slightly elevated. Drug toxicity can also be a cause, particularly chemotherapeutic drugs such as cisplatin and cyclosporine.[42]

PRES typically presents as patchy bilateral subcortical hypodensities on CT with predilection for the posterior aspects of the brain (parietal lobes, occipital lobes, and cerebellum).[43] PRES can less commonly involve the basal ganglia and brain stem. MR imaging demonstrates signal hyperintensity in these areas on T2-weighted and FLAIR sequences (Fig. 9). Diffusion restriction is not common and is an important differentiating finding between PRES and cerebral infarction. Enhancement is also not common, but when present is patchy. Normalization of blood pressure and/or removal of offending agents can lead to reversal of these imaging findings and improvement in the patient's condition. Delay in treatment may result in chronic neurologic morbidity.

Herpes encephalitis
NECT may appear normal early in the disease. Low attenuation can be seen in the medial temporal lobes and insula (Fig. 10). Mass effect may be present. Hemorrhage usually occurs later in the condition. MR imaging is the test of choice because imaging findings in this modality may be evident 24 hours earlier than in CT. The characteristic MR appearance is cortical swelling and mass effect within the bilateral temporal lobes with cortical and subcortical T2 hyperintensity (see Fig. 10). Diffusion restriction is also seen with possible patchy or gyriform enhancement. Imaging abnormalities may also affect the insula, subfrontal areas, and cingulate gyri.[44] Patients may progress to coma and death. Herpes encephalitis has a mortality rate ranging between 50% and

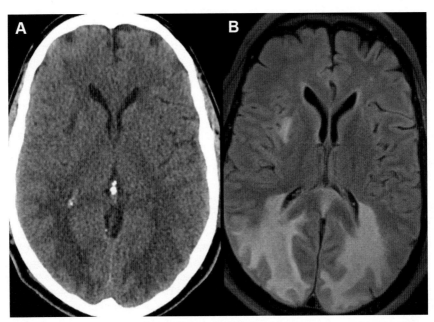

Fig. 9. Posterior reversible encephalopathy syndrome. NECT (*A*) demonstrates symmetric low attenuation within the bilateral parieto-occipital lobes. MR imaging FLAIR sequence (*B*) displays corresponding hyperintensity involving the bilateral parieto-occipital lobes.

75%. Rapid treatment gives the patient the best chance for recovery.

Progressive multifocal leukoencephalopathy

PML is caused by JC virus infection of oligodendrocytes resulting in demyelination. PML is usually seen in immunocompromized patients, such as patients with AIDS. This condition can also be seen in patients receiving natalizumab for treatment of multiple sclerosis.[45] Gadolinium-enhanced MR imaging is the modality of choice. PML is seen as multifocal T2 hyperintensity involving the subcortical white matter and usually extending into the deep white matter. These plaques can be variable in size ranging from focal subcortical lesions to confluent hemispheric regions. The subcortical U-fibers are involved with PML.[46] Diffusion restriction can occur with newer lesions. Enhancement is uncommon. Unfortunately, PML is a fatal disease with death usually occurring 6 to 8 months from diagnosis.

Venous infarct

As discussed earlier, cerebral venous infarction is within the differential diagnosis for lobar

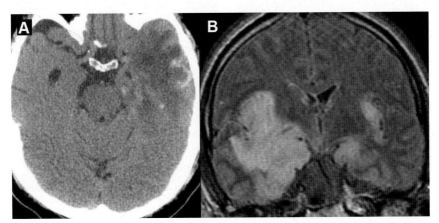

Fig. 10. Herpes encephalitis in 2 patients. NECT (*A*) demonstrates vasogenic edema of the left temporal lobe with petechial hemorrhage of the cortex. FLAIR-weighted MR imaging in the second patient (*B*) demonstrates bilateral hyperintense areas of the medial temporal lobes and insula, worse on the right.

hemorrhage (**Fig. 11**). Venous infarct can also present as vasogenic edema without hemorrhage. Parenchymal abnormalities are seen in over 50% of patients with cerebral venous thrombosis.[27] Parenchymal lesions are better seen on MR imaging. These parenchymal abnormalities can manifest as T2 hyperintensity, parenchymal swelling, or a combination of both (see **Fig. 11**).[27] ADC may be increased because of venous congestion or decreased possibly from cellular energy disruption. Parenchymal enhancement is variable and predominately involves the gyri.[27]

Key Points

- Cerebral infarct is a major differential diagnosis for PRES on NECT. Infarct demonstrates restricted diffusion but PRES typically does not.
- T2 hyperintensity within the temporal lobes with diffusion restriction raises high suspicion for herpes encephalitis. Rapid treatment may be lifesaving.
- The typical patient presenting with PML is immunosuppressed. PML involves the subcortical U-fibers, which can differentiate it from other demyelinating disorders.
- Venous infarct should be considered in patients with parenchymal edema that does not conform to a typical vascular distribution. Flame-shaped lobar hemorrhage can also be seen.

SCENARIO 5: HYDROCEPHALUS
Imaging Protocol

NECT is used emergently in the evaluation of patients with the common symptoms of hydrocephalus, headache and signs of increased intracranial pressure; however, multiplanar MR imaging is typically a better modality for determining the underlying cause of hydrocephalus. High-resolution, thin

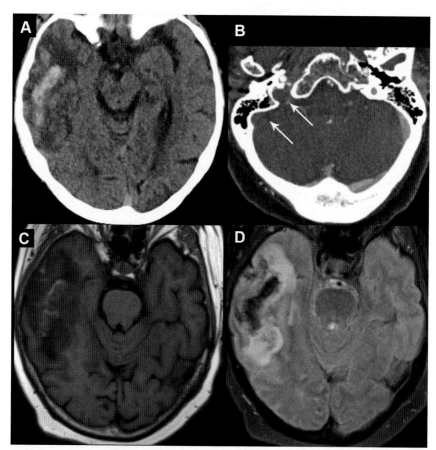

Fig. 11. Venous sinus thrombosis with intraparenchymal hemorrhage. NECT (*A*) shows right temporal vasogenic edema and intraparenchymal hemorrhage. CTA (*B*) demonstrates lack of luminal contrast within the right sigmoid sinus and jugular bulb (*arrows*) consistent with venous thrombosis. Corresponding T1-weighted MR (*C*) shows edema within the right temporal lobe with patchy T1 hyperintensity consistent with hemorrhage. MR FLAIR (*D*) further demonstrates the vasogenic edema and hemorrhage of the right temporal lobe.

T2-weighted sequences, provide superb details of the CSF spaces and may visualize subtle abnormalities such as obstructing webs or septa. Cine CSF flow sequences can be used to evaluate CSF flow at the aqueduct and craniocervical junction.

Findings

Imaging findings in hydrocephalus vary with severity and acuity of the condition. CT demonstrates enlarged lateral and third ventricles. The size of the fourth ventricle varies depending on the underlying cause. In acute intraventricular obstructive hydrocephalus (IVOH) low density may be seen in the surrounding periventricular white matter, which can be due to transependymal flow of CSF/periventricular edema.

The pattern of ventricular enlargement can indicate the location of the obstructing lesion. Triventricular hydrocephalus refers to enlargement of the lateral and third ventricles with a normal-sized fourth ventricle, which can be seen with stenosis of the cerebral aqueduct. Enlargement of all 4 ventricles is known as quadriventricular hydrocephalus. This enlargement can be caused by a fourth ventricular mass or obstruction of the fourth ventricular foramina. Rarely, unilateral hydrocephalus signifying enlargement of one of the lateral ventricles can be seen with obstruction at the foramen of Monro.

MR imaging demonstrates symmetric enlargement of the lateral ventricles. The third ventricle enlargement is revealed by the parallel or convex appearance of its lateral walls. The corpus callosum may have a thinned appearance on sagittal sequences. Transependymal CSF flow may be seen in acute IVOH as increased signal on T2-weighted sequences within the periventricular white matter, which usually does not suppress on FLAIR.

Differential Diagnosis

IVOH was known in past nomenclature as noncommunicating hydrocephalus; it describes an obstruction within the ventricular system proximal to or at the fourth ventricle foramina. IVOH may be congenital or acquired and acute or chronic. The most common cause of acquired IVOH is membranous obstruction from prior hemorrhage or inflammation, which most commonly occurs at the fourth ventricular foramina and the cerebral aqueduct. The second most common cause of acquired IVOH is an intraventricular mass. The type and prevalence of different masses depends on location. Colloid cysts are the most common obstructing mass at the foramen of Monro. Pineal masses and tectal plate gliomas can narrow the cerebral aqueduct.

Medulloblastomas are the most common fourth ventricle obstructing mass in children. Metastases, epidermoid cysts, hemangioblastomas, and choroid plexus papillomas can cause obstruction of the fourth ventricle in adults.[47]

Extraventricular obstructive hydrocephalus (EVOH) is also known as communicating hydrocephalus. Typically, the location of CSF obstruction lies outside the ventricular system. The most common causes of EVOH are SAH, meningitis, and diffuse extra-axial metastases.

Acute

Meningitis Inflammation and/or infection of the meninges can result in extraventricular obstruction because of dysfunction in absorption at the level of the arachnoid granulations. Hydrocephalus was the most common radiographic finding in one study of patients diagnosed with tuberculous meningitis.[48] Exudates within the subarachnoid space may cause the CSF to have an abnormal appearance of slightly increased T1 signal compared to normal CSF. Exudates may also exhibit increased T2 signal seen in FLAIR sequences. In the presence of frank pus, diffusion restriction can be seen. Enhancement of the meninges and enhancement within the sulci can occur with meningitis or carcinomatosis.[49]

Colloid cyst Colloid cysts are benign mucin-containing cysts of which about 99% are located at the foramen of Monro.[50] These cysts are derived from embryonic ectoderm like neurenteric and Rathke cleft cysts. Colloid cysts are typically well-circumscribed hyperdense cysts on NECT (**Fig. 12**). About two-thirds of colloid cysts are hyperintense on T1-weighted MR imaging.[51] T2 signal is more variable. Enhancement is uncommon, but rim enhancement can occasionally be seen.

A small proportion, about 10%, of colloid cysts can rapidly enlarge causing hydrocephalus, coma, and possibly death.[51] These colloid cysts usually show higher water content, therefore, the lesions to be more concerned about exhibit low T1 and high T2 signal on MR imaging.[50]

Subarachnoid hemorrhage SAH is the most common cause of EVOH. Hydrocephalus develops in about half of the cases of intraventricular hemorrhage. A greater degree of hemorrhage within the ventricular system increases the risk of developing hydrocephalus.[52] Hyperdensity with the sulci and CSF cisterns is evident on NECT with acute SAH. Almost 95% of NECT studies yield positive result for SAH within 24 hours with less than 50% yielding positive result at 1 week.[51] SAH can be seen as FLAIR hyperintensity on MR imaging; this is more sensitive than CT but less specific.

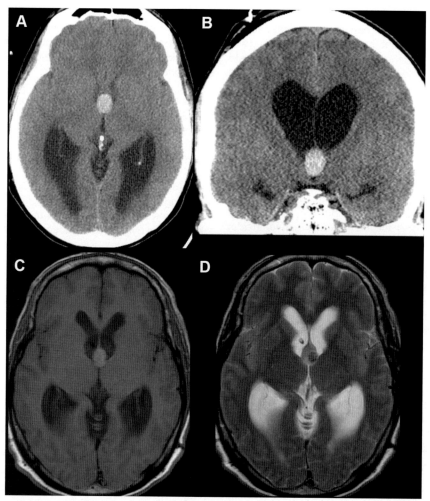

Fig. 12. Colloid cyst with hydrocephalus. NECT (*A, B*) demonstrates a well-circumscribed hyperdense mass at the foramen of Monro consistent with a colloid cyst. There is hydrocephalus with dilation of the posterior horns (*A*) and frontal horns (*B*) of the lateral ventricles. MR imaging of the cyst shows T1 hyperintensity (*C*) and T2 heterogeneity (*D*). Note the ventricular shunt catheter tip in the right frontal horn.

Hydrocephalus can occur early with SAH. Approximately 10% of patients with SAH require permanent CSF shunting.[53]

Chronic

Normal pressure hydrocephalus Normal pressure hydrocephalus (NPH) denotes ventriculomegaly with normal CSF pressure. There are no definitive evidence-based guidelines for the diagnosis or treatment of NPH at present. The classically described triad of NPH includes dementia, gait dysfunction, and urinary incontinence. The prevalence of NPH is approximately 5% in patients 80 years and older.[54] NPH can be designated as unlikely, possible, and probable based on a combination of clinical findings, imaging results, and response to high-volume lumbar puncture.[55]

NECT usually shows enlarged lateral and third ventricles. The fourth ventricle can be normal.

The Evans index, a ratio of the width of the frontal horns to the biparietal width of the brain, typically indicates ventriculomegaly when the value is greater than 0.30.[55] The sulci of the brain may show mild atrophy, but the ventricular enlargement is out of proportion to the degree of atrophy.

MR imaging also demonstrates ventriculomegaly out of proportion to sulcal widening. An exaggerated flow void may also be seen within the cerebral aqueduct. A small amount of increased T2 signal may be seen within the adjacent periventricular white matter. Indium-111 diethylene triamine pentaacetic acid (DTPA) scan with persistent ventricular activity at 24 hours is considered a reliable indicator of NPH.

Posterior fossa mass Medulloblastoma is the most common obstructing fourth ventricular mass in children. Metastases, epidermoid cysts, hemangioblastomas, and choroid plexus papillomas can cause obstruction of the fourth ventricle in adults (**Fig. 13**).

Medulloblastoma represents 30% to 40% of posterior fossa tumors in children. About 95% of patients with this tumor develop hydrocephalus.[51] Medulloblastoma often presents as a large hyperdense fourth ventricle mass on CT with variable intratumoral cysts or necrosis. The tumor heterogeneously enhances on CT and MR imaging. The tumor may also demonstrate diffusion restriction with low ADC on MR imaging because of the hypercellular nature of the mass.

Aqueductal stenosis There are various causes of aqueductal stenosis. Extraventricular pathology such as a tectal mass, vein of Galen malformation, or quadrigeminal cistern arachnoid cyst can obstruct the aqueduct. The obstructing pathologic condition may be within the aqueduct itself, as with an aqueductal web or fork. Prior inflammation of the periaqueductal tissues can also cause narrowing of the cerebral aqueduct.

CT and MR imaging demonstrate enlarged lateral and third ventricles with a normal-appearing fourth ventricle. Thinning of the corpus callosum may be seen. Tectal masses may not be evident on CT, but irregularity of the posterior third ventricle should prompt further evaluation with MR imaging.[56]

MR imaging is more sensitive to small tectal masses than CT. High-resolution, thin-section multiplanar MR imaging sequences are the best choice for visualizing webs within the cerebral aqueduct. The aqueduct may have a funnel-like shape, with dilatation of the portion of the aqueduct proximal to the web (**Fig. 14**). Aqueductal gliosis may be difficult to differentiate from congenital stenosis as both may manifest as narrowing of the aqueduct. T2*-weighted sequences can be helpful in determining the presence of prior hemorrhage, one potential cause of aqueductal gliosis.[51]

Key Points

- Determining the level of obstruction in hydrocephalus helps narrow the differential

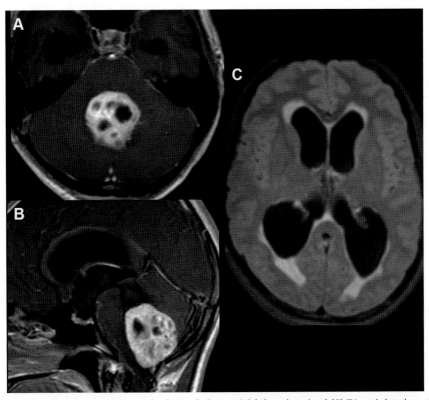

Fig. 13. Hemangioblastoma causing acute hydrocephalus. Axial (*A*) and sagittal (*B*) T1-weighted postgadolinium MR imaging demonstrates an avidly enhancing mass with intratumoral cysts within the fourth ventricle, which was proved to be a hemangioblastoma. There is enlargement of the lateral and third ventricles. Axial FLAIR MR image (*C*) shows T2 hyperintensity along the margins of the frontal and posterior horns of the lateral ventricles. This observation is consistent with transependymal flow of CSF and indicates acute hydrocephalus.

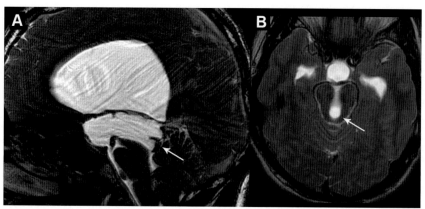

Fig. 14. Aqueductal stenosis. Sagittal MR T2 FIESTA sequence (A) demonstrates marked enlargement of the lateral and third ventricles. Fourth ventricle is normal in size. The cerebral aqueduct is dilated proximally with bowing of the tectum (*arrow*). This finding suggests distal obstruction within the aqueduct, possibly by a web or septation. Axial T2-weighted MR (B) illustrates the massive enlargement of the proximal cerebral aqueduct (*arrow*).

diagnosis. IVOH is due to obstruction within the ventricular system, possibly because of membranous web or intraventricular mass. EVOH is caused by obstruction outside the ventricles, typically due to previous hemorrhage or infection.

- NPH is a clinical diagnosis. Ventriculomegaly out of proportion to the size of the sulci on imaging can increase suspicion for the condition.
- Colloid cysts can have variable imaging characteristics on CT and MR imaging, and they are most commonly seen at the foramen of Monro. Cysts with a higher water content may be more prone to rapid enlargement, which could result in coma and death.

SUMMARY

Emergency neuroradiology can be challenging because of the wide range of conditions that present with acute neurologic symptoms or signs. NECT is almost always the most appropriate first imaging test and is extremely useful to exclude life-threatening conditions. The imaging findings of a variety of neurologic abnormalities overlap on NECT, however, and the differential diagnosis may be extremely broad. The first step to narrowing the differential diagnosis and providing imaging workup includes classifying the NECT findings into a broad category, as the authors have tried to do in this article. Based on the type of imaging abnormality, further imaging workup may include CTA, DSA, and/or MR imaging. Familiarity with specific imaging finding that suggest a specific diagnosis may help further facilitate appropriate clinical workup and treatment.

REFERENCES

1. Douglas AC, Wippold FJ 2nd, Broderick DF, et al. ACR Appropriateness Criteria Headache. J Am Coll Radiol 2014;11(7):657–67.
2. van der Wee N, Rinkel GJ, Hasan D, et al. Detection of subarachnoid haemorrhage on early CT: is lumbar puncture still needed after a negative scan? J Neurol Neurosurg Psychiatry 1995;58(3): 357–9.
3. van Gijn J, Kerr RS, Rinkel GJ. Subarachnoid haemorrhage. Lancet 2007;369(9558):306–18.
4. Greenberg ED, Fink KR, Gobin PY. Intracranial aneurysms and vasospasm: evidence-based diagnosis and treatment. In: Medina LS, Sanello PC, Jarvik JG, editors. Evidence-based neuroimaging diagnosis and treatment. New York: Springer; 2013. p. 239–59.
5. Donmez H, Serifov E, Kahriman G, et al. Comparison of 16-row multislice CT angiography with conventional angiography for detection and evaluation of intracranial aneurysms. Eur J Radiol 2011;80(2): 455–61.
6. Ruigrok YM, Rinkel GJ, Buskens E, et al. Perimesencephalic hemorrhage and CT angiography: a decision analysis. Stroke 2000;31(12):2976–83.
7. Marder CP, Narla V, Fink JR, et al. Subarachnoid hemorrhage: beyond aneurysms. AJR Am J Roentgenol 2014;202(1):25–37.
8. van Gijn J, van Dongen KJ, Vermeulen M, et al. Perimesencephalic hemorrhage: a nonaneurysmal and benign form of subarachnoid hemorrhage. Neurology 1985;35(4):493–7.
9. Velthuis BK, Rinkel GJ, Ramos LM, et al. Perimesencephalic hemorrhage. Exclusion of vertebrobasilar aneurysms with CT angiography. Stroke 1999; 30(5):1103–9.

10. Ducros A, Boukobza M, Porcher R, et al. The clinical and radiological spectrum of reversible cerebral vasoconstriction syndrome. A prospective series of 67 patients. Brain 2007;130(Pt 12):3091–101.

11. Marder CP, Donohue MM, Weinstein JR, et al. Multimodal imaging of reversible cerebral vasoconstriction syndrome: a series of 6 cases. AJNR Am J Neuroradiol 2012;33(7):1403–10.

12. Chang R, Friedman DP. Isolated cortical venous thrombosis presenting as subarachnoid hemorrhage: a report of three cases. AJNR Am J Neuroradiol 2004;25(10):1676–9.

13. Cordonnier C, Klijn CJ, van Beijnum J, et al. Radiological investigation of spontaneous intracerebral hemorrhage: systematic review and trinational survey. Stroke 2010;41(4):685–90.

14. Ciura VA, Romero JM. Nontraumatic acute intraparenchymal hemorrhage: algorithm for workup and differential diagnosis. Semin Roentgenol 2014;49(1):112–26.

15. Meretoja A, Strbian D, Putaala J, et al. SMASH-U: a proposal for etiologic classification of intracerebral hemorrhage. Stroke 2012;43(10):2592–7.

16. Ikram MA, Wieberdink RG, Koudstaal PJ. International epidemiology of intracerebral hemorrhage. Curr Atheroscler Rep 2012;14(4):300–6.

17. Zheng T, Wang S, Barras C, et al. Vascular imaging adds value in investigation of basal ganglia hemorrhage. J Clin Neurosci 2012;19(2):277–80.

18. Zhu XL, Chan MS, Poon WS. Spontaneous intracranial hemorrhage: which patients need diagnostic cerebral angiography? A prospective study of 206 cases and review of the literature. Stroke 1997;28(7):1406–9.

19. Martini SR, Flaherty ML, Brown WM, et al. Risk factors for intracerebral hemorrhage differ according to hemorrhage location. Neurology 2012;79(23):2275–82.

20. Romero JR, Preis SR, Beiser A, et al. Risk factors, stroke prevention treatments, and prevalence of cerebral microbleeds in the Framingham Heart Study. Stroke 2014;45(5):1492–4.

21. Knudsen KA, Rosand J, Karluk D, et al. Clinical diagnosis of cerebral amyloid angiopathy: validation of the Boston criteria. Neurology 2001;56(4):537–9.

22. Charidimou A, Jaunmuktane Z, Baron JC, et al. White matter perivascular spaces: an MRI marker in pathology-proven cerebral amyloid angiopathy? Neurology 2014;82(1):57–62.

23. Romero JM, Artunduaga M, Forero NP, et al. Accuracy of CT angiography for the diagnosis of vascular abnormalities causing intraparenchymal hemorrhage in young patients. Emerg Radiol 2009;16(3):195–201.

24. Meng G, Bai C, Yu T, et al. The association between cerebral developmental venous anomaly and concomitant cavernous malformation: an observational study using magnetic resonance imaging. BMC Neurol 2014;14:50.

25. Fink KR, Fink JR. Imaging of brain metastases. Surg Neurol Int 2013;4(Suppl 4):S209–19.

26. Kondziolka D, Bernstein M, Resch L, et al. Significance of hemorrhage into brain tumors: clinicopathological study. J Neurosurg 1987;67(6):852–7.

27. Leach JL, Fortuna RB, Jones BV, et al. Imaging of cerebral venous thrombosis: current techniques, spectrum of findings, and diagnostic pitfalls. Radiographics 2006;26(Suppl 1):S19–41 [discussion: S42–3].

28. Krüger S, Mottaghy FM, Buck AK, et al. Brain metastasis in lung cancer. Comparison of cerebral MRI and 18F-FDG-PET/CT for diagnosis in the initial staging. Nuklearmedizin 2011;50(3):101–6.

29. Yokoi K, Kamiya N, Matsuguma H, et al. Detection of brain metastasis in potentially operable non-small cell lung cancer: a comparison of CT and MRI. Chest 1999;115(3):714–9.

30. Schellinger PD, Meinck HM, Thron A. Diagnostic accuracy of MRI compared to CCT in patients with brain metastases. J Neurooncol 1999;44(3):275–81.

31. Davis PC, Hudgins PA, Peterman SB, et al. Diagnosis of cerebral metastases: double-dose delayed CT vs contrast-enhanced MR imaging. AJNR Am J Neuroradiol 1991;12(2):293–300.

32. Wang S, Kim S, Chawla S, et al. Differentiation between glioblastomas, solitary brain metastases, and primary cerebral lymphomas using diffusion tensor and dynamic susceptibility contrast-enhanced MR imaging. AJNR Am J Neuroradiol 2011;32(3):507–14.

33. Rath TJ, Hughes M, Arabi M, et al. Imaging of cerebritis, encephalitis, and brain abscess. Neuroimaging Clin N Am 2012;22(4):585–607.

34. Britt RH, Enzmann DR. Clinical stages of human brain abscesses on serial CT scans after contrast infusion. Computerized tomographic, neuropathological, and clinical correlations. J Neurosurg 1983;59(6):972–89.

35. Haimes AB, Zimmerman RD, Morgello S, et al. MR imaging of brain abscesses. AJR Am J Roentgenol 1989;152(5):1073–85.

36. Carpenter J, Stapleton S, Holliman R. Retrospective analysis of 49 cases of brain abscess and review of the literature. Eur J Clin Microbiol Infect Dis 2007;26(1):1–11.

37. Nathoo N, Nadvi SS, Narotam PK, et al. Brain abscess: management and outcome analysis of a computed tomography era experience with 973 patients. World Neurosurg 2011;75(5–6):716–26 [discussion: 612–7].

38. Koeller KK, Smirniotopoulos JG, Jones RV. Primary central nervous system lymphoma: radiologic-pathologic correlation. Radiographics 1997;17(6):1497–526.

39. Given CA 2nd, Stevens BS, Lee C. The MRI appearance of tumefactive demyelinating lesions. AJR Am J Roentgenol 2004;182(1):195–9.

40. Allen LM, Hasso AN, Handwerker J, et al. Sequence-specific MR imaging findings that are useful in dating ischemic stroke. Radiographics 2012;32(5):1285–97 [discussion: 1297–9].

41. Siddiqui TS, Irfan-ul-Haq, Rehman B, et al. Posterior reversible encephalopathy syndrome (PRES). J Coll Physicians Surg Pak 2012;22(3):168–70.

42. Güler T, Cakmak OY, Toprak SK, et al. Intrathecal methotrexate-induced posterior reversible encephalopathy syndrome (PRES). Turk J Haematol 2014; 31(1):109–10.

43. Hugonnet E, Da Ines D, Boby H, et al. Posterior reversible encephalopathy syndrome (PRES): features on CT and MR imaging. Diagn Interv Imaging 2013;94(1):45–52.

44. Taber KH, Hurley RA. Herpes encephalitis in the immunocompetent adult: advances in neuroimaging. J Neuropsychiatry Clin Neurosci 2010;22(2): 1 p preceding 125, 125–9.

45. Berger JR. The clinical features of PML. Cleve Clin J Med 2011;78(Suppl 2):S8–12.

46. Calabrese L. A rational approach to PML for the clinician. Cleve Clin J Med 2011;78(Suppl 2): S38–41.

47. Osborn AG. Osborn's brain: imaging, pathology, and anatomy. 1st edition. Salt Lake City (UT): Amirsys; 2013.

48. Sher K, Firdaus, Abbasi A, et al. Stages of tuberculous meningitis: a clinicoradiologic analysis. J Coll Physicians Surg Pak 2013;23(6):405–8.

49. Jearanaisilp S, Sangruji T, Danchaivijitr C, et al. Neoplastic meningitis: a retrospective review of clinical presentations, radiological and cerebrospinal fluid findings. J Med Assoc Thai 2014;97(8):870–7.

50. Osborn AG, Preece MT. Intracranial cysts: radiologic-pathologic correlation and imaging approach. Radiology 2006;239(3):650–64.

51. Osborn A, Salzman K, Barkovich A, et al. Diagnostic imaging: brain. 2nd edition. Salt Lake City (UT): Amirsys; 2010.

52. AlShardan MM, Mubasher M, Orz Y, et al. Factors that predict hydrocephalus following intraventricular hemorrhage. Br J Neurosurg 2014. [Epub ahead of print].

53. Bae IS, Yi HJ, Choi KS, et al. Comparison of incidence and risk factors for shunt-dependent hydrocephalus in aneurysmal subarachnoid hemorrhage patients. J Cerebrovasc Endovasc Neurosurg 2014;16(2):78–84.

54. Jaraj D, Rabiei K, Marlow T, et al. Prevalence of idiopathic normal-pressure hydrocephalus. Neurology 2014;82(16):1449–54.

55. Relkin N, Marmarou A, Klinge P, et al. Diagnosing idiopathic normal-pressure hydrocephalus. Neurosurgery 2005;57(3 Suppl):S4–16 [discussion: ii–v].

56. Barkovich AJ, Newton TH. MR of aqueductal stenosis: evidence of a broad spectrum of tectal distortion. AJNR Am J Neuroradiol 1989;10(3):471–6.

Index

Note: Page numbers of article titles are in **boldface** type.

Radiol Clin N Am 53 (2015) 891–901
http://dx.doi.org/10.1016/S0033-8389(15)00078-0
0033-8389/15/$ – see front matter © 2015 Elsevier Inc. All rights reserved.

Moving?

Make sure your subscription moves with you!

To notify us of your new address, find your **Clinics Account Number** (located on your mailing label above your name), and contact customer service at:

Email: journalscustomerservice-usa@elsevier.com

800-654-2452 (subscribers in the U.S. & Canada)
314-447-8871 (subscribers outside of the U.S. & Canada)

Fax number: 314-447-8029

Elsevier Health Sciences Division
Subscription Customer Service
3251 Riverport Lane
Maryland Heights, MO 63043

*To ensure uninterrupted delivery of your subscription, please notify us at least 4 weeks in advance of move.